SUPPORTING PET OWNERS THROUGH GRIEF

SUPPORTING PET OWNERS THROUGH GRIEF

A Veterinarian's Guide to Loss

Ryane E. Englar, DVM, DABVP
(Canine and Feline Practice)
Associate Professor of Practice
Executive Director, Clinical and Professional Skills
University of Arizona College of Veterinary Medicine
Oro Valley, AZ

Jill B. Englar, MSW, LCSW-C, CAGCS

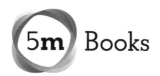

PART THREE: Accepting and Affirming That Healthcare Is Challenging: What it Takes to Rebuild the Veterinary Team

PART FOUR: Developing Reflective Practice

PART FIVE: Using the Literary Arts to Explore Grief: *Poems and Stories of Bereavement*

Preface

When I graduated from Cornell University in May 2008 as a full-fledged Doctor of Veterinary Medicine, I felt confident in only one aspect of my chosen career:

I didn't know everything that I thought I should. What I did know, I was unclear how to apply.

Don't get me wrong. I am grateful that I had the privilege learning from state-of-the-art training at the then #1 veterinary degree program in the United States.

I am immensely thankful to have had this opportunity when so many who desired it did not.

I am extraordinarily proud to be a part of a profession that has brought purpose and value to my day-to-day acts of service.

The truth is that gratitude and pride did not come overnight. Both took time to percolate as I learned – and relearned – over the better part of 15 years how to define and redefine myself outside of the office.

My training was the best in the country.

I had "participated" in root canals and open chest surgeries. I had learned the ins and outs of mechanical ventilation. I had been grilled and drilled on anything and everything that I could possibly be tested on and was essentially a walking encyclopaedia of knowledge by the end of fourth (clinical) year.

But, hiding behind my white coat as the newly minted doctor who could recite what was on page 762 of Ettinger's *Textbook of Veterinary Internal Medicine*, was a scared 21-year-old who felt wholeheartedly unprepared.

As much as my time at Cornell had been terrifyingly pumped full of rigor, I knew what to expect, from who, at all times.

Life was predictable back then.

Cornell had taught me my place, and like the good soldier I was, I fell into line and submitted all of me.

The world beyond those walls was predictably unpredictable, and I had not yet learned how to find comfort in the discomfort, how to be okay with not knowing, how to settle into the fact that everything from here on out would be essentially my "first":

- first appointment, alone
- first surgery, alone
- first emergency, alone
- first overnight shift, alone.

Sure, I had a team, but I didn't know then how to delegate or lean on other team members. So, it was truly by the grace of my support staff that I made it through that first day, first week, first month, and first year.

Graduation is a "make-it-or-break-it" transitional period for many veterinarians. I made it out alive, though not unscarred.

In those days, the only aspects of pet loss that I had been exposed to at Cornell were isolated, untrained, informal glimpses that clinicians glossed over in morning case prep.

In those days, we didn't have Morbidity and Mortality (M&M) rounds. Or, if we did, the students most certainly had not been invited.

In class and on rotation, we didn't talk about grief and grieving, death and dying, at least not in the ways that have been outlined here.

Death was highlighted only as a means of inducing fear.

We were told, again and again, that if we did "x" or if we didn't do "y", then our patient would, and I quote, "Stop breathing and die."

It was a reminder that was stamped into every fibre of my being, every time we were lectured to in critical care and anaesthesia pre-clinical sessions.

If I close my eyes, I can still hear those words jutting out to me in warning, as clear as day.

I had to be smarter, better, and bigger than death so that death did not find its way to me.

So began my run from death, because the only death we ever touched on in school was the death that you could cause through negligence.

That didn't mean death avoided us in the halls of the clinic. We encountered death. We just didn't talk about it.

I still remember the first patient that was euthanized by my own hand. Her name was Lefty.

She was a beautiful calico cat with a patch over her left eye that made her look a bit like a pirate, but the alluring orange of her coat was a fiery red that you might expect from a siren.

The first time that I met her was when she presented on Community Practice Service with a three-week history of progressive polyuria/polydipsia (PU/PD) and intermittent vomiting.

Her owners consented to a comprehensive work-up that diagnosed the underlying problem as chronic kidney disease (CKD). In those days, we called it chronic renal failure (CRF).

We worked in concert with her family to medically manage her the best we could until we couldn't, and that's when I saw her back nearly nine months later.

I remember walking into the exam room and not even recognizing the cat who laid before me.

In the months that had passed, she had lost her sheen. Her coat looked muted. Her eyes were dull. And her body spelled defeat.

Her bloodwork confirmed what we already knew: she had reached the end point of renal dysfunction.

We could have advised that she be admitted to the intensive care unit (ICU) for one last attempt at a Hail Mary.

And I did.

And then, I remember, her owners said, "No."

"No," followed by, "That wouldn't be fair."

I remember that those words took me by surprise because I had never heard them before in that context.

"Fair???" I asked, not quite catching their drift.

Lefty's owners could have gotten angry at me for questioning them.

Instead, one of her owners shared something that has stuck with me ever since.

Lefty's "mom" said:

You're asking us to take her away from home and family and everyone she loves for an End that is going to come anyway.

You're asking us to postpone the inevitable for what? A day? Two days? A week? Then what?

There's nothing that I would like more than that. We'd do anything to spend one more day, one more night with her.

That would be right for us.

But when we took her in, we promised to do right by her.

Doing right by her means making the choice for her, not us.

Making the choice means letting her go, even though letting her go is going to break us.

_____

I never forgot those words.

I remember filling up with tears in the back treatment area when I went to share the news with my colleagues and the attending clinician.

I remember relaying the client's wishes to the team.

And I remember someone on rotation saying, "So, they're giving up?"

I never forgot those words, either.

That's where clinical medicine and I went different ways.

To me, it wasn't about *giving up* on her.

It was about *accepting* the one and only choice that would make her whole again.

Life couldn't take away her pain and suffering, but death could.

I stopped running from death that day.

In those moments, death didn't seem so scary.

It seemed like a gift.

A gift that Lefty's family chose, for her, out of love.

It wasn't a decision that every family would have made. And that's okay.

It's not about cookie cutter treatment plans for cookie cutter cases.

Cases are more than cases. Patients are more than patients. Patients are individuals.

They are stories of lives that are as unique as fingerprints.

Each life, each story has a beginning, just as each life, each story has an ending.

Some ends may come before others.

And some ends we choose to rewrite, with love.

———————————————————

Since 2008, much has changed in the world of veterinary medical education, for the better. Curricular reform has been inspired by the accrediting bodies to identify, acknowledge, address, and remedy the proverbial elephant in the room: professional, communication-based, interpersonal skill deficiencies in graduates.

The American Veterinary Medical Association (AVMA) Council on Education (COE) now requires all accredited colleges of veterinary medicine to teach communication. Core curriculum includes communication in the British Isles and the Netherlands, and veterinary students at the Ontario Veterinary College (OVC) and the Royal Veterinary College of Veterinary Surgeons must demonstrate proficiency in communication skills to graduate. Other universities, such as the Atlantic Veterinary College of the University of Prince Edward Island, have built communication training into electives. In 2002, the North American Veterinary Medical Education Consortium was launched to develop guidelines for communication training. This momentum paved the way for U.S.-based colleges of veterinary medicine to modify pre-existing programs. Inaugural programs can draft professional skills into the curriculum from scratch, including the two programs for which I have served as founding faculty: Midwestern University College of Veterinary Medicine, which opened its doors in August 2014 to its inaugural class of 2018, and University of Arizona College of Veterinary Medicine, which opened its doors in August 2020 to its inaugural class of 2023.

At the University of Arizona, the Professional Skills coursework (VETM 802A, 802B, 802C, 802D, 815A, and 815B) represents six longitudinal semesters designed to introduce students to key occupational attributes that are required for success in the veterinary profession. Emphasis is placed on interpersonal and reflective skills that task students to consider:

- how they see themselves and each other
- how they establish and build onto their evolving professional identities
- how they define their roles in the profession as individuals and as colleagues
- how they communicate as team-members and as clinicians
- how they bolster connectivity within the veterinary team and practice relationship-centred care.

As students advance in the program, they actively engage in dialogue about:

- case management
- suboptimal patient outcomes
- client-centered goal setting
- unanticipated diagnoses and prognoses
- chronic illness
- terminal disease
- end-of-life: the medical aspects of euthanasia
- anticipatory grief and the interpersonal aspects of euthanasia
- euthanizing patients with treatable conditions
- economic euthanasia
- death notification
- unmet expectations for care
- boundary setting.

Emphasis is placed on how to engage in challenging conversations in clinical practice as students discover their voice as clinicians. With that voice comes the ability to make choices and to explain those choices to other members of the veterinary team. Not all cases have positive patient outcomes; not all cases are curable.

We frequently revisit case management from the perspective of suboptimal patient outcomes and encourage students to consider their interactions with clients as they engage in bad news delivery about patient diagnosis or prognosis, chronic illness, and terminal disease. We discuss what happens when there are unmet expectations for care and how to manage conflict within the veterinary team. This opens the door to entry-level discussions about how and when to set boundaries and how to reset ourselves as we reinvest in healthcare delivery to support the human-animal bond.

"One explicit goal is integration of medical content with intergroup dialogue skills and frameworks for critically reflective, life-long learning that originates from a place of cultural humility."(1)

Both as a profession and as a system by which we train the next generation of leaders, veterinary medicine has come so far.

We still have a significant way to go, as evidenced by a 2021 publication by Cooney et al. in the *Journal of Veterinary Medical Education*, which disclosed that:(2)

A survey of the 30 US veterinary schools was electronically mailed by the American Association of Veterinary Medical Colleges (AAVMC) in the fall of 2019, with a return rate of 10. Findings revealed that the average number of hours devoted to euthanasia methods and techniques was 2.8, yet euthanasia facilitation was considered a core competency by all schools responding. Not all veterinary students perform or are present for euthanasia. The most frequent method for teaching euthanasia was intracardiac and intravenous with dogs, cats, horses, livestock, and exotics. Whichever method of euthanasia is used, personnel performing euthanasia must be trained, knowledgeable, and proficient in the chosen techniques. The findings in this article suggest, however, that euthanasia techniques are inconsistent, and potentially incomplete, and that veterinary schools should consider incorporating more advanced euthanasia training programs into the curriculum.

This text aims to expand the breadth and depth of euthanasia education in colleges of veterinary medicine, so as to incorporate foundational understanding of grief and grieving, death and dying.

We owe it to Lefty's owners as much as we owe it to ourselves to acknowledge and affirm the inherent value of the human–animal bond and the resultant loss that takes place the day, the hour, the minute that earthly bond transitions.

Understanding the depth of loss and that loss is unique to all who experience it are foundational to the establishment and maintenance of veterinarian–client–patient relationships (VCPRs) that are long-lasting. VCPRs can survive death, but only when we fully commit ourselves to exploring and accepting the strength of the bond that was responsible for bringing us together.

References

1. Englar RE, Graham Brett T. Integrating communication skills, awareness of self and others, and reflective feedback into one inclusive anatomical representation of relationship-centered health care. J Vet Med Educ. 2023 (in press). Posted online 20 Dec 2022. https://doi.org/10.3138/jvme-2022-0060.
2. Cooney K, Dickinson GE, Hoffmann H. Euthanasia education in veterinary schools in the United States. J Vet Med Educ. 2021;48(6):706–9. https://doi.org/10.3138/jvme-2020-0050.

About the Authors

Ryane E. Englar

Ryane E. Englar, DVM, DABVP (Canine and Feline Practice) graduated from Cornell University College of Veterinary Medicine in 2008. She practiced as an associate veterinarian in companion animal practice before transitioning into the educational circuit as an advocate for pre-clinical training in primary care. She debuted in academia as a Clinical Instructor of the Community Practice Service at Cornell University's Hospital for Animals. She then transitioned into the role of Assistant Professor as founding faculty at Midwestern University College of Veterinary Medicine. While at Midwestern University, she had the opportunity to teach the inaugural Class of 2018, the Class of 2019, and the Class of 2020. While training these remarkable young professionals, Dr. Englar was awarded diplomate status by the American Board of Veterinary Practitioners (ABVP). She then joined the faculty at Kansas State University between May 2017 and January 2020 to launch the Clinical Skills curriculum.

In February 2020, Dr. Englar reprised her role of founding faculty when she returned "home" to Tucson to join the University of Arizona College of Veterinary Medicine. She serves as a dual appointment Associate Professor of Practice and the Executive Director of Clinical and Professional Skills.

Dr. Englar is passionate about advancing education for generalists by thinking outside of the box to develop new course materials for the hands-on learner. This text is preceded by six other labors of love that collectively provide students, clinicians, and educators alike with functional, relatable, and practice-friendly tools for success:

- *Performing the Small Animal Physical Examination* (John Wiley & Sons, Inc., 2017)
- *Writing Skills for Veterinarians* (5M Publishing, Ltd., 2019)
- *Common Clinical Presentations in Dogs and Cats* (John Wiley & Sons, Inc., 2019)

- *A Guide to Oral Communication in Veterinary Medicine* (5M Publishing, Ltd., 2020)
- *The Veterinary Workbook of Small Animal Clinical Cases* (5M Books Ltd, 2021)
- *Low-Cost Veterinary Clinical Diagnostics* (John Wiley & Sons, Inc., 2023).

Dr. Englar's students inspire her to write so that they have the resources they need to not just survive but thrive post-graduation.

When Dr. Englar is not teaching or advancing companion animal primary care, she trains in the art of ballroom dancing and competes nationally with her instructor, Lowell E. Fox.

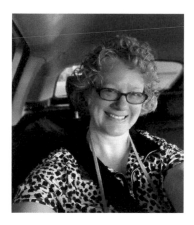 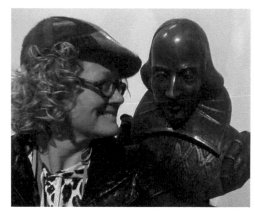

Jill B. Englar

Jill Englar, MSW, LCSW-C, CAGCS was a social worker for a local home healthcare agency when she attended a seminar on grief and bereavement by Dr. Alan Wolfelt. In that moment in time, her career path changed forever. His messaging that grief was individual and could not be carved out of a calendar resonated with her. There was no timeline for grief, which was defined by what and whom you had lost. Grief was about our internal processes – the bereaved's attempts to regain understanding of a world that had changed all around them. Having lost a brother and father three months apart in two separate accidents when she was 14, Jill was thrust back into school and told to return to normal living. Two months later, her mother was forced into bankruptcy and she lost their family home and floundered in the deep end of the ocean.

Everything that Dr. Wolfelt spoke about companioning the bereaved and allowing them to tell their grief story over and over again to process the pain of their loss made sense. That is when Jill decided to use her Master's degree in Social Work to become certified by the Association for Death Education and Counseling (ADEC) as a grief counselor and educator. Over the past 30 years at BridgingLife Hospice (formerly Carroll Hospice), she has journeyed with hundreds of bereaved individuals as they sought a "safe harbor" in which to share their story and have it honored.

Jill is proud to have co-authored this book with her daughter, Dr. Ryane Englar, who teaches veterinary students and colleagues how to communicate compassionate and informative end of life options and how to provide empathetic listening to the bereaved.

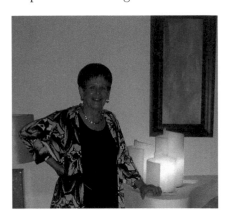 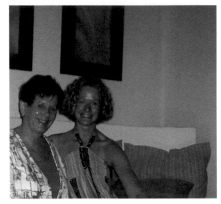

Teresa Graham Brett

Teresa Graham Brett, JD, leads efforts to fully integrate inclusion at the University of Arizona College of Veterinary Medicine. Along with Dr. Ryane Englar, she serves as course co-director of six consecutive semesters of the longitudinal Professional Skills coursework. They have

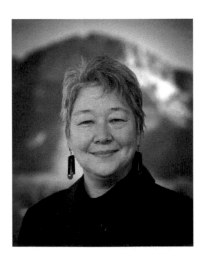

successfully integrated the development of skills for enhancing diversity and supporting inclusivity in veterinary medicine throughout the Professional Skills curriculum. Prior to being at the College of Veterinary Medicine, she served as Assistant Vice President for Diversity and Inclusion at the University of Arizona. Brett also served as Associate Vice President of Student Affairs and Dean of Students at the University of Texas at Austin, introducing intergroup dialogue coursework into the undergraduate curriculum. Prior to her time at UT, she served as Associate Dean and Co-Director of the Program on Intergroup Relations at University of Michigan, Ann Arbor. Brett provides consultation and training in the areas of intergroup dialogue, social justice education, and integration of equitable and inclusive content and learning processes into the curriculum.

Dedication

People talk about having a "heart dog." A heart dog has been described as many things by many different people:

- a once-in-a-lifetime dog
- a soulmate
- a game-changer and life-shaper
- a dog who influences who you are and who you become
- a dog who leaves a permanent mark on your soul.

It's much less common to hear about someone's "heart cat." Perhaps that's because of the age-old saying that a dog is man's best friend.

Yet, those of us who have been *chosen* by cats can attest to the fact that there is more to these creatures than their aloof reputation might suggest. Cats, like dogs, can also form secure attachments to their guardians. These attachments vary in terms of bond strength as is true of any relationship; however, there are those connections that transcend even death.

Some cats, special cats, can even knead their way into your hearts and in so doing, carve out a space that only they can occupy. It is a privilege that a select few humans come to know and depend upon.

It is an honor that my very own Bailey bestowed upon me.

I had grown up with cats underfoot. Before Bailey, there was Tiger and Pudding. Yet, as much as I loved my childhood cats and as much as I will forever be in their debt for inspiring my passion for veterinary medicine, their respective connections to me were not the same as mine and Bailey's.

From the moment I first laid my eyes on Bailey, before hers had even opened, something changed within me. It was as if from that moment forward, our lives were intricately, intimately woven together in a way that only we could ever understand.

She was truly *mine*. Not mine in the sense of ownership but rather, mine to look after, nourish, cherish, love, and protect.

She was *mine* to be forever responsible for in a way that I had never known. Perhaps that's how new parents feel when they hold their infant for the very first time. I don't know. I've never experienced that joy.

I just know that as I held Bailey in the palm of my hand, I felt complete. As though this little being who had only just met me would know me better than I knew myself in the days to come. There was a certain peace and comfort in knowing that. A certain sense of letting go of the walls that I had figuratively constructed and letting her in.

It's indescribable and unrelatable unless you yourself have experienced it, the pureness of a bond that has no reason for being. It just is. And, in that precarious state of existence somewhere between life and death, you for the first time ever truly find yourself. You learn to see yourself through another's lens and you recognize that the person you are, with them, is who you forever want to be.

Bailey's story is documented within this text, in Chapter 7. You'll come to see her through my own eyes and journal entries. What I hope you'll take away from the story of our journey together is that Bailey made me a better me.

Bailey was my "heart cat" in every way.

She was my baby.

She was an 18-year chapter of my life that I would not change a single page of.

After all, Bailey taught me what it meant to both live and love unconditionally.

She taught me how to love and how to let go; how to let someone in, and how to be my authentic self.

In Memoriam
Bailey's Crème Brûlée
April 12, 2004 – October 17, 2022

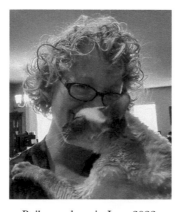

Bailey and me in June 2022.

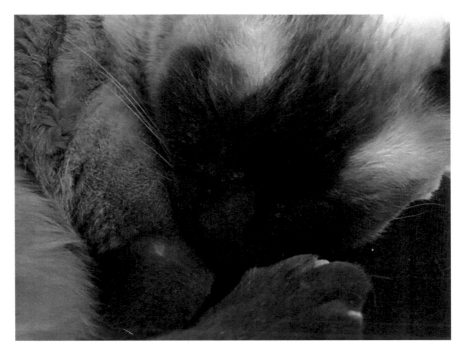

Bailey in January 2022.

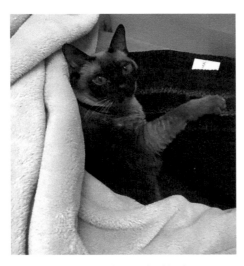

Bailey burrowing under blankets.

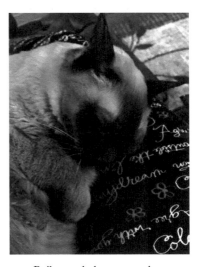

Bailey curled up on my lap.

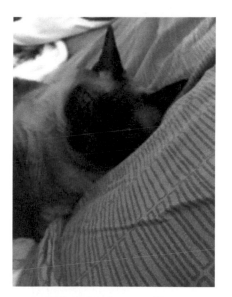

Bailey's head on my pillow.

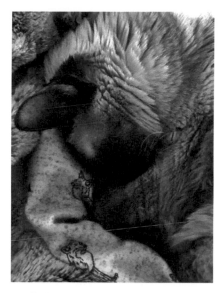

Bailey curled up on her fox blanket.

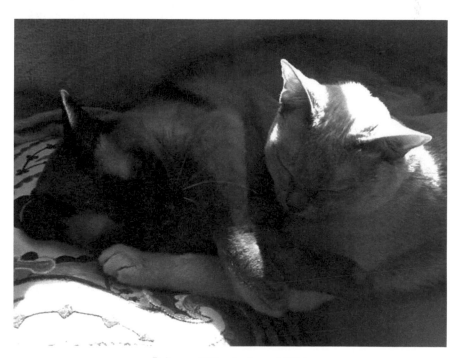

Bailey and Nina in August 2014.

Acknowledgments

Coaching On and Off the Dance Floor

Twelve weeks before writing this textbook, I unexpectedly sustained significant orthopedic trauma to my right knee. The inciting event had in fact occurred months prior, with the degree of damage unbeknownst to me. That single domino set into motion a chain reaction for which there could be only one end to the story: my right knee fell apart during a basic backstep action in foxtrot, and I collapsed into my dance instructor's frame.

The details of the grief that ensued have been penned into the body of Chapter 6, but the moment that surgical repair became a necessity, all I knew for sure was that my future in dance was uncertain.

To say that I was despondent in that snapshot of time was an understatement. Dance had become, over the years, my one consistent outlet, my one escape from the rigors of veterinary practice, and my one true source of self-expression. It was, after all, through dance that I had learned not to define myself by work alone. Dance had found a way to allow my authentic self to show the world what was inside my heart.

Yet, it wasn't dance alone that had changed me. It was more specifically my partnership in dance with instructor Lowell Fox of Arrowhead Arthur Murray (Peoria, Arizona). Lowell not only changed the way I felt about myself on the dance floor. Lowell changed the way I felt about me, period. Lowell became, by every measure, the best coach I had ever known because he told me what I needed to hear, when I needed to hear it, whether it was what I wanted to hear … or not!

By the time this text comes into print, we will have been dancing together for nine years. Nine years is a quarter of my life and most of my adulthood – at least, all the parts, post-college, that matter most. In that timeframe, Lowell managed to dig beneath my carefully constructed, protective walls to see the *real* me. There were times when I didn't recognize my own reflection or the person I was growing into, but he always did.

Lowell recognized and accepted and valued the *real* me and in doing so, he transformed my understanding of self and the way I related to the world around me. He taught me that I could be more than I ever imagined. His belief made me believe in me, too.

When surgical necessity required me to put aside my dance shoes, albeit transiently, I was stopped in my tracks, literally. Dance had become my sanctuary and I no longer knew who I was in its immediate absence. I struggled within myself and came to know exactly what Michael Jordan meant when he shared that "my body could stand the crutches, but my mind couldn't stand the sideline."

I wanted to be most where I couldn't and that stung.

Richard Bach once wrote that:(1)

Look in the mirror and one thing is sure: what we see is not who we are.

and

When you have come to the edge of all the light you have
And step into the darkness of the unknown
Believe that one of the two will happen to you
Either you'll find something solid to stand on
Or you'll be taught how to fly!(2)

Lowell brought both quotes to life as we navigated pre- and post-operative rehabilitation together. When I looked in the mirror, what I saw was adversity: a braced leg and the tortuous path of learning how to walk again.

When Lowell looked in my mirror, he saw tenacity and strength. He saw the me that I would grow into, when in that moment all I saw was the me caught between a rock and a hard place.

Lowell acknowledged my fears and affirmed them. At the same time, he worked overtime to reframe my mindset. He got me out of the habit of talking about my "bad" leg.

"The last I checked," he'd say to me, "You have two good legs, one just needed a leg up, literally," followed by a reminder that it was okay to ask for – and receive – help.

When I couldn't conceive of how he and our coach, Valentina Kostenko, would create our next routine, given that I had been benched, Lowell believed that "where there's a will, there's a way." They proceeded to bring to life the most breathtaking, beautiful piece of choreography that I have ever seen – an outside-of-the-box, exclusive upper body workout, with me seated at a bench and with Lowell as the figurative wind beneath my wings. The piece was written in my pre-operative period, yet chronicles my recovery, set to the tune of the Pentatonix version of "The Prayer."

When he had shared with me his plan to create our comeback routine, I couldn't imagine then how a piece on a bench could look anything but weak. Lowell knocked it out of the ballpark, times infinity. He and Valentina designed the most exquisitely radiant, powerful display of strength. He created what I needed to see, at a time when I needed it most, because he knew that I needed to see the End to know that it was just the Beginning.

When I regained my stability and was starting to take "baby steps," relearning how to put one foot in front of the other, Lowell reminded me that all steps, no matter how small, are still "forward progress."

When I talked about being "behind" at dance because I'd spent all my waking hours pouring into physical therapy, Lowell reminded me that PT was "how you get ahead."

When I couldn't visualize being back out there on the dance floor in the next chapter of life, Lowell reminded me of the dancer that I was *then* and the version 2.0 dancer that I was becoming *now*.

Lowell talked about our *next* competition until I finally believed that it could happen. He carried the torch of faith for me, for us, so that it could reignite the blaze within, that internal, confident, certain, and unwavering blaze that knew my journey in dance wasn't over; it was only just starting.

There are those in our lives because they have to be, and there are those in our lives because they want to be. That Lowell chooses to companion me in this journey of life – as my dance teacher, coach, and friend – is both a privilege and an honor. He is essential.

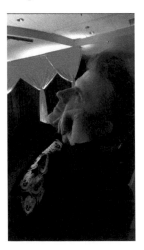

Lowell at the Nebraska Dance Festival
in November 2019.

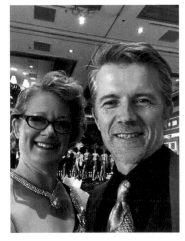

Lowell and me at the World Promotions
Event, Viva Las Vegas, in July 2022.

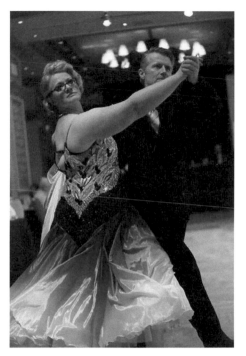

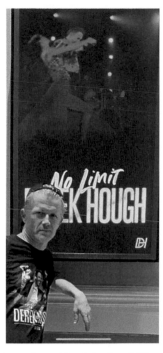

Lowell and me at the World Promotions Event, Viva Las Vegas, in July 2022.

Lowell outside of the Derek Hough show at the Summit Showroom at the Venetian Resort.

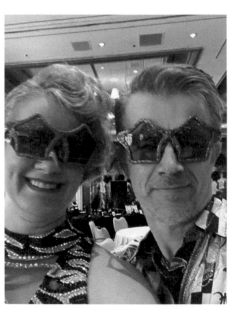

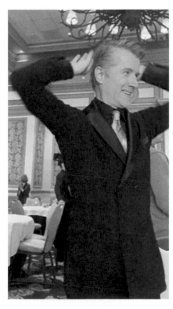

Lowell and me at the World Promotions Event, Viva Las Vegas, in July 2022.

Lowell Fox, demonstrating his "Fox-a-doble" creation.

Coaching On and Off the Lecture Circuit

It is often said that the veterinary profession is a small world. Veterinarians tend to operate under six degrees of separation or less. We are all just a friend of a friend of a friend, or so it seems.

The unexpected webs that link us to each other create a circle of relationships in which time stands still and geography knows no bounds. Classmates who have been apart for decades can be brought together again in unforeseen ways – through clients, through friends, or even family.

Colleagues are the unique family that we choose for ourselves. They understand us better than most because, simply put, they've been there, in our shoes, one too many times, more often than they can count. They recognize our professional challenges more than those on the periphery of our innermost circle, and they both see and honor our individual and collective struggles.

Through each other, we find strength, grace, and hope.

No one embodies that journey and the collaborative spirit that our profession strives to exude more than my very dear friend, Miguel Ángel Díaz Sánchez, Director of New Way Coaching.

Miguel Ángel, whom I know colloquially by his nickname Pancho, is an accomplished being. He is a pioneer who long ago recognized a need within our profession to broaden, expand, and deepen leadership training and coaching in communication.

It is in fact because of his passion for a team approach that our paths crossed years ago at one of Cindy Adams' interactive International Conferences on Communication in Veterinary Medicine (ICCVM). It may have been, for me, my first foray into the formalized world of veterinary communication training, yet Pancho welcomed me into the fold with open arms as if I were an old friend.

I recall being so in awe of his talent, his presence, and his evidence-based methodology that had pioneered successful partnerships with veterinarians, business owners, and entrepreneurs. I remember wanting to say so much to this inspirational leader, yet feeling like such a tadpole in this vast ocean of communication giants. Pancho picked up on my shyness from the start and when I explained my reluctance to share my ideas when I had so very little to contribute by comparison, he simply radiated a warm, sincere smile back at me and said, "We can be tadpoles together."

What he meant by that, and what he shared with me later, is that he was no "bigger" or "better" than me, and I was not "lesser." We both breathed the same air and swam in the same ocean.

I never forgot that moment in time. It has stuck with me all through the years as a reminder that we are all in the same boat, paddling forward, as one.

It's not about comparisons. It's about *connections*.

Pancho's humility is characteristic of a soul who uplifts others. Being in his presence is like reaching out and touching the sun. His warm zest for life is tangible. What I love most about him is that he rises to the occasion, always, to meet others where they are at, rather than expecting them to meet him at his tier.

The friendship that began that day is ever-present now and over the years we have found unexpected ways to reconnect. Our journey together to co-present in Prague in June 2022 was yet another testament to the fact that friendship has no expiration date.

Richard Bach once said: "Your friends will know you better in the first minute you meet than your acquaintances will know you in a thousand years."(3)

Such is Pancho's way and the beautiful harmony that he creates with others that share his journey.

Over the years, Pancho has taught me a great many life lessons, including the following:

- "Value yourself."
- "Ask yourself who you are and wait to hear the answer. You might surprise yourself."
- "There is no 'I' in teach. The best teachers transcend time and space because they ask the right questions: What is it that the student wishes to accomplish and how do you construct a path to get them there?"
- "Timelines are manmade constructs. Be open to possibilities you never forecast; even a weatherman gets it wrong. You don't have to be right to find your correct path. Even better yet, your correct path may change."
- "You don't have to be superhuman, you just have to be yourself."
- "Vulnerability is strength, you just have to see the world through the correct glasses."
- "Confront conflict with transparency: learn how to articulate 'What I want' and 'What I don't want.'"
- "Trade expectations for appreciation."
- "Know the difference between expectations and goals. You can expect sunny skies all you want, but the skies have their own will. Learn to lean on your own goals for you rather than your expectations for someone else. Expectations mislead; goals aspire."

Pancho's energy is like lightning on a mission – the right combination of strength and power with a touch of gentleness so as not to singe the rain.

He is inspirational and has influenced my reactions to life events in a way that has helped me to process them, on my own timeline, at my own pace.

I don't know that I will ever meet another Pancho, but I do know one thing for certain. The world is a much better place with him in it – someone I am honored to call a friend as well as the family that I choose for myself.

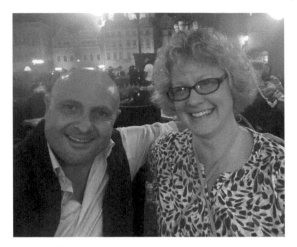

Pancho and me in Prague, June 2022.

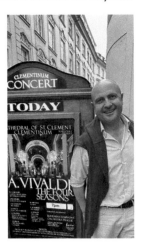

Pancho in Prague in 2022.

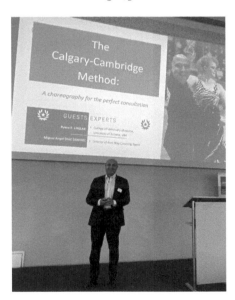

Pancho, my co-presenter, in Prague in 2022.

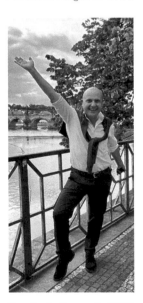

Pancho in Prague in 2022.

References

1. Bach R. The bridge across forever: a true love story. New York: William Morrow Paperbacks; 2006.
2. Bach R. Jonathan Livingston Seagull: a story. New York: Avon; 1973.
3. Bach R. Illusions: the adventures of a reluctant messiah. London: Arrow Books; reprint edition 2001.

Part One

The Human–Animal Bond, Grief, Grieving, Death, and Dying

CHAPTER I

Beyond Self

Animal–Animal Interactions, Human–Animal Interactions, and the Evolution of the Human–Animal Bond

The ability to stretch beyond self to establish connections with others is not unique to people. Such attachments within the animal kingdom were first researched with respect to the bond that forms between infant and mother, particularly among nonhuman primates(1, 2) and other mammalian species.(3) Early accounts postulated that "herd instinct" was innate rather than learned and that attachments between related animals formed only as a result of close proximity and physiologic state (e.g., lactation).(3) Subsequent research has disclosed that attachments can form between conspecifics in the absence of nursing and altriciality.

1.1 The Capacity for Animals to Recognize Members of the Same Species

Animals learn to recognize others through olfactory, vocal, and visual cues, and they use these cues to identify each other in the future.(4–11) Hermit crabs and lobsters have the capacity for individual recognition through scent(12, 13), and facial recognition is not unique to primates.(9, 11) Sheep and wasps also possess this ability.(7, 8)

Animals do not only recognize in the moment; some also have capacity for recall and remember conspecifics even when they have been apart for extended durations.(4) Despite two years of forced separation, sheep can identify previous flock mates(7), and a type of migratory songbird, the hooded warbler, recalls nesting neighbors from last year's breeding season.(14) Even more striking is the memory of the bottlenose dolphin, which can recognize the sound of podmates' whistles for two decades.(15) This is not unlike human affiliations: young adults commonly maintain connections across long distances for eight or more years.(16)

1.2 Interspecies Connections Between Non-Human Animals

Attachments are not unique to conspecifics. They can form between members of different species.(17–19) One or more species often overlap in terms of habitat and resources.(20) It is through this shared environment that symbiotic associations often form.(20–22) These relationships may be unilaterally beneficial, as in parasitism; helpful to one animal without impacting or harming the other, as in commensalism; or reflective of mutualism, in which both animals benefit from their interactions.(22) In some circumstances, mutualism is even obligate, in which animals (or species) are entirely dependent upon one another for survival.

Authors Surindar Paracer and Vernon Ahmadjian captured best the webs of connectivity that bridge species when they wrote that:(21)

No organism is an island – each one has a relationship to other organisms, directly or indirectly. Even humans bear a reminder of an ancient symbiosis – their cells contain mitochondria, organelles which once were symbiotic bacteria. In addition, each of us harbors several types of viruses and bacteria in our skin and intestinal tract. Similarly, chloroplasts in plant cells are organelles which have evolved from ancient symbiotic photosynthetic bacteria. Bacteria which form symbioses with higher forms of life are themselves host to symbiotic viruses. Satellite viruses depend on other viruses for their expression. It is difficult to imagine life and its evolutionary history without symbioses.

Connectivity to others is thought to be an evolutionarily sound strategy to combat predation through safety in numbers, as may be said of the aggregates of zebras and wildebeest that cohabitate on the plains of the Serengeti or the large mixed feeding groups of blackbirds and sandpipers.(23) Other examples exist in which there is reciprocity in predator warnings between species. Consider, for instance, the close associations between zebras and ostriches on the east African plains.(23) The superior vision of the ostrich paired with the zebra's superior olfaction are an example of behavioral opportunism that allows each to alert the other to potential danger.(20, 23, 24)

Interspecies connections may be motivated by survival, yet anecdotes spread through word of mouth, in the popular press, and via social media suggest that species interactions may be relational and involve close, enduring bonds.(25–31) Moreover, animals recognize each other's relationships and this knowledge drives their behaviors.(31) Animals react and respond to one another with respect to rank and status, but also with apparent friendship.(31)

1.3 Animal Friendships

Although some researchers have argued that friendships are human constructs, the neural and physiological mechanisms that underlie social bonds are not unique to humans.(4, 5, 32) The posterior pituitary-derived hormone, oxytocin, is present in all mammals and has been tied to sexual reproduction, parturition(33), and lactation.(34–37) Although oxytocin has been studied extensively with respect to the milk-ejection reflex, it is critical to note that oxytocin also exerts effects in males and non-lactating females.(37) Oxytocin is capable of inducing positive physiologic effects by acting as an anxiolytic, reducing blood pressure, and increasing nociceptive pain thresholds in both male and female rats.(38–42) Oxytocin can trigger maternal behavior in pup-less rats(43) and enhance social interactions.(37, 44) It has also been linked to pair-bonding.(20, 45)

Pair-bonding refers to a strong affinity that develops in some species, often among mating pairs. Such a bond is said to strengthen their commitment to each other as well as to the tasks of producing and rearing offspring by virtue of behavioral compatibility. Examples from the animal kingdom include the monogamy that is characteristic of prairie voles(46) and the majority of birds(47–50) as well as some insects(51, 52), lizards(53), and fish.(54–56)

Pair-bonding does not have to involve sexual relations. It can be more loosely defined as an intentional choice to establish and maintain a selective and enduring relationship between two unrelated beings. Social affiliation is an evolved trait that promotes individual and species survival, and is supported by neurobiology not only by means of oxytocin, but also vasopressin, corticotropin-releasing hormone (CRH), endogenous opioids, steroid hormones, and neuropeptides.(57)

Biology-enhanced bonding can also occur among heterospecifics, that is, individuals of different species. Reports of these are typically anecdotal, and most commonly among captive animals, although interspecies bonds among wildlife have been documented.(25–29) Such interspecies bonds have been reinforced and romanticized in children's literature. Consider, for instance, *The Wind in the Willows* (1908; mole–rat–badger–toad), *The Incredible Journey* (1961; cat–dogs), *Bambi* (1923; fawn–rabbit–skunk), *Winnie The Pooh* (1926; bear–piglet–donkey–tiger), *The Fox and the Hound* (1967), and *The Adventures of Milo and Otis* (1988; cat–dog).(58–63) The bonds between lead characters are presented as being analogous to human relationships with other humans. The depicted emotions and the emotional interplay that has been scripted within and between species resonates with those who see themselves and their relationships brought to life.

Perhaps no work is as substantial in capturing an unlikely friendship between two animals than E. B. White's enthralling tale, *Charlotte's Web* (1952), in which lonely spring pig Wilbur bonds with a barn-dwelling spider.(64) The story of Wilbur and Charlotte's friendship is rooted in sacrificial friendship. As winter draws nearer and Charlotte's life approaches its natural conclusion, she commits to a final act of web-messaging on Wilbur's behalf to save her friend from slaughter. As she lay dying, Wilbur is wrought with anticipatory loss:(64)

> *"Why did you do all this for me?" he asked. "I don't deserve it. I've never done anything for you."*

> *"You have been my friend," replied Charlotte. "That in itself is a tremendous thing."*

Friendship transcends death in that Charlotte's memory lives on, inside of Wilbur. The author concludes his tale with the following statement about grief and grieving, life and living:(64)

> *Wilbur never forgot Charlotte. Although he loved her children and grandchildren dearly, none of the new spiders ever quite took her place in his heart. She was in a class by herself. It is not often that someone comes along who is a true friend and a good writer. Charlotte was both.*

In this excerpt, E.B. White captures a certain sanctity about friendship as a bond that is inherently irreplaceable. Other connections can and may form, yet another spider can never replace Charlotte. Charlotte is, in essence, one of a kind.

1.4 Human–Animal Interactions

Many people search for and desire the kind of depth that such intimate emotional attachment to others offers, and often find these experiences in non-human animals.(65) Those who have experienced this articulate that these bonds promote security, stability, and unconditional positive regard. (66–68) Yet, emotionally deep connections between humans and animals are not unique to the present day, though the growing significance of this so-called human–animal bond was slow to be recognized by the scientific community.(69)

History tells us that ancient peoples and cultures came to depend upon and value their close proximity to animals.(70) In those early civilizations, animals functioned as sources of food (through hunting, herding, or fishing), clothing (through hides, wool, or hair), footwear (as in leather), shelter (as in teepees), flooring (as through the use of dung to prepare plaster floors), heat and fuel (as through the burning of dung), fertilizer (as through the use of dung to support agronomy), pest control (through mousers), and alarm bells (through the barking of guard dogs) that warned of impending danger.(20, 71–74) In some cultures and communities, animals were seen as links to human spirituality or guiding spirits.(75)

Human–animal interactions and specifically human–animal connections have in many ways shaped our development as a species around the world.(73) Prehistoric peoples were aware of and attuned to non-human animals and depicted them in some of the earliest works of art, cave drawings.(71, 72) Archeological evidence discloses that ancestors of the dog associated closely with human settlements over 14,000 years ago, 2000 years or so before their domestication.(70, 76) Wolves are depicted in cave paintings as being seated around campfires in the company of people.(75) It is presumed that they were valued as guardians, hunters, fishers, and herders.(76, 77)

1.5 The History of Domestication

Domestication of the dog took place at least 12,000 years ago.(17) Cats began their association with humans, primarily as a means of rodent control, between 9000 and 12,000 years ago, in the Fertile Crescent.(70) Egyptians came across lions, panthers, and jungle cats in the wild, and grew accepting of those smaller cats that patrolled their granaries. The dual nature of cats – gracefully swift and gentle, yet potentially aggressive and dangerous – piqued the human interest. The rise of cats in ancient Egypt was attributed to the human perception that they were made in the image of goddess Bastet. Daughter of the sun god, Ra, and protector and bringer of good health, Bastet was depicted as having the head of a cat and a slender female body. By day, Bastet was said to watch over Ra as his boat pulled the sun through the sky. At night, Bastet was said to transform into a cat to protect Ra from his serpentine enemy, Apep.

Companion dogs were also valued in ancient Egypt. When they died, they were said to guide the afterlife. Owners openly mourned deceased canine companions by shaving off their eyebrows and muddying their hair as a sign of respect.(70) Those with financial means embalmed and mummified companion dogs in preparation for burial within sacred necropolises.(70, 75, 78) Some companion dogs were even buried within their owners' tombs.(75)

Companion dogs were also a part of the histories of the early Greek and Roman empires.(70, 79) Dogs were respected for their perceived loyalty, which was written into *The Odyssey* when Homer paid tribute to the fictitious dog, Argos, who after years of forced separation from master, Odysseus, was the only one to recognize him in disguise upon his return:(80)

> *As they spoke, a dog who was lying there lifted his head*
> *and pricked up his ears. It was Argos, Odysseus' dog;*
> *he had trained him and brought him up as a puppy, but never*
> *hunted with him before he sailed off to Troy.*
> *In earlier times the young men had taken him out*
> *with them to hunt for wild goats and deer and hares,*
> *but he had grown old in his master's absence, and now*
> *he lay abandoned on one of the heaps of mule*
> *and cattle dung that piled up outside the front gates*
> *until the farmhands could come by and cart it off*
> *to manure the fields. And so the dog Argos lay there,*
> *covered with ticks. As soon as he was aware*
> *of Odysseus, he wagged his tail and flattened his ears,*
> *but he lacked the strength to get up and go to his master.*
> *Odysseus wiped a tear away.*
>
> (Translated, from the Greek, by Stephen Mitchell)

The timeless connection between Odysseus and Argos reflects the times. Much like ancient Egypt, early Greek and Roman empires affirmed the importance of companion animals through their burials, and owners' epithets are expressive of the sorrow that was felt at time of death.(70) The paired skeletal remains of a child and dog Delta – identified by his silver engraved collar – at the ruins of Pompeii emphasize the degree to which humans bonded with their companion animals.(70) Animal burial sites have been uncovered in other parts of the world, including Peru, where preserved bodies of the early Chiribaya people have been buried with food alongside their dogs, wrapped in blankets.(70, 81)

During the Middle Ages, there was a shift in public perception towards cats in Europe. They were transiently rejected as a symbol of Satan and associated with witchcraft.(17, 70)

After the Middle Ages, there was a rise in the popularity of purebred animals.(70) Certain breeds became status symbols as they were owned by the wealthy elite and/or the ruling class.(70) Some dogs belonging to the aristocracy in Asia were assigned their own servants.(70) In China, the Pekingese dog was bred by royalty for royalty.(70) The mark of a good palace dog was one that was small enough to be able to fit into an empress' sleeve.(70) In Japan, dogs were housed in the royal family's private quarters for warmth and security.(70) Lap dogs were also popularized by Queen Victoria during the 19th century.(70)

At the same time, there was a push for the growing middle class to acquire "aristocratic" animals to elevate their status and/or appear affluent.(70) "Best in show" events were a way to emulate the rich as dogs continued to work their way into the home and become a central part of family life.(70) Meanwhile, it was not until the 19th century in Western culture that cats' popularity resurfaced.(17)

1.6 The Beginnings of Animal-Assisted Therapy and Service Animals

In addition to providing guardianship and companionship, animals were beginning to receive recognition as therapeutic agents. The concept that animals could fulfill this role was not new: equine-assisted therapy was routinely used in ancient Greece for disabled soldiers.(75, 82)

Animal-assisted therapy was first formally documented in England at a Quaker Hospital, the Retreat, at York in 1792. Founded by William Tuke, the Retreat commonly paired rabbits with patients to reduce the use of physical restraints.(75) This marked a significant transitional period in the field of mental health. Prior to the opening of the Retreat, mental health patients had been housed in asylums. The Retreat humanized those in need and provided resources, including small mammals, that fostered connections between patients and the world around them rather than reinforce isolation.

Over the next 100 years, animals continued to be introduced to institutional care facilities to support the physically and mentally disabled. (75, 79, 83, 84) During psychotherapy sessions in the late 1800s and early 1900s, Sigmund Freud's dogs often made themselves present, particularly Jofi, the Chow Chow.(75) The dogs had been initially brought in by Freud to function as a source of comfort for him until he recognized the positive impact that they had on his patients.(75, 79) Thereafter, he maintained them in his practice.

Dogs were not formally implemented into therapeutic settings in the United States until 1919, when they made their debut at St. Elizabeth's Hospital in Washington, D.C., to companion psychiatric care residents. (75) Animal-assisted therapy expanded during World War II as a means to support soldiers who had endured physical and psychological trauma, long before the discovery of post-traumatic stress disorder (PTSD) as a diagnosis in 1980.(75, 83) Specifically, Dr. Charles Mayo, the Founder of the Mayo Clinic and the Commanding Officer of the Pawling Army Air Force Convalescent Hospital, brought Smoky, his Yorkshire Terrier, to the wards. Smoky was so popular that his therapy work continued for 12 years after World War II.(75, 79)

In addition to contributing to the service of therapy, dogs can also be trained to perform a service role. Although the first guide dog training school was founded in Germany after World War I, the formal use of service dogs is relatively new. The requirement that public institutions provide reasonable accommodations for service dogs was written into law in 1990 in the Americans with Disabilities Act (ADA).(75) The ADA identifies service dogs as "any animal individually trained to do work or perform tasks for the benefit of a person with a disability including a physical, sensory, psychiatric, intellectual, or other mental disability" (CRF:36:104). (75) Service dogs can be viewed as adaptive interventions for those with a wide range of needs, including people with sight, hearing, or physical impairments.(75)

Although not classified as service animals under the ADA, dogs can also serve as emotional support animals (ESA).(75) An ESA may not be specifically trained to perform tasks that assist with disabilities, yet its presence has been associated with the provision of comfort, reduction of depression, and increased motivation to interact with others.(75)

Support and service animals provide unique roles. These animals are often said to give people back their lives by promoting independence, personal autonomy, self-ownership, and/or self-determination. It is not uncommon for strong attachments to form between support and service animals and their handlers, and for these animals to be seen as companioning their handlers through life in a way that no one else can replicate.

1.7 Enhancers of the Human–Animal Bond

Indeed, companionship – whether in the form of a service dog, ESA, or, simply put, a best friend in a non-human animal body – is prized by many in today's world. Attachments can form between people and any animal, whether domestic or wild. Among companion animals, people most often bond with dogs, cats, horses, llamas, pigs, goats, birds, fish, reptiles, and small mammals.(17) Such bonds are said to be enhanced by anthropomorphism, neoteny, and allelomimetic behaviors.(17)

Anthropomorphism refers to the assignment of human characteristics to anyone other than a human being, as opposed to personification, which applies human traits to inanimate objects.(17, 65) For instance, an anthropomorphized cat may be said to display empathy if the cat is perceived to be considerate of the owner's emotional plight. Likewise, an anthropomorphized dog may be said to exhibit a guilty disposition if the owner catches the dog after it inappropriately eliminated in the home. In fact, in a 2007 study by Morris et al., nearly three-fourths of dog-owning participants reported their perception that their dogs were capable of feeling "guilt."(65, 85) Social media posts about companion animals frequently ascribe human-like traits. A parrot that is bobbing its head may be described as dancing. A howling dog may be depicted as singing.

Neoteny is the retention of juvenile traits into adulthood.(17, 86) These features in animals may be physical, as in rounded foreheads, large eyes, and foreshortened muzzles.(86) Brachycephalic canine and feline breeds, for instance the Pomeranian dog and the Persian cat, have maximized these infantile characteristics.(17) Neotenic features may also be behavioral. Consider, for instance, the play behavior and high-pitched, often frequent vocalizations in adult domesticated dogs as compared with wolves. (17, 86) Juvenile behaviors facilitate handling when it comes to production animals. Domesticated animals are in this way more tractable than their non-domesticated counterparts.(20) Juvenile behaviors, among companion animals, may also elicit care-giving responses, which in turn may serve as reinforcement for displaying them.(17)

The cinema is rich with examples of neoteny. Consider the classic animated cartoon character, Mickey Mouse, who was co-created in 1928 by Walt Disney and Ub Iwerks. Between his initial creation and 1979, when Dr. Stephen Jay Gould published his insights about neoteny in an article in *Natural History* magazine, Mickey Mouse underwent significant changes in his head and facial feature proportions:

> *Mickey's eye size increased from 27 to 42% of head length; his head length increased from 42.7 to 48.1% of body length; and his nose to front ear (cranial vault) from 71.7 to 95.6% of nose to rear ear. He is evolving towards his young nephew Morty. With more juvenile form comes more juvenile behavior, and over the years, Mickey, like Morty, has become more affable and vulnerable and less cunning.(20)*

The same fate has transformed the teddy bear. Today's toy bears little resemblance to the original model, "Teddy's Bear," named after the then president Theodore Roosevelt, and designed in 1903 by the Ideal Toy Company.(20, 87) This shift reflects the pervasive trend towards marketing for cuteness rather than realism. Evidence-based research consistently points to the human preference for features that are exaggerated and/or infantile.(20)

The depiction of infantile features is a key influencer of human emotion. Neotenic features in the 1942 Disney motion picture, *Bambi*, influenced an entire generation's perception of hunting.(20, 88, 89) In the words of author Shane Mahoney, penned in *Sports Afield*:(90)

> *For hunters, the film has long been seen as emblematic of, and perhaps as the instigator of, antihunting sentiment. While the latter is not true (opposition to hunting long predates this film), there is no doubt that Bambi launched an alternative worldview upon the American (and eventually the global) consciousness where animals share virtually every human capacity and virtue but no human vice, and where man is definitely a foreboding presence and a villain seeking an end to the ideals of peaceful coexistence.*

The neotenic face is a powerful storyteller and driver of emotion, whether we are consciously or unconsciously aware of it.(20) Even the 1982 American science fiction film, *E.T.*, produced and directed by Steven Spielberg, managed to inspire an alternate, gentler view of extra-terrestrial life by outfitting the main character with rounded, enlarged eyes, communicative facial expressions, including a recognizable smile, and an erect humanoid stance.(17)

In addition to neoteny, allelomimetic behaviors are also said to intensify the bond that many of us share with companion animals. Such behaviors are a fancy way of describing actions that are likely to be replicated. In other words, exhibiting one or more behaviors is likely to inspire another animal to do the same. Such copycat or imitative behavior can occur in any species, but most often occurs in those who reside within social groups. It is thought to have evolutionarily developed as a safety mechanism. For instance, if one animal flees, the others take note and follow suit.(20) This synchrony of behavior is essential for survival and is characteristic of prey animals, such as the white-tailed deer. When this species is alarmed, the tail goes up. The color of the tail, white, is a visual cue to the others in the area that danger has arrived and it's best to run.

1.8 The Evolving Roles of Companion Animals

As companion animals, particularly dogs, have ventured into the home to take on new roles as family members, their social group has in many ways become our own. Dogs see us as a part of their pack. As such, they often exhibit allomimetic behaviors towards us. The same can be said of psittasines, many of which have the capacity to mimic human speech.(20) When they do, we are apt to anthropomorphize them. We are more likely to believe that they comprehend precisely what we have conveyed through words, non-verbal cues, or both, and that perception of mutual communication strengthens our bond.(20)

The social support that is afforded via attachments to one or more companion animals has historically been overlooked and/or undervalued, yet more recent recognition of its significance has revolutionized the practice of veterinary medicine, specifically its move towards relationship-centered care.(69)

Companion animals are now considered to be members of the family by 85%–99% of pet owners.(17, 65, 69, 91–93) Many perceive their pet to be almost human and identify love as the foundation of their bond. (94) This distinction emphasizes the value that is placed upon dog- and cat- "ownership." Many describe their role as parent or guardian rather than owner. Within the family structure, pets may be seen as children or sibling figures to human children.(95–99) Their inherent value has risen, prompting their owners to increasingly take on the added responsibility of advocating for their pets.(100, 101) This newfound role of advocacy requires the veterinary client to take a lead role in presenting the patient, relaying patient history, and initiating dialogue about a particular presenting complaint.(100–103) The veterinary consultation becomes a joint effort or partnership, rather than a dictation or monologue.(104) Decision-making is thus shared, requiring veterinarians to identify, understand, and ultimately connect with owners if they are to advance patient care.(65, 69, 104–106)

The numbers of pet owners and owned pets, many of which reside in multi-pet households, continue to climb.

According to the 2022 **PDSA Animal Wellbeing (PAW) Report**, United Kingdom (U.K.) households collectively owned 10.2 million pet dogs, 11.1 million pet cats, and 1 million pet rabbits.(107) These figures represent an annual increase in 0.4 million dogs and 0.9 million cats, and a decrease by rabbits on the order of 100,000 as compared with the figures from the 2021 PDSA Animal Wellbeing (PAW) Report.(107) One out of every two households owns a pet in the U.K.(65), and roughly one in two adults in the U.K. own at least one pet.(107) Dogs and cats are owned by 27% and 24% of U.K. adults, respectively.(107)

According to the American Veterinary Medical Association (AVMA), American households collectively owned 76.8 million dogs, 58.4 million cats, 7.5 million birds, and 1.9 million horses in 2017–2018.(108) These figures represent a significant increase of nearly 7 million dogs from 2001, yet a decrease of 15.6 million cats, 0.8 million birds, and 3 million horses from 2001.(108) In 2017–2018, roughly 38% of U.S. households owned dogs as compared with the 25.4% that owned cats; however, there were on average more cats per cat-owning household (1.8) than dogs per dog-owning household (1.6).(108)

According to a 2020 study by Applebaum et al. that examined U.S. pet ownership using the General Social Survey, women are more likely to own multiple pets and dogs than men.(109) Also more likely to own pets are middle-aged adults, whites, and nonurban residents.(109)

Industry surveys provide a starting point; however, such reports demonstrate discrepancies in estimates of U.S. pet ownership.(109) The American Pet Products Association (AAPA) estimated that 67% of households owned at least one pet in 2019 as compared with AVMA-derived data (57%) and Simmons National Consumer Study-derived data (53%) in 2019.(109)

1.9 The Impact of Global Pandemic on the Human–Animal Bond

The emergence of the COVID-19 as a global pandemic in spring 2020, in response to soaring infections with severe acute respiratory syndrome coronavirus 2 (SARS-CoV-2) appreciably impacted the veterinary industry and other healthcare professions.(110) Out of respect for safety in the face of so much uncertainty, veterinary clinics had to initiate significant changes in operations and standard operating procedures (SOPs) to continue the provision and delivery of services while mitigating safety risks.(110) Many practices implemented curbside care in response to the need for social distancing and/or had to cancel or limit appointments.(110, 111)

Despite reduced availability of veterinary care, the estimated dog population and the proportion of dog-owning adults climbed in the U.K. between February 2020, just prior to the onset of the pandemic, and the present day.(107) U.K. pet owners also reported an increase in the number of pets that they acquired from abroad.(107) Globally, public interest in adopting pets and/or providing foster care also increased.(112–115) The surge in adoption interest and/or requests has been attributed to the implementation of social distancing measures that enabled remote work from home options and/or unemployment, resulting in increased time spent at home. (114, 116, 117) Research suggests that the companion animals act as stress-reducing agents during times of uncertainty, so it is likely that the pandemic strengthened bonds between owners and their pets.(114, 115, 118, 119) Pet-ownership was one means by which people were able to survive in the face of the social isolation that many found themselves experiencing.

What is it about pets that is so nurturing, particularly during times of uncertainty? In other words, what makes us look outside of our own kind to find support in companion animals?

Research points to the third tier of Abraham Maslow's hierarchy of needs, the human need for love.(120) Humans seek out and desire companionship, emotional support, and a sense of belonging that they can find in bonded relationships with animals.(95, 121–123) Such bonds are often described as being reliable and free of judgment, qualities that are especially welcome during times of stress or adversity.(95, 124–127)

1.10 The Human–Animal Bond and Wildlife

Literary works and motion pictures do not limit this bond to companion animals, but broaden the scope to include wildlife. One of the most famous passages in Antoine Saint-Exupery's 1943 masterpiece, *Le Petit Prince*, emphasizes the bond between a boy and a fox. The boy tamed the fox and when it came time for the boy to depart from the fox's planet, the fox spoke of tears. The Little Prince suggested that it was the fox's fault for having felt so deeply, as the boy had not wanted the fox to be harmed in any way. When the fox said that he would cry, the Little Prince suggested that this bond between them had done the fox no good. The fox disagreed and proclaimed:(128)

> *"It has done me good," said the fox, "because of the color of the wheat fields." And then he added:*
>
> *"Go and look again at the roses. You will understand now that yours is unique in all the world. Then come back to say goodbye to me, and I will make you a present of a secret."*
>
> *The little prince went away, to look again at the roses.*
>
> *"You are not at all like my rose," he said. "As yet you are nothing. No one has tamed you, and you have tamed no one. You are like my fox when I first knew him. He was only a fox like a hundred thousand other foxes. But I have made him my friend, and now he is unique in all the world."*

A more recent celebration of the human–animal bond can be found in the 1993 motion picture, *Free Willy*, about a foster child named Jesse who befriends an orca whale. The movie is based loosely on the real-life killer whale, Keiko, whose Japanese name translates into "Lucky One."(129, 130) Keiko had been captured from the wild near Iceland in 1979 to serve as entertainment at several aquatic parks before starring in the motion picture.(129, 130) Keiko was ultimately released into the wild, as was the movie's lead character; however, Keiko died one year after he was granted freedom.(129, 130)

In the movie, character Jesse is caught vandalizing an adventure park. (131) As penance, he is required to scrub the walls to remove his graffiti. (131) While doing so, he becomes enamored with Willy, the park's recently captured orca.(131) One night, when Jesse runs away from home, he finds himself sitting in the moonlight near Willy's tank.(131) Willy appears to react to the sound of Jesse playing the harmonica.(131) So begins their connection. Both appear to bond over having been cut off from their families – Willy, on account of his capture, and Jesse, because he feels abandoned by his birth mother.(131)

At one point in the movie, Jesse accidentally falls into Willy's tank and Willy saves Jesse from drowning.(131) Jesse's adult friend, handyman Randolph, responds by saying: "Willy doesn't like visitors in his tank. What the heck were you doing out there?"(131)

Jesse responds: "Came to say goodbye. Job was almost up. Didn't wanna say goodbye."(131)

Their dialogue continues:(131)

> Randolph: "Well, just maybe…
> Randolph gets up and briefly takes an orca carving out of Jesse's hands.
> Randolph: "Orcas. Ever look into Willy's eyes? Those eyes discovered the stars long before man was even a whisper on Mother Earth. Can look into a man's soul if they want."
> Randolph gives the carving back to Jesse.
> Randolph: "Willy? He won't look at Rae or me. Maybe he sees you."

The implication is that Jesse and Willy formed a bond that is unlike any other. It is ultimately this bond that leads Willy to trust Jesse as Jesse conjures up a plan to release him back into the ocean.

Movies such as this one humanize wildlife because they portray the connection between man and animal to be equivalent, if not stronger, than connections between two or more people.

1.11 The Human–Animal Bond and Companion Animals

The bonds that form between companion animals and their guardians tend to be intensified by the fact that dogs, cats, and other pets have transitioned into many households as family.(132, 133) Although not everyone within the home may have the same affinity for the pets that are housed within(134), pets are less often viewed as objects or property and more often seen as partners, best friends, confidantes, children or child-substitutes, and/or siblings.(17, 132, 135)

In 2007, the AVMA reported that over 70% of homes with children aged six or older had at least one pet.(132) Elementary-age children tend to interact with pets primarily through touch.(132) Petting and hugging animals in these early years can be soothing for the child. Sometimes this is termed the "pet effect."(135) Although it is not unique to children – adults who engage in human–animal bonds may also experience it – positive touch may condition relaxation and mediate autonomic responses to stress.(135–137)

Positive touch can also teach healthy physical interactions with living beings.(132) It is thought that youth may be able to apply lessons learned to future social relationships with other people.(132) Evidence shows that those who had pets growing up are more likely to recognize the non-verbal cues of others, and they are more likely to connect to peers, family, and their surrounding communities.(132) Because of this propensity to promote social engagement, pets have been termed "transitional objects" to human relationships (135, 138) or "social lubricants."(75, 123) Children who engage with pets exhibit greater empathy and self-esteem, and are more likely to partake in team sports or social events.(70)

As children grow into adolescence, they may still benefit from emotional support and physical touch; however, they are more apt to incorporate bonds with companion animals into their goals.(132) For instance, a teenager with an interest in pursuing a veterinary medicine degree may see their relationship with a pet as having a higher purpose in terms of preparing them for a career in healthcare. In this respect, pets become one of the ways that people may define themselves.(135) In other words, they find their identities within pets. They may, for instance, come to view themselves as nurturing, but only because they see that quality in the way that they have tended to their pets.(135, 139)

Adults who have an affinity for pets tend to view them as significant "people."(140) Adults may even express a preference for pets over family – or consider pets to be family – in large part because pets are seen to love unconditionally, without care for material goods or social constructs, such as social status.(75, 96) In this respect, pets offer personal safety, that is, the freedom to be ourselves.(75, 141) Sue-Ellen Brown expressed it best when she wrote that "a child may be able to show sadness only in front of the family dog. The child's sense of self is affirmed by the dog's perceived attentiveness and acceptance of her emotion."(142)

Because pets appear to celebrate us as we are, many of us reciprocate and celebrate them. It is not unusual for us to celebrate their birthdays(75) and/or incorporate them into holiday plans. Close proximity breeds familiarity. Sharing living quarters and in some cases bedrooms and even beds elevate pets' status within the family.

The presence of pets in our lives also offers consistency. Pets may companion us through schooling, career offers, and career changes. Pets may see us through other transitions, such as the death of loved ones or significant transitions in life. As Dr. Froma Walsh shared in her manuscript with respect to the relational significance of companion animals:(70)

> *Companion animals meet relational needs for consistent, reliable bonds and facilitate transitions through disruptive life changes. As one woman remarked, "My cat Max has been with me through two marriages, divorce, and widowhood as the one relationship I can always count on." These attachments are especially strong for growing numbers of adults who are remaining single or are living on their own for extended periods of time. Some view their pet as their "significant other" and even their "soul mate."*

Affirming Walsh's reflection above, the American Animal Hospital Association (AAHA) found that 40% of pet owners within the U.S. felt that their pet was a better listener than their partner.(75) This is reminiscent of the key theme of 1961–1966 television series, *Mister Ed*, in which the equine star talks to his master, Wilbur Post. Wilbur in fact spends so much time at the barn that Wilbur's wife, Carol, believes that he loves Mister Ed more than he loves her.

1.12 Portrayal of the Human–Animal Bond by the Arts

Our love for companion animals and their reciprocal affection for us has long been romanticized by the arts – whether literature, film, or television – in the same way that such emotions were roused towards wildlife in *Le Petit Prince*. However, because many homes have dogs rather than talking foxes, human–animal bond stories that involve domesticated species or companion animals are more relatable and more likely to "stick." *Lassie* was one of the earliest American television series to capture the bond between a female Collie dog and her boy, Timmy Martin. So popular was this show that it was televised from 1954 to 1973.

Two years after *Lassie* first aired, author Fred Gibson published *Old Yeller*. Winning the Newbery Honor in 1957, *Old Yeller* is a timeless tale of love that develops between a stray mongrel dog and Travis, the eldest son of a Texas rancher who has been tasked with looking after his mother and younger brother Arliss while his father is off on a cattle drive. Travis reluctantly accepts the dog after the dog proves his worth: the dog saves

Arliss from a bear and Travis from wild hogs. Old Yeller ultimately contracts rabies while protecting the family from a rabid wolf. Because of the wounds that Old Yeller sustained during the altercation, Travis's mother fears the potential for rabies transmission not only to the dog, but also to the family. To mitigate the risk, Travis is called upon to shoot Old Yeller.

Following Old Yeller's death, Travis grieves deeply for the friendship that cannot be replaced. Gibson writes in the first-person, from the perspective of Travis:(143)

> *Days went by, and I couldn't seem to get over it. I couldn't eat. I couldn't sleep. I couldn't cry. I was all empty inside, but hurting. Hurting worse than I'd ever hurt in my life. Hurting with a sickness there didn't seem to be any cure for. Thinking every minute of my big yeller dog, how we'd worked together and romped together, how he'd fought the she bear off Little Arliss, how he'd saved me from the killer hogs, how he'd fought the mad wolf off Mama and Lisbeth. Thinking that after all this, I'd had to shoot him the same as I'd done the roan bull and the Spot heifer. Mama tried to talk to me about it, and I let her. But while everything she said made sense, it didn't do a thing to that dead feeling I had. Lisbeth talked to me. She didn't say much; she was too shy. But she pointed out that I had another dog, the speckled pup. "He's part Old Yeller," she said. "And he was the best one of the bunch." But that didn't help any either. The speckled pup might be part Old Yeller, but he wasn't Old Yeller. He hadn't saved all our lives and then been shot down like he was nothing.*

Literary and cinematic depictions of friendship, love, and loss continue to pique our curiosity and are named as such with respect to the emotions that the human–animal bond inspires. In 1961, just five years after *Old Yeller* was published, Wilson Rawls wrote *Where the Red Fern Grows*. The tale begins with a boy, Billy Coleman, who buys and trains two Coonhounds for hunting. The dogs ultimately save Billy from a mountain lion attack, but one of the dogs, Old Dan, subsequently succumbs to his injuries. Within days, the second dog, Little Ann, loses her will to live and dies on top of Old Dan's grave. Billy is heartbroken. Several of the statements that Billy makes in the aftermath of his dogs' deaths evoke strong emotions. The first memorializes friendship: "I looked at his grave and, with tears in my eyes, I voiced these words: 'You were worth it, old friend, and a thousand times over.'"(144)

A second statement acknowledges that life without his dogs will never be the same: "I buried Little Ann by the side of Old Dan. I knew that was where she wanted to be. I also buried a part of my life along with my dog."(144)

Fellow hunter Mr. Kyle says it best when he names the connection that binds dogs to humankind:

People have been trying to understand dogs ever since the beginning of time. One never knows what they'll do. You can read every day where a dog saved the life of a drowning child, or lay down his life for his master. Some people call this loyalty. I don't. I may be wrong, but I call it love–the deepest kind of love.(144)

Cats appear less frequently in literary works as reflections of the human–animal bond, perhaps because dogs have historically been labeled as "man's best friend," whereas cats have classically been thought of as aloof and independent. Yet, perhaps no tale of feline friendship is as poignant as the third book in a trilogy by Peter Gethers, *The Cat Who'll Live Forever: The Final Adventures of Norton, the Perfect Cat, and His Imperfect Human.* Gethers had been a self-proclaimed cat-hater until he was gifted six-week-old Norton, a Scottish Fold kitten. In the weeks, months, and years that followed, Norton and Gethers became inseparable, transforming Gethers' precon-ceived notions about cats in *The Cat Who Went to Paris* and *A Cat Abroad.* The last text in the series chronicles Norton's final cross-country trip and ultimately his passing. Gethers reflects upon Norton's death as follows: "The thing that eventually strikes you about the death of someone you love is the permanence. When that hits, there is an overpowering sense of loneliness and aloneness. Those wounds do not remain raw, not forever, but they do remain."(145)

The someone that Gethers loved was a cat, but not just any cat. Norton was the cat that Gethers swore he would hate.

1.13 Defining the Human–Animal Bond

Indeed, animals work their way into our lives and into our hearts in mys-terious and at times inexplicable ways. The human–animal bond has been defined by the AVMA as: "the mutually beneficial and dynamic relation-ship between people and other animals that is influenced by behaviors that are essential to the health and wellbeing of both."(95, 146)

The AVMA considers this bond to be inclusive of physical, emotional, and psychological elements.(146) Such a definition appears too scientific, too clinical, and too cold for the warmth that underlies those connections that seem bigger than life. At the same time, the definition seems too basic to describe something so complex, particularly given that human–animal bond research is an evolving field that has proposed several disparate, rather than unified, theories.(66)

In addition to its provision of social support, the human–animal bond has been proposed to exist owing to attachment theory or the biophilia hypothesis.(17, 20, 66, 73, 77, 147–152)

Attachment theory was developed by John Bowlby in the 1950s. (20, 147–150) Bowlby was heavily influenced by studies of imprinting by animal ethnologist Konrad Lorenz.(20) Attachment theory suggests that infants are biologically programmed to connect to caregivers – typically their mothers – at birth.(20, 147–150) This innate parent–child attachment serves as the foundation of all future relationships because this first connection establishes the child's expectations surrounding caregiver roles and responsibilities.(147, 153) Times of uncertainty and stress activate the child's need to look to attachment figures for support.(147, 148) As the child matures, the child shifts focus from the primary attachment figure onto transitional objects, such as blankets or stuffed toys, as a means of engaging with their environment.(20) These more portable, totable objects can provide comfort even in the absence of the primary attachment figure.(20, 154, 155) Although pets are not traditional transitional objects, they can be viewed by children as meeting the same need.(20, 138) Pets teach children to seek comfort outside of themselves and their immediate support system, their bond with parental figures.(20)

Attachments may be strengthened by one or more of the following perceptions by pet owners:(17)

- they rescued the pet
- the pet rescued them
- the pet is their sole source of support
- the pet is a link to a person, animal, relationship, or lifestage (e.g., childhood) that ceases to exist.

In addition to attachment theory, the biophilia hypothesis has been put forward as a means by which to better understand human attraction to and bonding with animals. According to proponents of this theory, the energy that the natural world exudes draws us in because we have an innate appreciation for life and that which is life-like.(20, 156, 157) This inherent attraction to nature has been correlated with positive patient health outcomes.(157, 158) Viewing a garden during post-operative recovery as opposed to a brick wall resulted in shorter hospital stays.(20, 158) Surgical patients who had the garden view also required fewer analgesics to manage their post-operative pain.(20, 158)

1.14 Evaluating the Benefits of the Human–Animal Bond and Their Implications

Interactions with live animals have also been correlated with positive health effects, including, but not limited to:

- reduced depression and enhanced morale in cancer patients(159, 160)
- reduced blood pressure(20, 70, 161, 162) and heart rate(163)
- reduced plasma cholesterol and triglyceride values(70, 135)
- reduced risk of death from heart attacks(135)
- improved cardiopulmonary function(164)
- increased independence for those with disabilities(75, 135)
- increased one-year survival rates among patients who suffered myocardial infarction(165)
- reduced anxiety(132)
- increased levels of oxytocin, which is involved in the development and display of affection and empathy(135)
- decreased levels of the stress hormone, cortisol(135, 166)
- increased sense of self and purpose(66, 135, 139, 142, 167)
- increased social support and companionship(17, 70, 75)
- facilitated communication and expression of ideas(73)
- facilitated transitions at end of life for those in hospice care(168)
- increased exercise, playtime, and/or relaxation(17, 169–173)
- increased acceptance during emotionally challenging times, such as serious illness and/or the death of a loved one.(17, 71, 95)

The biophilia hypothesis proposes that conscious or unconscious self-interest drives our conservation of nature. It has been said that "the human brain was structured to pay selective attention to other kinds of life"(174) in order to experience elevated levels of well-being.(73, 174) Being attuned to the needs of animals does not necessarily mean that the human instinct towards them is to be kind.(73) However, awareness is the first step towards a better understanding of others and is thought to lay the groundwork for building relationships that lead to strong and solid, lasting bonds.

In retrospect, human–animal interactions have come a significant way from their beginnings involving ancient peoples, cultures, and civilizations. Yet, there is much to be discovered about the human–animal bond and its significance. We must continually remind ourselves that the human–animal bond has been defined as a mutually beneficial relationship. Often when we consider this bond, we focus on how companion animals benefit human well-being.(65)

We may not always be aware of or open to considering the welfare needs of our companion animals.(65) We are still in the process of understanding those needs and demystifying animal minds. They are much like onions. We have only just begun to peel back the first few layers. At times, we may not even know where to begin. We have many more layers left to explore and much more to understand about the animals who choose to companion us through life. We are only just beginning to comprehend the complexities of animal behavior and the many ways our companion animals communicate with us and with each other.

Human–animal bond researchers are actively engaging in studies to make sense of the apparent emotions and "personalities" of our companion animals. The presence of these traits confers sentience and moves us towards a better understanding of welfare and quality of life with the intent to alleviate suffering.(175)

At time of graduation, new Doctor of Veterinary Medicine (DVM) graduates of AVMA-accredited colleges pledge an oath that incorporates considerations of welfare:(176)

Being admitted to the profession of veterinary medicine, I solemnly swear to use my scientific knowledge and skills for the benefit of society through the protection of animal health and welfare, the prevention and relief of animal suffering, the conservation of animal resources, the promotion of public health, and the advancement of medical knowledge.

I will practice my profession conscientiously, with dignity, and in keeping with the principles of veterinary medical ethics.

I accept as a lifelong obligation the continual improvement of my professional knowledge and competence.

Veterinary medicine is indeed a profession of lifelong learning. One never reaches the pinnacle. As advocates for animals, veterinarians and pet owners must work together to continually clarify our understanding of animals and their needs so that our at times unilaterally beneficial relationships with animals broaden.

We must strive for reciprocity.

If we are to rise to the occasion to meet the needs of all animals, including our beloved companions, then we must expand the evidence base that facilitates perspective-taking to view the world through their lens. Only when we do so can we fully appreciate animals' contributions to our lives and communities.

These contributions are made in life and through death, and those impacted most deeply in the process are forever changed.

The remainder of this text is about those changes that take place inside of us as we grieve the loss of a companion animal. It is about moving us towards a better understanding of bereavement so that we can companion ourselves and each other through that grueling and at times brutal journey through grief.

Grief is something that impacts all who live, not just veterinarians, although those within our profession bear witness to it with far greater frequency that most other humans do.

Our accrediting bodies, such as the AVMA, have tasked us to navigate quality of life and end of life discussions, grief and grieving, and to see human–animal relationships as integral to client and community health. (146) This requires us as practitioners to come to a better, clearer understanding about not only what companion animals need, but also what our clients need from us.

Moreover, veterinarians must learn how client perceptions, experiences, emotions, and perspectives shape and influence patient outcomes. Relationship-centered care requires us to tune into how our clients react to healthcare news and how we in turn deliver such news so that we and our clients can move forward and partner to find solutions to patient care.

Nowhere in veterinary practice is this more essential than in consultations involving end of life, as death is final and severs the physical here-and-now aspect of the human–animal bond.

References

1. Harlow HF, Harlow MK. Effect of various mother-infant relationships on rhesus monkey behavior. In: Foss BM, editor. Determinants of infant behavior IV. New York: John Wiley & Sons; 1969. p. 34–60.
2. Harlow HF, Zimmermann RR. Affectional responses in the infant monkey: orphaned baby monkeys develop a strong and persistent attachment to inanimate surrogate mothers. Science. 1959;130(3373):421–32. https://doi.org/10.1126/science.130.3373.421, PMID 13675765.
3. Cairns RB. Attachment behavior of mammals. Psychol Rev. 1966;73(5):409–26. https://doi.org/10.1037/h0023691, PMID 5341659.
4. Brent LJ, Chang SW, Gariépy JF, Platt ML. The neuroethology of friendship. Ann N Y Acad Sci. 2014;1316(1):1–17. https://doi.org/10.1111/nyas.12315, PMID 24329760.
5. Broad KD, Curley JP, Keverne EB. Mother-infant bonding and the evolution of mammalian social relationships. Philos Trans R Soc Lond B Biol Sci. 2006;361(1476):2199–214. https://doi.org/10.1098/rstb.2006.1940, PMID 17118933.
6. Tibbetts EA, Dale J. Individual recognition: it is good to be different. Trends Ecol Evol. 2007;22(10):529–37. https://doi.org/10.1016/j.tree.2007.09.001, PMID 17904686.
7. Kendrick KM, da Costa AP, Leigh AE, Hinton MR, Peirce JW. Sheep don't forget a face. Nature. 2001;414(6860):165–6. https://doi.org/10.1038/35102669, PMID 11700543.

8. Tibbetts EA. Visual signals of individual identity in the wasp Polistes fuscatus. Proc Biol Sci. 2002;269(1499):1423–8. https://doi.org/10.1098/rspb.2002.2031, PMID 12137570.

9. Parr LA, Winslow JT, Hopkins WD, de Waal FB. Recognizing facial cues: individual discrimination by chimpanzees (Pan troglodytes) and rhesus monkeys (Macaca mulatta). J Comp Psychol. 2000;114(1):47–60. https://doi.org/10.1037/0735–7036.114.1.47, PMID 10739311.

10. Bruce V, Young A. Understanding face recognition. Br J Psychol. 1986;77(3):305–27. https://doi.org/10.1111/j.2044–8295.1986.tb02199.x, PMID 3756376.

11. Tsao DY, Moeller S, Freiwald WA. Comparing face patch systems in macaques and humans. Proc Natl Acad Sci USA. 2008;105(49):19514–9. https://doi.org/10.1073/pnas.0809662105, PMID 19033466.

12. Gherardi F, Tricarico E, Atema J. Unraveling the nature of individual recognition by odor in hermit crabs. J Chem Ecol. 2005;31(12):2877–96. https://doi.org/10.1007/s10886–005–8400–5, PMID 16365711.

13. Karavanich C, Atema J. Individual recognition and memory in lobster dominance. Anim Behav. 1998;56(6):1553–60. https://doi.org/10.1006/anbe.1998.0914, PMID 9933553.

14. Godard R. Long-term-memory of individual neighbors in a migratory songbird. Nature. 1991;350(6315):228–9. https://doi.org/10.1038/350228a0.

15. Bruck JN. Decades-long social memory in bottlenose dolphins. Proc Biol Sci. 2013;280(1768):20131726. https://doi.org/10.1098/rspb.2013.1726, PMID 23926160.

16. Johnson AJ, Becker JAH, Craig EA, Gilchrist ES, Haigh MM. Changes in friendship commitment: comparing geographically close and long-distance young-adult friendships. Commun Q. 2009;57(4):395–415. https://doi.org/10.1080/01463370903313430.

17. Lagoni L, Hetts S, Butler C. The human-animal bond. In: Lagoni L, Hetts S, Butler C, editors. The human-animal bond and grief. Philadelphia: Saunders; 1994. p. 3–28.

18. Harlow HF. The nature of love. Am Psychol. 1958;13(12):673–85. https://doi.org/10.1037/h0047884.

19. Igel GJ, Calvin AD. The development of affectional responses in infant dogs. J Comp Physiol Psychol. 1960;53:302–5. https://doi.org/10.1037/h0049308, PMID 13852617.

20. Beck AM. The biology of the human-animal bond. Anim Front. 2014;4(3):32–6. https://doi.org/10.2527/af.2014–0019.

21. Paracer S, Ahmadjian V. Symbiosis: an introduction to biological associations. 2nd ed. Vol. xi. New York: Oxford University Press; 2000.

22. Gontier N. History of symbiosis. In: Kliman RM, editor. Encyclopedia of evolutionary biology. 4. Oxford: Academic Press; 2016. p. 272–81.

23. Terborgh J. Mixed flocks and polyspecific associations: costs and benefits of mixed groups to birds and monkeys. Am J Primatol. 1990;21(2):87–100. https://doi.org/10.1002/ajp.1350210203, PMID 31963979.

24. Grzimek B, MacLeod N, Archibald JD, Levin PS. Grzimek's animal life encyclopedia: extinction. 2 volumes (xv, 964 pages) Detroit: Gale/Cengage Learning; 2013.

25. Holland JS. Unlikely friendships: 47 remarkable stories from the animal kingdom. New York: Workman Publishing. Vol. xiii; 2011.

26. Holland JS. The dog and the piglet: and four other true stories of animal friendships. New York: Workman Publishing; 2012.
27. Holland JS. The leopard and the cow: and four other true stories of animal friendships. New York: Workman Publishing; 2012.
28. Holland JS. Unlikely friendships: dogs: 37 stories of canine compassion and courage. New York: Workman Publishing; 2016.
29. Holland JS, Holland JS. The monkey and the dove: and four other true stories of animal friendships. New York: Workman Publishing; 2012.
30. Dagg AI. Animal friendships. Vol. viii. New York: Cambridge University Press; 2011.
31. Seyfarth RM, Cheney DL. The evolutionary origins of friendship. Annu Rev Psychol. 2012;63:153–77. https://doi.org/10.1146/annurev-psych-120710-100337, PMID 21740224.
32. Chang SW, Brent LJ, Adams GK, Klein JT, Pearson JM, Watson KK, et al. Neuroethology of primate social behavior. Proc Natl Acad Sci USA. 2013;110;Suppl 2:10387–94. https://doi.org/10.1073/pnas.1301213110, PMID 23754410.
33. Lee HJ, Macbeth AH, Pagani JH, Young WS, 3rd. Oxytocin: the great facilitator of life. Prog Neurobiol. 2009;88(2):127–51. https://doi.org/10.1016/j.pneurobio.2009.04.001, PMID 19482229.
34. Algers B, Rojanasthien S, Uvnäs-Moberg K. The relationship between teat stimulation, oxytocin release and grunting rate in the sow during nursing. Appl Anim Behav Sci. 1990;26(3):267–76. https://doi.org/10.1016/0168-1591(90)90142-Z.
35. Leng G, Caquineau C, Sabatier N. Regulation of oxytocin secretion. Vitam Horm. 2005;71:27–58. https://doi.org/10.1016/S0083-6729(05)71002-5, PMID 16112264.
36. Lincoln DW, Wakerley JB. Electrophysiological evidence for the activation of supraoptic neurones during the release of oxytocin. J Physiol. 1974;242(2):533–54. https://doi.org/10.1113/jphysiol.1974.sp010722, PMID 4616998.
37. Uvnäs-Moberg K, Johansson B, Lupoli B, Svennersten-Sjaunja K. Oxytocin facilitates behavioural, metabolic and physiological adaptations during lactation. Appl Anim Behav Sci. 2001;72(3):225–34. https://doi.org/10.1016/s0168-1591(01)00112-5, PMID 11311416.
38. Petersson M, Alster P, Lundeberg T, Uvnäs-Moberg K. Oxytocin causes a long-term decrease of blood pressure in female and male rats. Physiol Behav. 1996;60(5):1311–5. https://doi.org/10.1016/s0031-9384(96)00261-2, PMID 8916187.
39. Petersson M. ALster P, Lundeberg T, Uvnäs-Moberg K. Oxytocin increases nociceptive pain thresholds in a long-term perspective in female and male rats. Neurosci Lett. 1996;212(2):87–90.
40. Argiolas A, Gessa GL. Central functions of oxytocin. Neurosci Biobehav Rev. 1991;15(2):217–31. https://doi.org/10.1016/s0149-7634(05)80002-8, PMID 1852313.
41. Uvnäs-Moberg K. Oxytocin linked antistress effects--the relaxation and growth response. Acta Physiol Scand Suppl. 1997;640:38–42. PMID 9401603.
42. Uvnäs-Moberg K. Antistress pattern induced by oxytocin. News Physiol Sci. 1998;13:22–5. https://doi.org/10.1152/physiologyonline.1998.13.1.22, PMID 11390754.
43. Pedersen CA, Prange AJ. Induction of maternal behaviour in virgin rats after intracerebroventricular administration of oxytocin. Proc Natl Acad Sci U S A. 1979;76(12):6661–5. https://doi.org/10.1073/pnas.76.12.6661, PMID 293752.

44. Witt DM, Winslow JT, Insel TR. Enhanced social interactions in rats following chronic, centrally infused oxytocin. Pharmacol Biochem Behav. 1992;43(3):855–61. https://doi.org/10.1016/0091-3057(92)90418-f, PMID 1448480.

45. Young LJ, Wang Z. The neurobiology of pair bonding. Nat Neurosci. 2004;7(10): 1048–54. https://doi.org/10.1038/nn1327, PMID 15452576.

46. Carter CS, DeVries AC, Getz LL. Physiological substrates of mammalian monogamy: the prairie vole model. Neurosci Biobehav Rev. 1995;19(2):303–14. https://doi.org/10.1016/0149-7634(94)00070-h, PMID 7630584.

47. Lack D. Ecological adaptations for breeding in birds. London: Methuen; 1968.

48. Silver R, Andrews H, Ball GF. Parental care in an ecological perspective: a quantitative analysis of avian subfamilies. Am Zool. 1985;25(3):823–40. https://doi.org/10.1093/icb/25.3.823.

49. Silver R. Biparental care in birds: mechanisms controlling incubation bout duration, hormones and behaviour in higher vertebrates. Horm Behav Higher Vertebr. 1983:451–62.

50. Mainwaring MC, Griffith SC. Looking after your partner: sentinel behaviour in a socially monogamous bird. PeerJ. 2013;1:e83. https://doi.org/10.7717/peerj.83, PMID 23761856.

51. Nalepa CA, Jones SC. Evolution of monogamy in termites. Biol Rev. 1991;66(1): 83–97. https://doi.org/10.1111/j.1469-185X.1991.tb01136.x.

52. Jaffé R, Pioker-Hara FC, Dos Santos CF, Santiago LR, Alves DA, de M P Kleinert A, et al. Monogamy in large bee societies: a stingless paradox. Naturwissenschaften. 2014;101(3):261–4. https://doi.org/10.1007/s00114-014-1149-3, PMID 24463620.

53. Bull CM. Monogamy in lizards. Behav Processes. 2000;51(1–3):7–20. https://doi.org/10.1016/s0376-6357(00)00115-7, PMID 11074308.

54. DeWoody JA, Fletcher DE, Wilkins SD, Nelson WS, Avise JC. Genetic monogamy and biparental care in an externally fertilizing fish, the largemouth bass (Micropterus salmoides). Proc Biol Sci. 2000;267(1460):2431–7. https://doi.org/10.1098/rspb.2000.1302, PMID 11133034.

55. Morley JI, Balshine S. Faithful fish: territory and mate defence favour monogamy in an African cichlid fish. Behav Ecol Sociobiol. 2002;52(4):326–31. https://doi.org/10.1007/s00265-002-0520-0.

56. Whiteman EA, Côte IM. Monogamy in marine fishes. Biol Rev Camb Philos Soc. 2004;79(2):351–75. https://doi.org/10.1017/s1464793103006304, PMID 15191228.

57. Carter CS, Keverne EB. The neurobiology of social affiliation and pair bonding. In: Pfaff DW, editor. Hormones, brain, and behavior. 2nd ed. Amsterdam, Boston: Academic Press; 2009.

58. Grahame K, Rogers B. Pforzheimer Bruce Rogers collection. The Wind in the Willows. Library of Congress. New York: Charles Scribner's Sons; 1908.

59. Burnford SE, Burger C. The incredible journey. 1st ed. Boston: Little; 1961.

60. Mannix DP, Schoenherr J. The fox and the hound. 1st ed. New York: Dutton; 1967.

61. Saltzman M. The adventures of Milo & Otis. New York: Morrow Junior Books; 1988.

62. Salten F, Woods MJ. Bambi: a life in the woods. New York: Simon & S. Books for Young readers; 1923.

63. Milne AA. Winnie-the-pooh. London: Methuen & Comp; 1926.

64. White EB, Williams G, Rosenwald EG, Lessing J. Rosenwald collection. Charlotte's web. 1st ed. New York: Library of Congress; Harper & Brothers; 1952.

65. Wensley SP. Animal welfare and the human-animal bond: considerations for veterinary faculty, students, and practitioners. J Vet Med Educ. 2008;35(4):532–9. https://doi.org/10.3138/jvme.35.4.532, PMID 19228905.

66. Hill L, Winefield H, Bennett P. Are stronger bonds better? Examining the relationship between the human-animal bond and human social support, and its impact on resilience. Aust Psychol. 2020;55(6):729–38. https://doi.org/10.1111/ap.12466.

67. Cobb S. Presidential Address-1976. Social support as a moderator of life stress. Psychosom Med. 1976;38(5):300–14. https://doi.org/10.1097/00006842–1976090 00–00003, PMID 981490.

68. Collis GM, McNicholas J. A theoretical basis for health benefits of pet ownership. In: Wilson CC, Turner DC, editors. Companion animals in human health. Thousand Oaks: SAGE; 1998. p. 105–22.

69. Martin F, Ruby KL, Deking TM, Taunton AE. Factors associated with client, staff, and student satisfaction regarding small animal euthanasia procedures at a veterinary teaching hospital. J Am Vet Med Assoc. 2004;224(11):1774–9. https://doi.org/10.2460/javma.2004.224.1774, PMID 15198261.

70. Walsh F. Human-animal bonds I: the relational significance of companion animals. Fam Process. 2009;48(4):462–80. https://doi.org/10.1111/j.1545–5300.2009.01296.x, PMID 19930433.

71. Staats S, Sears K, Pierfelice L. Teachers' pets and why they have them: an investigation of the human animal bond. J Appl Soc Psychol. 2006;36(8):1881–91. https://doi.org/10.1111/j.0021–9029.2006.00086.x.

72. Robinson I, Waltham Centre for Pet Nutrition. The Waltham book of human-animal interaction: benefits of pet ownership. 1st ed. Vol. xiii. New York: Pergamon Press; 1995.

73. Fine AH, Tedeschi P, Elvove E. Forward thinking: the evolving field of human-animal interactions. In: Fine AH, editor. Handbook on animal-assisted therapy: foundations and guidelines for animal-assisted interventions. 4th ed. Amsterdam; Boston: Elsevier Academic Press; 2015. p. 21–35.

74. Smith A, Oechsner A, Rowley-Conwy P, Moore AMT. Epipalaeolithic animal tending to Neolithic herding at Abu Hureyra, Syria (12,800–7,800 calBP): deciphering dung spherulites. PLOS ONE. 2022;17(9):e0272947. https://doi.org/10.1371/journal.pone.0272947, PMID 36103475.

75. Silcox D, Castillo YA, Reed BJ. The human animal bond: applications for rehabilitation professionals. J Appl Rehabil Couns. 2014;45(3):27–37. https://doi.org/10.1891/0047–2220.45.3.27.

76. Serpell J. In the company of animals: a study of human-animal relationships. Cambridge. New York: Cambridge University Press; 2008.

77. Fine AH. Beck AM. Understanding our kinship with animals: input for health care professionals interested in the human-animal bond. In: Fine AH, editor. Handbook on animal-assisted therapy: foundations and guidelines for animal-assisted interventions. 4th ed. Amsterdam; Boston: Elsevier Academic Press; 2015. p. 3–10.

78. Ikram S. Divine creatures: animal mummies in ancient Egypt. Cairo. 2005.

79. Coren S. The pawprints of history: dogs and the course of human events. Vol. xiii. New York: Free Press; 2002.

80. Homer MS. The odyssey. Vol. xlv. New York: Atria Books; 2013.

81. Lange KE. Heir of the dog. Natl Geogr. 2007;31.

82. Beck AM, Katcher AH. Between pets and people: the importance of animal companionship. Vol. xviii. West Lafayette, IN: Purdue University Press; 1996.

83. Altschiller D. Animal-assisted therapy. Santa Barbara, CA: Greenwood Publishing Group; 2011.

84. Serpell JA. Animal-assisted interventions in historical perspective. In: Fine A, editor. The handbook of animal assisted therapy. 3rd ed. London: Elsevier Academic Press; 2010. p. 17–32.

85. Morris PH, Doe C, Godsell E. Secondary emotions in non-primate species? Behavioural reports and subjective claims by animal owners. Cogn Emot. 2007;21(1):3–25.

86. Grandin T, Deesing M. Behavioral genetics and animal science. In: Grandin T, Deesing M, editors. Genetics and the behavior of domestic animals. 2nd ed. London: Academic Press, Elsevier; 2014. p. 1–40.

87. Hinde RA, Barden LA. The evolution of the teddy bear. Anim Behav. 1985;33(4): 1371–3. https://doi.org/10.1016/S0003–3472(85)80205–0.

88. Lutts RH. The trouble with Bambi: Walt Disney's Bambi and the American vision of nature. For Conserv Hist. 1992;36(4):160–71. https://doi.org/10.2307/3983677.

89. Cartmill M. The Bambi syndrome. Nat Hist. 1993;102(6):6–12.

90. Mahoney S. Are you afraid of Bambi? Walt Disney's famous movie was more than an antihunting film—it posed a dangerous and unrealistic vision of nature. Sports Afield. 2014;237(3).

91. Brown JP, Silverman JD. The current and future market for veterinarians and veterinary medical services in the United States. J Am Vet Med Assoc. 1999;215(2): 161–83. PMID 10416465.

92. Bustad LK, Hines LM, Leathers CW. The human-companion animal bond and the veterinarian. Vet Clin North Am Small Anim Pract. 1981;11(4):787–810. https://doi.org/10.1016/s0195–5616(81)50086–6, PMID 6977933.

93. Voith VL. Attachment of people to companion animals. Vet Clin North Am Small Anim Pract. 1985;15(2):289–95. https://doi.org/10.1016/s0195–5616 (85)50301–0, PMID 3872510.

94. Bradshaw JWS, Casey RA. Anthropomorphism and anthropocentrism as influences in the quality of life of companion animals. Anim Welf. 2007;16(S1):149–54. https://doi.org/10.1017/S0962728600031869.

95. Applebaum JW, MacLean EL, McDonald SE. Love, fear, and the human-animal bond: on adversity and multispecies relationships. Compr Psychoneuroendocrinol. 2021;7. https://doi.org/10.1016/j.cpnec.2021.100071, PMID 34485952.

96. Hirschman EC. Consumers and their companions. J Consum Res. 1994;20(4):616. https://doi.org/10.1086/209374.

97. Cassels MT, White N, Gee NR, Hughes C. One of the family? Measuring early adolescents' relationships with pets and siblings. J Appl Dev Psychol. 2017;49:12–20. https://doi.org/10.1016/j.appdev.2017.01.003.

98. Laurent-Simpson A. "They make me not wanna have a child": effects of companion animals on fertility intentions of the childfree. Sociol Inq. 2017;87(4):586–607. https://doi.org/10.1111/soin.12163.

99. Laurent-Simpson A. Considering alternate sources of role identity: childless parents and their animal "kids". Sociol Forum. 2017;32(3):610–34. https://doi.org/10.1111/socf.12351.

100. Englar RE. Common clinical presentations in dogs and cats. Hoboken, NJ: Wiley/Blackwell; 2019.

101. Shaw JR, Adams CL, Bonnett BN, Larson S, Roter DL. Use of the roter inter-action analysis system to analyze veterinarian-client-patient communication in companion animal practice. J Am Vet Med Assoc. 2004;225(2):222–9. https://doi.org/10.2460/javma.2004.225.222, PMID 15323378.

102. Gillis J. The history of the patient history since 1850. Bull Hist Med. 2006;80(3): 490–512. https://doi.org/10.1353/bhm.2006.0097, PMID 17147133.

103. Gillis J. Taking a medical history in childhood illness: representations of parents in pediatric texts since 1850. Bull Hist Med. 2005;79(3):393–429. https://doi.org/10.1353/bhm.2005.0105, PMID 16184015.

104. Tarrant C, Stokes T, Colman AM. Models of the medical consultation: opportunities and limitations of a game theory perspective. Qual Saf Health Care. 2004;13(6):461–6. https://doi.org/10.1136/qhc.13.6.461, PMID 15576709.

105. Charles C, Gafni A, Whelan T. Shared decision-making in the medical encounter: what does it mean? (or it takes at least two to tango). Soc Sci Med. 1997;44(5): 681–92. https://doi.org/10.1016/s0277–9536(96)00221–3, PMID 9032835.

106. Elwyn G, Edwards A, Kinnersley P. Shared decision-making in primary care: the neglected second half of the consultation. Br J Gen Pract. 1999;49(443):477–82. PMID 10562751.

107. PDS. A animal wellbeing (PAW) report. Available from: https://www.pdsa.org.uk/what-we-do/pdsa-animal-wellbeing-report/paw-report-2022; 2022.

108. U.S. Pet ownership statistics. American Veterinary Medical Association; 2017–2018. Available from: https://www.avma.org/resources-tools/reports-statistics/us-pet-ownership-statistics.

109. Applebaum JW, Peek CW, Zsembik BA. Examining U.S. pet ownership using the General Social Survey. Soc Sci J. 2023;60(1):110–9. https://doi.org/10.1080/03623319.2020.1728507.

110. Kogan LR, Erdman P, Bussolari C, Currin-McCulloch J, Packman W. The initial months of COVID-19: dog owners' veterinary-related concerns. Front Vet Sci. 2021;8:629121. https://doi.org/10.3389/fvets.2021.629121, PMID 33604366.

111. COVID-19. American Veterinary Medical Association. Available from: https://www.avma.org/resources-tools/one-health/covid-19.

112. Powell L, Houlihan C, Stone M, Gitlin I, Ji X, Reinhard CL, et al. Animal shelters' response to the COVID-19 pandemic: a pilot survey of 14 shelters in the Northeastern United States. Animals (Basel). 2021;11(9). https://doi.org/10.3390/ani11092669, PMID 34573635.

113. Szydlowski M, Gragg C. An overview of the current and potential effects of COVID-19 on U.S. animal shelters. AIJR Prepr. 2020.

114. Ho J, Hussain S, Sparagano O. Did the COVID-19 pandemic spark a public interest in pet adoption? Front Vet Sci. 2021;8:647308. https://doi.org/10.3389/fvets.2021.647308, PMID 34046443.

115. Morgan L, Protopopova A, Birkler RID, Itin-Shwartz B, Sutton GA, Gamliel A et al. Human-dog relationships during the COVID-19 pandemic: booming dog adoption during social isolation. Humanit Soc Sci Commun. 2020;7(1). https://doi.org/10.1057/s41599–020–00649-x.

116. Dhama K, Patel SK, Sharun K, Pathak M, Tiwari R, Yatoo MI et al. SARS-CoV-2 jumping the species barrier: zoonotic lessons from SARS, MERS and recent advances to combat this pandemic virus. Travel Med Infect Dis. 2020;37:101830. https://doi.org/10.1016/j.tmaid.2020.101830, PMID 32755673.

117. Dhama K, Khan S, Tiwari R, Sircar S, Bhat S, Malik YS, et al. Coronavirus disease 2019-COVID-19. Clin Microbiol Rev. 2020;33(4). https://doi.org/10.1128/CMR.00028–20, PMID 32580969.

118. Bowen J, García E, Darder P, Argüelles J, Fatjó J. The effects of the Spanish COVID-19 lockdown on people, their pets, and the human-animal bond. J Vet Behav. 2020;40:75–91. https://doi.org/10.1016/j.jveb.2020.05.013, PMID 32837452.

119. Hoy-Gerlach J, Rauktis M, Newhill C. Nonhuman animal companionship: a crucial support for people during the COVID-19 pandemic. Soc Regist. 2020;4(2):109–20. https://doi.org/10.14746/sr.2020.4.2.08.

120. Maslow AH. A theory of human motivation. Psychol Rev. 1943;50(4):370–96. https://doi.org/10.1037/h0054346.

121. Laing M, Maylea C. "They burn brightly, but only for a short time": the role of social workers in companion animal grief and loss. Anthrozoös. 2018;31(2):221–32. https://doi.org/10.1080/08927936.2018.1434062.

122. Risley-Curtiss C. Social work practitioners and the human-companion animal bond: a national study. Soc Work. 2010;55(1):38–46. https://doi.org/10.1093/sw/55.1.38, PMID 20069939.

123. Morley C, Fook J. The importance of pet loss and some implications for services. Mortality. 2005;10(2):127–43. https://doi.org/10.1080/13576270412331329849.

124. Collins EA, Cody AM, McDonald SE, Nicotera N, Ascione FR, Williams JH. A template analysis of intimate partner violence survivors' experiences of animal maltreatment: implications for safety planning and intervention. Violence Against Women. 2018;24(4):452–76. https://doi.org/10.1177/1077801217697266, PMID 29332521.

125. McDonald SE, Cody AM, Collins EA, Stim HT, Nicotera N, Ascione FR, et al. Concomitant exposure to animal maltreatment and socioemotional adjustment among children exposed to intimate partner violence: a mixed methods study. J Child Adolesc Trauma. 2018;11(3):353–65. https://doi.org/10.1007/s40653–017–0176–6, PMID 32318161.

126. McDonald SE, Collins EA, Nicotera N, Hageman TO, Ascione FR, Williams JH, et al. Children's experiences of companion animal maltreatment in households characterized by intimate partner violence. Child Abuse Negl. 2015;50:116–27. https://doi.org/10.1016/j.chiabu.2015.10.005, PMID 26520828.

127. McDonald SE, Matijczak A, Nicotera N, Applebaum JW, Kremer L, Natoli G, et al. "He was like, my ride or die": sexual and Gender Minority Emerging Adults' Perspectives on Living with Pets during the Transition to Adulthood. Emerg Adulthood. 2022;10(4):1008–25. https://doi.org/10.1177/21676968211025340.

128. Saint-Exupéry Ad WK, Mamoulian R. Collection. Library of Congress. The little prince. New York: Reynal & Hitchcock; 1943.

129. Copyright Collection (Library of Congress). Keiko: the untold story of the star of Free Willy. 2014.

130. Markwell K. Animals and tourism: understanding diverse relationships. Bristol, UK. Buffalo: Channel View Publications; 2015.

131. Wincer S, Richter JJ, Petty L, Ironside M (Library of Congress). Free Willy. Warner Bros; 1993.

132. Mueller MK, Fine AH, O'Haire ME. Understanding the role of human-animal interaction in the family context. In: Fine AH, editor. Handbook on animal-assisted therapy: foundations and guidelines for animal-assisted interventions. 4th ed. Amsterdam; Boston: Elsevier Academic Press; 2015. p. 237–48.

133. Albert A, Bulcroft K. Pets, families, and the life course. Journal of Marriage and the Family. 1988;50(2):543–52. https://doi.org/10.2307/352019.

134. Fine AH. Our faithful companions: exploring the essence of our kinship with animals. Loveland, CO: Alpine; 2014.

135. Horowitz S. The human-animal bond: health implications across the lifespan. Altern Complement Ther. 2008;14(5):251–6. https://doi.org/10.1089/act.2008.14505.

136. Virués-Ortega J, Buela-Casal G. Psychophysiological effects of human-animal interaction: theoretical issues and long-term interaction effects. J Nerv Ment Dis. 2006;194(1):52–7. https://doi.org/10.1097/01.nmd.0000195354.03653.63, PMID 16462556.

137. Vormbrock JK, Grossberg JM. Cardiovascular effects of human-pet dog interactions. J Behav Med. 1988;11(5):509–17. https://doi.org/10.1007/BF00844843, PMID 3236382.

138. Triebenbacher SL. Pets as transitional objects: their role in children's emotional development. Psychol Rep. 1998;82(1):191–200. https://doi.org/10.2466/pr0.1998.82.1.191, PMID 9520553.

139. Fine AH, Beiler PF. Therapists and animals: demystifying animal-assisted therapy. In: Strozier AL, Carpenter J, editors. Introduction to alternative and complementary therapies. New York: Haworth Press; 2008. p. 223–8.

140. Gunter B, Furnham A. Pets and people: the psychology of pet ownership. Vol. vi. London: Whurr Publishers; 1999.

141. Risley-Curtiss C, Holley LC, Wolf S. The animal-human bond and ethnic diversity. Soc Work. 2006;51(3):257–68. https://doi.org/10.1093/sw/51.3.257, PMID 17076123.

142. Brown S. The human-animal bond and self psychology: toward a new understanding. Soc Animals. 2004;12(1):67–86. https://doi.org/10.1163/156853004323029540.

143. Gibson F. Old Yeller. New York: Harper; 1956.

144. Rawls W. Where the red fern grows; the story of two dogs and a boy. 1st ed. Garden City, NY: Doubleday Publishing; 1961.

145. Gethers P. The cat who'll live forever: the final adventures of Norton, the perfect cat, and his imperfect human. 1st ed. New York: Broadway Books; 2001.

146. Human-animal bond. American Veterinary Medical Association. Available from: https://www.avma.org/one-health/human-animal-bond.

147. Rockett B, Carr S. Animals and attachment theory. Soc Animals. 2014;22(4):415–33. https://doi.org/10.1163/15685306–12341322.

148. Bowlby J. Attachment and loss: Vol. 1. Attachment. London: Pimlico; 1969.

149. Bowlby J. Attachment and loss: Vol. 2. Separation: anxiety and anger. London: Pimlico; 1973.

150. Bowlby J. The nature of the child's tie to his mother. Int J Psychoanal. 1958;39(5):350–73. PMID 13610508.

151. Beck L, Madresh EA. Romantic partners and four legged friends: an extension of attachment theory to relationships with pet. Anthrozoös. 2008;21(1):43–56. https://doi.org/10.2752/089279308X274056.

152. Meehan M, Massavelli B, Pachana N. Using attachment theory and social support theory to examine and measure pets as sources of social support and attachment figures. Anthrozoös. 2017;30(2):273–89. https://doi.org/10.1080/08927936.2017.1311050.

153. Bowlby J. A secure base: parent-child attachment and healthy human development. Vol. xii. New York: Basic Books; 1988.

154. Winnicott DW. [Transitional objects and transitional phenomena. A study of the first not-me possession]. Psyche (Stuttg). 1969;23(9):666–82. PMID 5824774.

155. Winnicott DW. The use of an object. Int J Psychoanal. 1969;50(4):711–6.

156. Wilson EO. Biophilia. Cambridge, MA: Harvard University Press; 1984.

157. Kellert SR, Wilson EO. The Biophilia hypothesis. Washington, DC: Island Press; 1993.

158. Ulrich RS. View through a window may influence recovery from surgery. Science. 1984;224(4647):420–1. https://doi.org/10.1126/science.6143402, PMID 6143402.

159. Orlandi M, Trangeled K, Mambrini A, Tagliani M, Ferrarini A, Zanetti L, et al. Pet therapy effects on oncological day hospital patients undergoing chemotherapy treatment. Anticancer Res. 2007;27(6C):4301–3. PMID 18214035.

160. Wu AS, Niedra R, Pendergast L, McCrindle BW. Acceptability and impact of pet visitation on a pediatric cardiology inpatient unit. J Pediatr Nurs. 2002;17(5): 354–62. https://doi.org/10.1053/jpdn.2002.127173, PMID 12395303.

161. Friedmann E, Katcher AH, Thomas SA, Lynch JJ, Messent PR. Social interaction and blood pressure. Influence of animal companions. J Nerv Ment Dis. 1983;171(8):461–5. https://doi.org/10.1097/00005053–198308000–00002, PMID 6875529.

162. Katcher AH, Friedmann E, Beck AM, Lynch JJ. Looking, talking and blood pressure: the physiological consequences of interaction with the living environment. In: Katcher AH, Beck AM, editors. New perspectives on our lives with companion animals. Philadelphia: University of Pennsylvania Press; 1983. p. 351–9.

163. Allen K, Blascovich J, Mendes WB. Cardiovascular reactivity and the presence of pets, friends, and spouses: the truth about cats and dogs. Psychosom Med. 2002;64(5):727–39. https://doi.org/10.1097/01.psy.0000024236.11538.41, PMID 12271103.

164. Cole KM, Gawlinski A, Steers N, Kotlerman J. Animal-assisted therapy in patients hospitalized with heart failure. Am J Crit Care. 2007;16(6):575–85; quiz 86; discussion 87–8. https://doi.org/10.4037/ajcc2007.16.6.575, PMID 17962502.

165. Friedmann E, Thomas SA. Pet ownership, social support, and one-year survival after acute myocardial infarction in the Cardiac Arrhythmia Suppression Trial (CAST). Am J Cardiol. 1995;76(17):1213–7. https://doi.org/10.1016/s0002–9149(99)80343–9, PMID 7502998.

166. Odendaal JS, Meintjes RA. Neurophysiological correlates of affiliative behaviour between humans and dogs. Vet J. 2003;165(3):296–301. https://doi.org/10.1016/s1090–0233(02)00237-x, PMID 12672376.

167. Bradley L, Bennett PC. Companion-animals' effectiveness in managing chronic pain in adult community members. Anthrozoos. 2015;28(4):635–47. https://doi.org/10.1080/08927936.2015.1070006.

168. Geisler AM. Companion animals in palliative care: stories from the bedside. Am J Hosp Palliat Care. 2004;21(4):285–8. https://doi.org/10.1177/104990910402100411, PMID 15315191.

169. Anderson WP, Reid CM, Jennings GL. Pet ownership and risk factors for cardiovascular disease. Med J Aust. 1992;157(5):298–301. https://doi.org/10.5694/j.1326–5377.1992.tb137178.x, PMID 1435469.

170. Yabroff KR, Troiano RP, Berrigan D. Walking the dog: is pet ownership associated with physical activity in California? J Phys Act Health. 2008;5(2):216–28. https://doi.org/10.1123/jpah.5.2.216, PMID 18382031.

171. Cutt H, Giles-Corti B, Knuiman M. Encouraging physical activity through dog walking: why don't some owners walk with their dog? Prev Med. 2008;46(2):120–6. https://doi.org/10.1016/j.ypmed.2007.08.015, PMID 17942146.
172. Cutt H, Giles-Corti B, Knuiman M, Timperio A, Bull F. Understanding dog owners' increased levels of physical activity: results from RESIDE. Am J Public Health. 2008;98(1):66–9. https://doi.org/10.2105/AJPH.2006.103499, PMID 18048786.
173. Cutt HE, Giles-Corti B, Knuiman MW, Pikora TJ. Physical activity behavior of dog owners: development and reliability of the Dogs and Physical Activity (DAPA) tool. J Phys Act Health. 2008;5;Suppl 1:S73–89. https://doi.org/10.1123/jpah.5.s1.s73, PMID 18364529.
174. Wilkes J. The role of companion animals in counseling and psychology: discovering their use in the therapeutic process. Springfield, IL: Charles C. Thomas Publishing Ltd.; 2009.
175. Wemelsfelder F. How animals communicate quality of life: the qualitative assessment of behaviour. Anim Welf. 2007;16(S1):25–31. https://doi.org/10.1017/S0962728600031699.
176. Veterinarian's oath. American Veterinary Medical Association. Available from: https://www.avma.org/resources-tools/avma-policies/veterinarians-oath.

CHAPTER 2

The Circle of Life and Loss

An Introduction to Grief and Grieving

The circle of life is a concept that we are introduced to early in our lives, in the classroom, if not through personal experience. As early as elementary school, we are trained in the name of science to identify the interdependence of organisms upon one another within one or more ecosystems.(1, 2) As we map out the various webs of life into visual displays, we consider the food chains by which life survives. A food web is one of the earliest ways that we become socialized to the concept that life feeds upon life, literally and figuratively.(3) We learn, for instance, that the sun's energy is harnessed by a seed that then grows into a plant. The grains from that plant are ultimately consumed by a mouse, who is destined by the circle of life to feed the owl. In this respect, every species has their place, just as every animal comes into being and one day dies. We know this to be true and we romanticize it in feature films, such as in the opening song to the 1994 animated Disney hit, *The Lion King*.(4)

From the day we arrive on the planet
And, blinking, step into the sun
There's more to see than can ever be seen
More to do than can ever be done.
There's far too much to take in here
More to find than can ever be found
But the sun rolling high
Through the sapphire sky
Keeps great and small on the endless round.
It's the circle of life
And it moves us all
Through despair and hope
Through faith and love
'Til we find our place
On the path unwinding

In the circle
The circle of life.

Yet, particularly in Western culture, we tend to keep death at an arm's length.(5–11) We acknowledge that death happens on paper, within our webs of life. We bear witness to it in the theaters – *Bambi*(12–15) and *All Dogs Go to Heaven*(16) come to mind – and we are exposed to death in age-appropriate fiction.(17–21) However, until we experience it personally, death seems at best a figurative construct – something that we know happens to others, but never us – and never to those within our innermost sphere. Death is, in this way, perceived as distant and is often described as just another stage of life. This suits us just fine, so long as it happens to someone else – someone we don't love or even know.

When we do confront death face-to-face, as the bereaved, we tend to replace open dialogue with euphemisms.(6) Among Western societies, it is common to outsource care for the deceased.(6) We hire others – funeral directors and morticians – to do the work associated with death for us, thus decreasing our exposure to a fate to which we will all one day succumb.(6)

2.1 The Overarching Impact of Loss

When loss does happen, it is a shock to the system. Like a stone dropping into a pond, there's significant disruption in the surface tension that glues the water molecules together and the water line literally falls apart. We fall apart. Only, it's not a one-time disruption. It's a disruption that begins at our core, like the epicenter of an earthquake, and ripples out.

Sometimes there is a fault line along which the ground surface breaks. The rest of the world can see and hear and feel our outward expressions of loss.

On other occasions, the ground shifts deep beneath the surface, under-ground, and the surface does not break. We break somewhere within, our inner screams drowned out by the silence and the shock and the pain that cannot find its way to the surface to be spoken.

Novelist Katharine Weber describes the connection between life and loss in her 2011 novel, *The Music Lesson*, when she writes that: "Life seems sometimes like nothing more than a series of losses, from begin-ning to end. That's the given. How you respond to those losses, what you make of what's left, that's the part you have to make up as you go."(22)

2.2 Examples of Non-Death Loss

Weber's words ring true in that loss is an expected part of life. As the living, we experience loss, to varying degrees, every day. Examples of non-death loss include:(23–28)

- time: as time passes, we lose the present day to the past
- seasons: as seasons change, we lose summer's greenery to leafless trees against a backdrop of snow and ice
- innocence: as we make the transition from childhood into adulthood
- unity: homes divided by discord and/or divorce
- parents and siblings: for those who are placed in foster care
- shifts in relationships and power dynamics as the child–parent relationship morphs into a relationship between two adults
- friendship: friends may come and go; friends may become separated geographically or by choice
- partners: relationships and unions may come to a halt; lovers may choose to move on, move away, and/or get divorced
- loss of a familiar place
- loss of a home to housing insecurity
- loss of satiety because of food insecurity
- loss of safety or security, to abuse
- loss of aspirations: a college athlete may come to realize that they are not skilled enough to play a professional sport
- change in daily schedule or routine
- major life change: for example, a grown child may move out of the house and onto college; a grown child may move out of state
- moving cross-country or overseas
- changing country of citizenship: feeling as though one is breaking ties with one's homeland
- employment: we may lose what was once a fulfilling job or we may choose to depart one workplace for another; our position or title may change; we may get demoted
- co-workers and/or employers may move on, leading to a shift in the workplace culture and a "new normal"
- estrangement with friends or family
- infertility
- adoptions that do not materialize
- biological parents: for those who experienced closed adoptions and never had the opportunity to meet one or both birth parents
- loss of material goods or possessions

- loss of trust
- loss of mobility
- loss of physical health
- loss of mental health or cognitive function.

In addition to the aforementioned losses, we may grieve:

- the unknown: uncertainty with respect to the future may be unsettling
- social isolation: living alone may precipitate feelings of loneliness
- loss of normalcy: we may long for the normalcy of ordinary moments with those who are no longer with us.

2.3 The Permanence of Loss Through Death

Life events, among other life changes, are losses in their own right.

Some losses are more tangible than others. Some losses are more relatable to us than others. Some losses affect us more deeply than others.

All losses leave some kind of memory, an impact, or an imprint inside of us.

Death is often said to be the most powerful of our losses because it is *permanent.*(29–32)

Have you ever dreamed that you are searching for someone, a loved one, whom you could not find?

Death is the moment that nightmare becomes a reality and your life is forever changed.(32)

Your mind and heart may play tricks on you. You may talk yourself into believing that your loved one is still with you.

You may continue to search for the one you love but come up empty-handed.(33–37)

The permanence of loss is an indescribable sting that stings and stings and stings again.

Some deaths sting more than others. No loss is insignificant, but some may appear to be more bearable than others. Other losses rock us to our core.

Some deaths are untimely, and we do not have time to prepare.

Even when we anticipate death(38, 39), we cannot always predict our response to it.

The relationships that we shared with the deceased are unique.(31, 40) So, too, is our response to their deaths. No two individuals grieve the same way, for the same being, for the same period of time.(31, 40)

2.4 The Uniqueness of Grief

Our journey through grief is ours and ours alone.(31, 40)

Author Mitch Albom, of *Tuesdays with Morrie* and *The Five People You Meet in Heaven*, conceptualized the yearning that is associated with life after loss when he wrote the following passage in his 2008 book, *For One More Day*:(41)

> *Have you ever lost someone you loved and wanted one more conversation, one more chance to make up for the time when you thought they would be here forever? If so, then you know you can go your whole life collecting days, and none will outweigh the one you wish you had back.*

Albom's words may have been confined to the pages of a novel, yet if you have ever loved and lost, you may find that his haunting message of bereavement resonates within.

Albom's messaging is clear and on point: life without those we love is forever changed and no matter what or who comes after the death of a loved one, we cannot ever get back to what we once shared.

We may add to our network and broaden our reach, but we are acutely aware of a deficit, a void that can never be filled.

These are normal, natural reactions to loss. These reactions are what we refer to as *grief*.(31, 40, 42, 43)

2.5 Defining Grief

Grief has many definitions.

Some have likened grief to the ebb and flow of the tide, or a rollercoaster of emotions.(23, 44) The tide captures the variation in feelings that come and go, yet the prescribed intervals by which the tide appears and recedes do always fit the erratic nature of grief's emotional rollercoaster. The imagery of the rollercoaster may more accurately reflect the overarching loss of control and the unpredictability of the experience.(44)

Some have described grief as a river that we must wade through to get to the other side, or the deep end of the ocean.(45) Others compare grief to an errant boat or canoe.(44, 46) When author John Bramblett experienced the death of his son, he described grief as such:(46)

> *I found my path of discovery was not always straight. I was like the canoeist who sets his sights on a point on the distant shore only to paddle a frustrating,*

zigzagging course as the elements of wind, water, and errant paddle strokes work against him. He may occasionally even lose sight of his goal as mists rise up between him and his destination, obscuring the shoreline he is moving toward.

Bramblett is able to create a visual image of the grief-associated confusion and disorientation that can be challenging to articulate.(44, 46)

In her book, *Eat, Pray, Love,* author Elizabeth Gilbert compares grief to "a specific location, a coordinate on a map of time."(47) She exquisitely captures the solitude of the bereaved when she shares that "when you are standing in that forest of sorrow, you cannot imagine that you could ever find your way to a better place."(47)

Some relate grief to losing part of oneself, yet having that perpetual, gnawing sensation that the missing body part is ever-present. Grief has, in this way, been likened to a phantom limb.(48)

For others, grief is a monster or a beast that symbolizes the conflict that is stirred up by not only physical death, but also the emotional end of an era, a chapter of life, or a pattern of behavior.(42) Gould describes the *grief octopus* as having many tentacles that grab and disorient the bereaved as they flail around helplessly, trying to make sense of a world that has been turned on its head.(44)

Perhaps no on-stage musical captures the metaphor of the beast better than *Les Miserables*, in which character Fantine grieves the life she knew before loss:(49, 50)

I dreamed a dream in time gone by,
When hope was high and life worth living.
I dreamed that love would never die.
I prayed that God would be forgiving.

Then I was young and unafraid,
And dreams were made and used and wasted.
There was no ransom to be paid,
No song unsung, no wine untasted.

Grief stole the life that Fantine had envisioned for herself. She acknowledges this loss when she sings:(49, 50)

But the tigers come at night,
With their voices soft as thunder,
As they tear your hopes apart,
And they turn your dreams to shame.

Fantine goes on to describe the conflict that has become her life:(49, 50)

And still I dream he'll come to me,
That we would live the years together,
But there are dreams that cannot be,
And there are storms we cannot weather.

I had a dream my life would be,
So different from this hell I'm living,
So different now from what it seemed.
Now life has killed the dream, I dreamed.

In this portrait of grief, grief has been presented as a thief that takes away what ought to have been. Grief steals the life we knew, and finds us, the bereaved, on a journey to find ourselves again.

2.6 Grief as a Journey

Grief is a journey that makes us long for what we had. That journey makes us question ourselves, our past actions, and our present pursuits.

We may search for meaning as we attempt to make sense of what cannot be.

In this quest for meaning, we may search for the one we have "lost." Country singer-songwriter Toby Keith affirms this "search" in his 2009 hit, *Cryin' for Me*, written as a tribute to his friend Wayman Tisdale:(51)

I got up and dialed your number.
Your voice came on the line,
That old familiar message,
I have heard a thousand times.
It just said, sorry that I missed you.
Leave a message and God bless.
I know that you think I am crazy,
But I just had to hear your voice I guess.

I'm going to miss that smile.
I'm going to miss you my friend.
Even though it hurts the way it ended up,
I'd do it all again.

2.7 Grief as a Process

Grief is clearly many things to many people.

Irrespective of which analogy resonates with you, or if you hold tight to your own metaphor, grief is a *process*. Grief is the mind, body, and heart coming to terms with the reality that who you want and need cannot, after death, return to you in the flesh, ever.

The permanence of death is not something that sinks in overnight. It is predictably unpredictable and leaves us wanting more, as if we could just go back in time and live life again. American country music band, Diamond Rio, describes this yearning best in the lyrics to *One More Day*:(52)

Last night I had a crazy dream.
A wish was granted just for me,
It could be for anything.
I didn't ask for money
Or a mansion in Malibu.
I simply wished for one more day with you.

One more day, one more time,
One more sunset, maybe I'd be satisfied.
But then again, I know what it would do,
Leave me wishing still for one more day with you.

For some, the process of grief may seem straightforward or even easy. Others may feel primed to push back, as if refusal to accept it can undo death and restore what once was.

What is critical to both acknowledge and to honor is that grief is not a clear-cut path from A to B. It is also not a race. The finish line of acceptance comes only after hard work is put in, and even then, one is never truly "over" grief.

You never "move on" from grief. You learn to "move with" grief or rather, grief learns to "move with" you.

In this respect, grief may ebb and flow for days, weeks, months, or years. Grief may also return to you unexpectedly, years after it has apparently passed, when you recall a name, a person, or an event that linked them to you.

A word, statement, gesture, written card, letter, or fragrance may trigger a memory, a reminder of the one we once loved. And in that moment, we are carried back in time to what once was.

In those moments, it is not that grief is pulling us backwards; it is not that we are regressing. It is not that we have failed to "move on."

We are remembering. And in remembering, we relive grief, at times, all over again.

2.8 The Stages of Grief

Although we all grieve differently, our grief maps share some of the same coordinates. These coordinates can remind us that what we are experiencing is normal and expected.

There is often comfort in knowing that we are not alone when we feel or react a certain way.

Many of the bereaved experience grief in stages. Stages of grief were first introduced in 1969 by Elisabeth Kübler-Ross in her now famous book, *On Death and Dying*.(53) These stages were not intended to be a recipe, but rather a guide based upon her experiences exploring death through the lenses of terminally ill patients.(53)

Although not everyone experiences every stage, knowing what others before you have faced may provide reassurance that you are "on track." These so-called stages make grief predictable despite its uniqueness and that may in and of itself provide comfort to the bereaved.

The first stage of grief is denial. Denial can be thought of as going into "survivor mode." In order to survive the initial impact, our minds shield us from fully absorbing the enormity of the loss.

We cannot believe what we have just heard or seen. We cannot absorb that death has occurred. It seems surreal. It does not seem possible. Life as we know it has turned on its head. We may feel that we are spinning our wheels in place, trying to make sense of a topsy-turvy world that has lost its meaning.

Denial is powerful. It shields us from pain with numbness. This numbness helps us to "power through" each minute, each hour, each day.

Denial is, in a sense, the pause button on life. It is a time-out. It is our mind slowing down what we understand to be true so that our heart has time to catch up.

Denial is the Band-Aid on a deep and painful wound. We are aware of the wound but cannot appreciate its depth. The Band-Aid shields us from full knowledge when we are not yet ready to process it.

We may not only deny that death has happened, we also may go to great lengths to avoid it. Avoidance is a way for us to protect ourselves and conserve our energy as we prepare for the grief work that is up ahead.

The second stage of grief is anger. As denial fades, it takes the brakes off our emotions and we begin to feel again. When these feelings surface, one of the strongest to take hold may be anger.

We may cast blame at anyone and everyone in our way, especially those we love most.

We may be angry with the one who died for leaving us behind.

We may be angry with the medical team, particularly if trauma took the life of our loved one before we were "ready" to say goodbye.

Maybe we did not get to say goodbye.

Maybe things went unsaid at the bedside.

Maybe we regret what we said or maybe we regret thinking what we did.

We may be angry with ourselves.

We may be angry with others in our close circle who may not understand the enormity of our loss.

We may be angry with those who expect us to move on before we are ready.

If we are spiritual, we may be angry at our faith.

We may feel that faith let us down.

We may feel let down by life, too, or by those with whom we surround ourselves.

Anger is a way to lash out against that empty feeling of nothingness.

Anger may not be rational. Anger may not be logical. It does not have to be either.

Anger provides us with something to cling tight to. Anger provides us with purpose, something to do.

Anger is a way for us to feel that we have control over an event in which we are powerless.

Anger is not the only emotion to arise from death, but it is inherently strong.

It cannot bring the deceased back to life, but it ties us to them in death.

The third stage of grief is bargaining. Bargaining is a way of negotiating the hurt.

Sometimes we bargain with a higher power.

Sometimes we bargain with the living.

Sometimes we bargain with ourselves: We may say aloud or silently, to ourselves, "I will do ___[insert task]___ if only ___[insert name of deceased]___can come back to me."

Sometimes we wish we could trade our life for theirs.

Bargaining is yet another attempt to regain control over the situation. It makes us feel powerful when in fact we are powerless.

We may play the "what if" game or "if only."

- "What if we could go back in time?"
- "What if I had said I was sorry?"

- "What if I had not said … ?"
- "If only she had seen a doctor sooner."
- "If only he had been diagnosed six months earlier."
- "If only I had been a better sister …"
- "If only I had known that our time together was limited."
- "If only we had discussed what to do in the event that the unthinkable happened."

Bargaining gives us the illusion that we have the power to go back in time, the power to reverse death.

Like anger, bargaining ties us to our loved one and to the past.

Bargaining is also often tied to guilt. We may hold ourselves accountable for words and actions that were beyond our control.

We may feel guilty that we didn't do more, even if we did all we could.

We often relive our memories and/or those final moments. We pick apart our words and actions. We think about what we would have said and done differently, as if do-overs are possible.

At some point, we stop living in the past and again become mindful of the present.

The fourth stage of grief is depression. We become intensely aware of how our loved one's death impacts the present-day. We sink into the emptiness that loss brings. We are also acutely aware that we may find ourselves at a loss for words. It is difficult to find meaning when we no longer understand the world around us.

We may experience intense feelings of sadness and despair.

We may feel isolated and alone as others move on with their lives without us.

We may feel as if we are living life in slow motion. The rest of the world goes on, but we may feel "stuck."

For some, life transiently loses meaning. One might question the point of life, the purpose behind them still being here. Others might question their fit within family, their circle of friends, or community.

It is normal to question where to go from here, or how to go on with life without the one we love.

Anguish and despair are normal emotions that may leave us feeling raw or wounded.

Memories may intensify or reawaken these feelings just when we think we have overcome them. They pull us back in for a second or third round.

Consider that grief comes in waves as new aspects of loss are realized:(54)

When someone you love dies, and you're not expecting it, you don't lose her all at once;
you lose her in pieces over a long time — the way the mail stops coming, and her scent

fades from the pillows and even from the clothes in her closet and drawers. Gradually, you accumulate the parts of her that are gone. Just when the day comes — when there's a particular missing part that overwhelms you with the feeling that she's gone, forever — there comes another day, and another specifically missing part.

The final stage of grief is acceptance. Acceptance does not mean that grief is over. Acceptance does not mean that you have forgotten your loved one. Acceptance does not mean that you are "alright" or "back to normal." Your life is never going to be "back to normal." You are living the "new normal."

In that way, acceptance is not about moving beyond the loss. Acceptance is about learning how to live with loss.

Acceptance is about adjusting to this new life, without the one you love.

Acceptance is about restructuring life to find new meaning in it.

Acceptance is about reinvesting in the present and planning for the future.

You honor the memory of your loved one by living.

You still remember your loved one, but memories hurt less. Memories feel warm and welcome. They are reminders that your loved one is still a part of who you are and all that you do.

Acceptance is a new beginning, a new chapter. Just like a book, the new chapter does not replace the old. Instead, the new chapter represents additional pages – opportunities to grow onward and upward from here.

In that way, we emerge from our shell of grief like a butterfly emerges from a cocoon. We are forever changed by what we have experienced, but the final product is whole. We are, in a sense, ready to participate in life again.

Each grief journey is a process: it takes time to grieve. We each grieve in our own way. There are no shortcuts through grief. "When you experience loss, people say you'll move through the 5 stages of grief … Denial, Anger, Bargaining, Depression, Acceptance … What they don't tell you is that you'll cycle through them all every day."(55)

Some people take less time in their grief journey than others. There is no way to predict this.

Some stages of grief may be fleeting. Others may make us feel "stuck" for a while. Some stages may feel like forever.

Some people may try to rush us through our grief. They may think that by doing so, they can help us to skip over our pain and overwhelming sense of despair.

What we need to understand, what we need others to understand, is that there is no fast-forward button for grief. Skipping steps of the process, whether intentional or not, does not facilitate healing. Only time heals, and that timeline is up to the bereaved.

2.9 Beyond the Stages of Grief

Despite the fact that grief is universal, "the lack of widely accepted guidelines as to what constitutes 'normal' grieving results in mourning being a common experience with little universality."(56)

Although Kübler-Ross' staging of grief was intended to be descriptive, critics express concern that it has become prescriptive.(53) When applied too stringently, as though grief adheres to a rigid linear timeline, the bereaved can feel as though they are grieving incorrectly if and when they do not react in the prescribed manner.(53)

Concern has also been raised that the audience for this model has inappropriately been applied to caregivers and the bereaved when in fact Kübler-Ross aimed to describe the emotional and behavioral journey of the terminally ill, dying patient.(53) Caregivers who ascribe to this model may believe that their responsibility is to shuttle the patient through each stage.(53) In fact, hastening patients towards acceptance before they are truly "ready" deprives them of experiencing grief in their own unique way.(53) This conscious or unconscious attempt to fast-track the process can complicate grief.(53)

In an attempt to broaden the model for understanding grief and loss, and highlight that grief is experienced fluidly rather than linearly, others have developed their own constructs.(53) These include, but are not limited to:(53)

- The Four Phases of Grief by Bowlby and Parkes
- Worden's Four Basic Tasks in Adapting to Loss
- Wolfelt's Companioning Approach to Grieving
- Neimeyer's Narrative and Constructivist Model.

During the 1980s, Bowlby and Parkes reformulated the stages of grief as four phases:(53, 57)

- shock and disbelief
- searching and yearning
- disorganization and repair
- rebuilding and healing.

Bowlby and Parkes intended to capture the initial numbness that the bereaved feel, followed by the quest to "find" the lost person. When that search comes up empty-handed and yearning is unfulfilled, there is initial despair. It takes time to process that despair. Bowlby and Parkes emphasized that grief is an adaptive process and the timeline for the bereaved varies before they can commit to rebuilding life and healing from their loss.(58) Reemergence into life implies acceptance of their new reality as well as their "renewed sense of identity."(53) The bereaved are, in a sense, taking back control of their life and how they desire to live out what remains of it.

William Worden also developed his own unique model on grief and loss based upon an 18-year collaboration with Harvard psychiatrist Avery Weisman at the Massachusetts General Hospital. They collectively studied life-threatening illness and life-threatening behaviors, such as suicidal ideation, with financial support from the National Institute of Health (NIH). Worden was asked to develop training for mental health professionals in bereavement. As he developed his course, he elected to borrow terminology from psychology and replace the terms, stages, or phases, with tasks. Just as there are developmental tasks to complete as prescribed by developmental psychology, there are tasks that the bereaved must complete to adjust to life without a loved one. These tasks are not linear.(53) They can occur in any order. It is ultimately up to the bereaved to decide how and when to complete the tasks.(53) Tasks can be worked on simultaneously or independently, and tasks may be approached intermittently until complete.(53)

Worden summarized his work as four basic tasks in adapting to loss:(33, 53)

- accepting the reality of the loss
- experiencing the pain of grief
- adjusting to the environment
- redirecting emotional energy.

The first two tasks, accepting the reality of the loss and experiencing the pain of grief, are self-explanatory.

Adjusting to the environment implies coping and reengagement with one's surroundings.(53) The bereaved learn how to reinvest in daily routines and may even find comfort in them.(53) Hobbies or work may resume.(53)

The final task, redirecting emotional energy, is a reconfiguring of focus onto new activities that may offer enjoyment.(53) It is an outward expression that the bereaved are ready to re-invest, to test out new experiences, and to find joy even in the absence of their loved ones.(53)There is a shift of energy from focusing on the suffering that is associated with loss to learning how to live again.(53)

Additional theories on grief and grieving ground themselves less in stages, phases, or tasks, and more in experiential and narrative methods.(53)

Dr. Alan Wolfelt, of the Center for Loss and Life Transition, developed 11 tenets of companioning the bereaved.(59)

- **Tenet One:**
  "Companioning is about being present to another person's pain; it is not about taking away the pain."
- **Tenet Two:**
  "Companioning is about going to the wilderness of the soul with another human being; it is not about thinking you are responsible for finding the way out."
- **Tenet Three:**
  "Companioning is about honoring the spirit; it is not about focusing on the intellect.
- **Tenet Four:**
  "Companioning is about listening with the heart; it is not about analyzing with the head."
- **Tenet Five:**
  "Companioning is about bearing witness to the struggles of others; it is not about judging or directing these struggles."
- **Tenet Six:**
  "Companioning is about walking alongside; it is not about leading."
- **Tenet Seven:**
  "Companioning is about discovering the gifts of sacred silence; it is not about filling up every moment with words."
- **Tenet Eight:**
  "Companioning is about being still; it is not about frantic movement forward."
- **Tenet Nine:**
  "Companioning is about respecting disorder and confusion; it is not about imposing order and logic."
- **Tenet Ten:**
  "Companioning is about learning from others; it is not about teaching them."
- **Tenet Eleven:**
  "Companioning is about compassionate curiosity; it is not about expertise."

The companioning approach by Wolfelt paints a different portrait of grief. Grief is viewed as an extension of love.(53) Rather than avoiding grief or focusing on "fixing" it, the bereaved can lean into grief as something to be embraced, experienced, and expressed.(53) They should be encouraged to feel what they feel because healing is about learning how to incorporate grief into lives that continue on.(53)

Those who support the bereaved bear witness to this journey and in this way walk beside them.(53) Best described in Wolfelt's words, as Tenet Two: "Companioning is about going to the wilderness of the soul with another human being; it is not about thinking you are responsible for finding the way out."(53, 60, 61)

Self-compassion, and self-care are essential aspects of the grieving process as the bereaved relearn how to identify themselves in a world without the physical presence of their loved ones.(53, 60)

Narrative is one way in which the bereaved can explore their new identities.(53) Neimeyer's Narrative and Constructivist Model emphasizes that grief is about meaning-making.(53, 62, 63) Loss changes our reality and our core-beliefs.(64) Loss forever altes what we thought we understood about the world.(64) It is through loss that we come to understand life's fragility and that permanence is but a construct. Nothing and no one is truly forever.

Our understanding of the world around us and therefore what we choose to find meaning in is challenged and re-shaped by loss.(64) To survive loss, we must learn how to reconstruct meaning and/or find new meaning that allows us to continue our life story in the absence of who we miss.(62)

According to Neimeyer, the bereaved can learn to:(64)

> … assimilate *the loss experience into their pre-loss beliefs and self-narratives, in effect maintaining consistency with who they previously were … Alternatively, individuals can attempt to* accommodate *to the loss by reorganizing, deepening, or expanding their beliefs and self-narrative to embrace the reality of the loss, often seeking validation for a changed identity in connection with a new field of social relationships.*

The search to find meaning and create purpose is not a new theme. It is one that was asserted by Victor Frankl in his influential book, *Man's Search for Meaning*, which chronicles his experiences imprisoned within Nazi concentration camps during World War II. Frankl credited his survival with identifying purpose and channeling that purpose to envision the desired outcome. In the words of Frankl: "When we are no longer able to change a situation, we are challenged to change ourselves."(65)

In applying this theme to bereavement, internal change by the bereaved is precipitated by an active investment in reorganizing oneself. (66) There is an attitude shift in terms of willingness to adapt to a new life story.(53, 66–68) This paves the way to not only survive loss, but also potentially thrive in spite of it.(53, 60, 68)

Narrative retelling of the death and/or reflective writing can support this process as the bereaved take ownership of their experience.(64) In the words of Neimeyer:(64)

> ... *therapies that emphasize a fuller re-telling of the narrative of the death under conditions of safety(69) can provide a measure of social validation for the account, and redress the empathic failure or silence with which many of the bereaved are met, especially when their losses or their responses to them are non-normative. (70) Importantly, such retelling—specifically focusing on the hardest parts of the experience and "staying with" them until the associated images and meanings can be held with less anguish— plays a pivotal part in demonstrably efficacious treatments for complicated grief.(69) As with exposure-based therapies for other forms of traumatic events, re-narration of the loss promotes mastery of difficult material and helps counteract avoidance coping. Equally important, it can help identify aspects of the experience for which further meaning-based processing is necessary.*

In addition to re-telling their story or writing about it, the bereaved may choose to write a letter to the deceased to share what they wished they had shared when that individual was still alive.(53) Others who are grieving may find comfort in exploring how they feel through visualization activities and metaphors.(53, 64) Language is powerful and imagery can put a name on something that is otherwise challenging to articulate. For instance, if someone were to compare themselves to fish in a fishbowl, they may be articulating a sense of isolation.(64) They are likely expressing that they are feeling walled off from others and being observed from the outside in.(64)

Imagery can be vivid and/or abstract. It requires active listening by those who are companioning the bereaved through grief to ensure that there is shared understanding and that the bereaved have effectively conveyed what it is that they wanted others to hear.

2.10 Religious and Cultural Perspectives on Death and Dying

Death is universal. However, the way in which we conceptualize death and what happens when someone dies varies significantly across cultures, religions, and communities.(72) For some people, there is no core belief in life after death. Death is seen as the ultimate end, in which life ceases to exist.(72) For others, death implies rebirth or a transition from a physical to a spiritual state of existence.(72) Others believe that the deceased coexist with the living and influence their well-being.(72)

Cultural and religious conceptions about death and dying also dictate what it means to die well.(72–77) In 1990, Kellahear defined what is meant by an "acceptable" death as compared with a "good" death.(78) Kellahear's findings can be summarized as follows:(72)

> *An acceptable death is said to be non-dramatic, disciplined, and with very little emotion. This is the atmosphere that seems to exist in structured settings such as hospitals in the West where most people die. On the other hand, a good death is said to be one that allows for social adjustments and personal preparation by the dying person and his or her family.*

A good death is often perceived as one in which there is ample time for saying goodbye.(72) Both the dying person and their family are able to prepare for life without that individual.(72) Yet, a good death means different things to different people. Gire explains that:(72)

> *Among the Kwahu-Tafo of Ghana, a good death is one in which the dying person has accomplished most of what he or she set out to do and has made peace with others before dying.(77) In Nigeria, death of one that has lived a long, and for the most part a successful, life can often be inferred from the nature of the captions in their obituaries. In such cases, the preambles go along the lines of "with gratitude to God for a life well spent …" captions that would never be seen for one that has died an early death or death that has occurred under very tragic circumstances. Yet in other societies, a good death may be one in which a person dies in service of his country or religion; in other words, the person is regarded as a martyr.(80)*

Cultural and religious conceptions about death and dying are significant influencers of the ways in which people live their lives and whether they fear death or choose to embrace it.(72) Some cultures have been described as death-affirming.(72) Others, classically Western societies, trend towards death-denying or death-defying.(5, 6, 72) Death may be depicted as the enemy or something to resist(72, 81), in stark contrast to many Eastern cultural beliefs, which promote death acceptance as a part of life.(72)

After the death of a loved one, cultural and religious conceptions about grieving influence how those left behind choose to live out the reminder of their lives. Walker A Bristol, M.Div., a Humanist Chaplain, explains that:(82)

Religion and culture are intertwined with how grief is processed, both outwardly and inwardly ... Philosophical beliefs about the nature of life and death greatly influence the meaning of the dying process. Religions encapsulate the practices that facilitate the safe passage of a soul from this plane to another—or, for those traditions without a belief in the afterlife, affirm and cherish the memory of someone lost in the world of the living. Culture similarly creates, or limits, the space in which a person is allowed or encouraged to grieve, and offers tools for undergoing the grief journey.

It is beyond the scope of this text to outline all cultural and religious conceptions. The goal is not to be comprehensive, rather to acknowledge that there are many perspectives when it comes to death and dying. These perspectives are shaped by so many facets of who we are and by what and who have influenced us. This is significant when it comes to healthcare delivery and provider-patient relationships. Specifically, in the realm of veterinary practice, the veterinarian–client-patient relationship is perhaps put to the test most often when it comes to decision making about euthanasia. In these situations, it is essential to move towards understanding when it comes to our clients' beliefs, thoughts, concerns, and perspectives. Providing a safe, supportive space in which to engage in dialogue and perspective-taking can be valuable in helping clients navigate those decisions within the framework of their belief and value system.

References

1. Gallegos L, Jerezano ME, Flores F. Preconceptions and relations used by children in the construction of food chains. J Res Sci Teach. 1994;31(3):259–72. https://doi.org/10.1002/tea.3660310306.
2. Finley FN, Stewart J, Yarroch WL. Teacher's perceptions of important difficult science content. Sci Educ. 1982;66(4):531–8. https://doi.org/10.1002/sce.3730660404.
3. Brumby MN. Student's perceptions of the concept of life. Sci Educ. 1982;66(4): 613–22. https://doi.org/10.1002/sce.3730660411.
4. John E, Rice T, Zimmer H, Twillie C, ML, Weaver J, et al. Lion King: original songs [performed music]; Burbank, CA: Walt Disney Records; 2014.
5. Palgi P, Abramovitch H. Death: a cross-cultural perspective. Annu Rev Anthropol. 1984;13(1):385–417. https://doi.org/10.1146/annurev.an.13.100184.002125.
6. Robert M, Tradii L. Do we deny death? I. A genealogy of death denial. Mortality. 2019;24(3):247–60. https://doi.org/10.1080/13576275.2017.1415318.
7. Faunce WA, Fulton RL. The sociology of death: a neglected area of research. Soc Forces. 1958;36(3):205–9. https://doi.org/10.2307/2573805.
8. Feifel H. The meaning of death. New York: McGraw-Hill; 1959.
9. Zimmermann C, Rodin G. The denial of death [thesis]: sociological critique and implications for palliative care. Palliative Medicine; 2004;18(2):121–8.

10. Kellehear A. Are we a death-denying society? A sociological review. Soc Sci Med. 1984;18(9):713–23. https://doi.org/10.1016/0277-9536(84)90094-7, PMID 6729531.

11. McKay RC. From denial toward integration of death in Western culture. S Afr J Sociol. 1992;23(3):89–95. https://doi.org/10.1080/02580144.1992.10520114.

12. Sobchack VC. The violent dance: a personal memoir of death in the movies. J Popul Film. 1974;3(1):2–14. https://doi.org/10.1080/00472719.1974.10661713.

13. Laderman G. The Disney way of death. J Am Acad Relig. 2000;68(1):27–46.

14. Lutts RH. The trouble with Bambi: Walt Disney's Bambi and the American vision of nature. For Conserv Hist. 1992;36(4):160–71. https://doi.org/10.2307/3983677.

15. Hastings AW. Bambi and the hunting ethos. J Popul Film Telev. 1996;24(2):53–9. https://doi.org/10.1080/01956051.1996.9943714.

16. O'Neill K. The afterlife in popular culture: heaven, hell, and the underworld in the American imagination. Santa Barbara, CA: Greenwood Publishing Group; 2022.

17. White EB, Williams G, Rosenwald EG, Lessing J. Rosenwald collection. 1st ed. Library of Congress. Charlotte's web. New York: Harper & Brothers; 1952.

18. Homer MS. The odyssey. Vol. XLV. New York: Atria Books; 2013.

19. Gipson F. Old Yeller. New York: Harper; 1956.

20. Rawls W. Where the red fern grows; the story of two dogs and a boy. 1st ed. Garden City, NY: Doubleday Publishing; 1961.

21. Burnford SE, Burger C. The incredible journey. 1st ed. Boston: Little; 1961.

22. Weber K. The music lesson. 1st ed. New York: Crown Publishing Group Publishers; 1998.

23. McGahan K. Only gone from your sight: Jack McAfghan's little guide to pet loss and grief. Kate McGahan; 2018.

24. Gitterman A, Knight C. Non-death loss: grieving for the loss of familiar place and for precious time and associated opportunities. Clin Soc Work J. 2019;47(2):147–55. https://doi.org/10.1007/s10615-018-0682-5.

25. Harris DL. Non-death loss and grief: context and clinical implications. New York: Routledge; 2020.

26. Mitchell MB. "No one acknowledged my loss and hurt": non-death loss, grief, and trauma in foster care. Child Adolesc Soc Work J. 2018;35(1):1–9. https://doi.org/10.1007/s10560-017-0502-8.

27. Harris DL. Counting our losses: reflecting on change, loss, and transition in everyday life. New York: Taylor & Francis Group, LLC; 2011.

28. Smith PH, Delgado H. Working with non-death losses in counseling: an overview of grief needs and approaches. Adultspan J. 2020;19(2):118–27. https://doi.org/10.1002/adsp.12100.

29. O'Connor K, Barrera M. Changes in parental self-identity following the death of a child to cancer. Death Stud. 2014;38(6–10):404–11. https://doi.org/10.1080/07481187.2013.801376, PMID 24666147.

30. Niemiec RM, Schulenberg SE. Understanding death attitudes: the integration of movies, positive psychology, and meaning management. Death Stud. 2011;35(5):387–407. https://doi.org/10.1080/07481187.2010.544517, PMID 24501852.

31. Wolfelt A. Understanding grief: helping yourself heal. Vol. xvi. Muncie, IN: Accelerated Development Inc; 1992.

32. Wolfelt A. The journey through grief: reflections on healing. Fort Collins, CO: Companion Press; 1997.

33. Worden JW. Theoretical perspectives on loss and grief. In: Stillion JM, Attig J, editors. Death, dying, and bereavement: contemporary perspectives, institutions, and practices. Springer Publishing Company; 2014. p. 91–103.

34. White C, Fessler DMT. An evolutionary account of vigilance in grief. Evol Med Public Health. 2018;2018(1):34–42. https://doi.org/10.1093/emph/eox018, PMID 29492265.

35. Eisma MC, Stroebe MS. Emotion regulatory strategies in complicated grief: a systematic review. Behav Ther. 2021;52(1):234–49. https://doi.org/10.1016/j.beth.2020.04.004, PMID 33483120.

36. Stroebe MS, Schut H, Stroebe W. Trauma and grief: a comparative analysis. In: Harvey JH, editor. Perspectives on loss: a sourcebook. Philadelphia: Taylor & Francis; 1998. p. 81–98.

37. Worden JW. Grief counseling and grief therapy: a handbook for the mental health practitioner. New York: Springer Publishing Company, LLC; 2018.

38. Sweeting HN, Gilhooly ML. Anticipatory grief: a review. Soc Sci Med. 1990;30(10):1073–80. https://doi.org/10.1016/0277-9536(90)90293-2, PMID 2194293.

39. Coelho A, Barbosa A. Family anticipatory grief: an integrative literature review. Am J Hosp Palliat Care. 2017;34(8):774–85. https://doi.org/10.1177/1049909116647960, PMID 27151972.

40. Humphrey KM. Counseling strategies for loss and grief. Vol. xv. Alexandria, VA: American Counseling Association; 2009.

41. Albom M. For one more day. 1st ed. New York: Hyperion; 2006.

42. Friedman R, James C, James JW. The grief recovery handbook for pet loss. Vol. xi. Lanham: Taylor Trade Publishing; 2014.

43. Howarth R. Concepts and controversies in grief and loss. J Ment Health Couns. 2011;33(1):4–10. https://doi.org/10.17744/mehc.33.1.900m56162888u737.

44. Gould JB. "A picture is worth a thousand words": a strategy for grief education. Death Stud. 1994;18(1):65–74. https://doi.org/10.1080/07481189408252643.

45. Englar J. Please be gentle; 1999. Available at: https://griefforwardblog.wordpress.com/2019/12/20/after-loss-creed/.

46. Bramblett J. When goodbye is forever. New York: Ballantine Book Company; 1991.

47. Gilbert E. Eat, pray, love: one woman's search for everything across Italy, India and Indonesia. New York: Viking Press; 2006.

48. Ratcliffe M. Grief and phantom limbs: a phenomenological comparison. In: Ratcliffe M, editor. The new yearbook for phenomenology and phenomenological philosophy. New York: Routledge; 2019.

49. Anthony J. I dreamed a dream [performed music]. Hollywood, CA: GNP crescendo Records; 1988.

50. Broadway's greatest hits. Vol. I [sound recording]. Roswell, GA: Platinum Entertainment; 1998.

51. Keith T. American ride [sound recording]. Nashville, TN, Universal City, CA.: Show Dog Nashville; Manufactured and distributed by Universal; 2009.

52. Rio D. One more day [sound recording]. New York, NY: Arista Nashville; 2000.

53. Tyrrell P, Harberger S, Schoo C, Siddiqui W. Kubler-Ross stages of dying and subsequent models of grief. StatPearls. Treasure Island, FL; 2022.

54. Irving H. A prayer for Owen Meany. Boston: Mariner Books Classics; 2014.

55. Suzuki R. The longest night: a collection of poetry from a life half lived. Illustrated edn. Ranata Suzuki; 2018.

56. Maples MR. Mental ghosts and the process of grief. J Personal Interpers Loss. 1998;3(2):217–31. https://doi.org/10.1080/10811449808414443.

57. Bowlby J. Attachment and loss. Vol. 3. London: Pimlico; 1980.

58. Parkes CM. The first year of bereavement. A longitudinal study of the reaction of London widows to the death of their husbands. Psychiatry. 1970;33(4):444–67. https://doi.org/10.1080/00332747.1970.11023644, PMID 5275840.

59. Wolfelt A. Eleven tenets of companioning the bereaved: center for loss and life transition; 2019. Available from: https://www.centerforloss.com/2019/12/elev en-tenets-of-companioning/.

60. Bruce CA. Helping patients, families, caregivers, and physicians, in the grieving process. J Am Osteopath Assoc. 2007;107(12);Suppl 7:ES33–40. PMID 18165376.

61. Schuelke T, Crawford C, Kentor R, Eppelheimer H, Chipriano C, Springmeyer K, et al. Current grief support in pediatric palliative care. Children (Basel). 2021;8(4). https://doi.org/10.3390/children8040278, PMID 33916583.

62. Neimeyer RA. Reauthoring life narratives: grief therapy as meaning reconstruction. Isr J Psychiatry Relat Sci. 2001;38(3–4):171–83. PMID 11725416.

63. Gillies J, Neimeyer RA. Loss, grief, and the search for significance: toward a model of meaning reconstruction in bereavement. J Constr Psychol. 2006;19(1):31–65. https://doi.org/10.1080/10720530500311182.

64. Neimeyer RA, Burke LA, Mackay MM, van Dyke Stringer JG. Grief therapy and the reconstruction of meaning: from principles to practice. J Contemp Psychother. 2010;40(2):73–83. https://doi.org/10.1007/s10879-009-9135-3.

65. Frankl VE. Man's search for meaning: an introduction to logotherapy. Boston: Beacon Press; 1963.

66. Alves D, Mendes I, Gonçalves MM, Neimeyer RA. Innovative moments in grief therapy: reconstructing meaning following perinatal death. Death Stud. 2012;36(9):795–818. https://doi.org/10.1080/07481187.2011.608291, PMID 245 63928.

67. Neimeyer RA. Searching for the meaning of meaning: grief therapy and the process of reconstruction. Death Stud. 2000;24(6):541–58. https://doi. org/10.1080/07481180050121480, PMID 11503667.

68. Neimeyer RA, Baldwin SA, Gillies J. Continuing bonds and reconstructing meaning: mitigating complications in bereavement. Death Stud. 2006;30(8):715–38. https:// doi.org/10.1080/07481180600848322, PMID 16972369.

69. Rynearson EK. Violent death. New York: Routledge; 2006.

70. Neimeyer RA, Jordan JR. Disenfranchisement as empathic failure: grief therapy and the co-construction of meaning. In: Doka K, editor. Disenfranchised grief. Champaign, IL: Research Press; 2002. p. 95–117.

71. Shear K, Frank E, Houck PR, Reynolds CF, 3rd. Treatment of complicated grief: a randomized controlled trial. JAMA. 2005;293(21):2601–8. https://doi.org/10.1001/ jama.293.21.2601, PMID 15928281.

72. Gire J. How death imitates life: cultural influences on conceptions of death and dying. Online readings in psychology and culture 6(2). https://doi.org/10.9707/ 2307-0919.1120.

73. Cain CL, McCleskey S. Expanded definitions of the "good death"? Race, ethnicity and medical aid in dying. Sociol Health Illn. 2019;41(6):1175–91. https://doi. org/10.1111/1467-9566.12903, PMID 30950077.

74. Broom A, Cavenagh J. Masculinity, moralities and being cared for: an exploration of experiences of living and dying in a hospice. Soc Sci Med. 2010;71(5):869–76. https://doi.org/10.1016/j.socscimed.2010.05.026, PMID 20573434.

75. Carr DA. "Good death" for whom? Quality of spouse's death and psychological distress among older widowed persons. J Health Soc Behav. 2003;44(2):215–32. https://doi.org/10.2307/1519809, PMID 12866391.

76. Zimmermann C. Denial of impending death: a discourse analysis of the palliative care literature. Soc Sci Med. 2004;59(8):1769–80. https://doi.org/10.1016/j.socscimed.2004.02.012, PMID 15279932.

77. Zimmermann C. Acceptance of dying: a discourse analysis of palliative care literature. Soc Sci Med. 2012;75(1):217–24. https://doi.org/10.1016/j.socscimed.2012.02.047, PMID 22513246.

78. Kellahear A. Dying of cancer: the final year of life. London: Harwood Academic Publishers; 1990.

79. van der Geest S. Funerals are for the living: conversations with elderly people in Kwahu, Ghana. Afr Stud Rev. 2000;43(3):103–29. https://doi.org/10.2307/525071.

80. Rosenblatt PC. Grief across cultures: a review and research agenda. In: Stroebe MS, Hansson RO, Schut H, Stroebe W, editors. Handbook of bereavement research and practice: advances in theory and intervention. Washington, DC. American Psychological Association; 2008. p. 207–22.

81. Kalish RA, Reynolds DK. Death and ethnicity: a psychocultural study. Farmingdale, NY: Baywood Publishing; 1984.

82. Bristol WA. Religion and the care, treatment, and rights of animals. Tufts University; 2019.

CHAPTER 3

The Multifaceted Impact of Grief

Normal Reactions and Responses Among the Bereaved

The preceding chapter described grief as a journey throughout which the bereaved can be companioned.(1–4) In this respect, those who companion the bereaved are like the figurative footprints in the sand, who walk beside and accompany those who navigate the stages, phases, or tasks of grieving.

3.1 The Transience of Life and the Permanence of Loss

No matter how many companions support the bereaved along the way, the reality is that those who grieve must experience and work through much of the process on their own. Although the footprints may be visible for a short period of time, they are inevitably washed away by the rising tide. Life goes on in the birth-death-rebirth sequence that can be ascribed to the rhythmic, predictable patterning of the rising-falling tide. Life is transient, while loss of life is permanent. This imagery is captured in "The Tide Rises, The Tide Falls," one of many in the 1880 collection of poems by American poet Henry Wadsworth Longfellow, *Ultima Thule*:(5)

> *The tide rises, the tide falls,*
> *The twilight darkens, the curlew calls;*
> *Along the sea-sands damp and brown*
> *The traveller [sic] hastens toward the town,*
> *And the tide rises, the tide falls.*
>
> *Darkness settles on roofs and walls,*
> *But the sea, the sea in the darkness calls;*
> *The little waves, with their soft, white hands,*
> *Efface the footprints in the sands,*
> *And the tide rises, the tide falls.*

The morning breaks; the steeds in their stalls
Stamp and neigh, as the hostler calls;
The day returns, but nevermore
Returns the traveller [sic] to the shore,
And the tide rises, the tide falls.

Longfellow's poem reads as a metaphor for the fleeting nature of life and the mystery of death. Death is inevitable and final, yet something that one cannot fully wrap one's head around.

Grief is the natural reaction to our internal struggle with loss.(6–10) Grief is in many ways how we wrestle within ourselves to make sense of what and who we lost and why.(10, 11)

We may search for meaning because our worlds were disrupted and torn apart.(10, 11)

The physical absence of our loved ones may prompt us to reconsider our identities and our worldviews.(11) In the words of Neimeyer and Burke:(11)

> ... *the simplest routines of daily living require painful review and revision, as when we no longer need to wake to nurse a baby that has died of sudden infant death syndrome, or when in our widowhood we go to bed alone. These and a hundred other violations of the 'micro-narratives' of our everyday lives can ultimately vitiate our capacity to make sense of the larger 'macro-narrative' of the loss and our existence in its wake, launching a search for meaning that may find few simple answers.*

Attempts to make sense of loss are particularly common among those who experience the loss of a child.(12)

Violent and/or otherwise traumatic, unexpected deaths complicate the process.(12)

3.2 Defining Impact

As the bereaved cope with their losses, they are impacted by their respective grief journeys.

When I think of the word, *impact*, mechanics – the field of study within the discipline of physics – comes to mind. I recall the definition of impact as being significant force that is applied when two or more bodies collide. (13–16) The kinetic energy of the projectile that strikes another object must go somewhere.(13–16) It may be changed into heat and sound energy(13), resulting in the struck object becoming deformed and/or riddled with vibrations. Or, if the impact is high velocity, there is insufficient time for such changes to occur, and the struck object fractures.(17, 18)

3.3 The Many Impacts of Grief

Grief is impactful.(19–22) Grief that is not anticipatory hits us out of left field. It barrels into us full force whether we have time to brace ourselves for the impact or not. When it hits, grief creates internal and/or external changes.

Much like a high velocity impact, grief may shatter us in the figurative sense. We may feel broken.

Whether outsiders perceive it or not, we are forever changed.

Impact provokes one or more reactions. A reaction is a survival-oriented,(23) spontaneous impulse that is driven by the unconscious mind.(24) It is what we display when we say or do something "without thinking."

Reactions occur without consideration of the long-term effects of our actions. They are the basis of instinct.(25)

Some might refer to reactions as being knee-jerk, likening them to pure reflex. Consider the patellar reflex, for instance. Quadriceps muscle contraction and resultant lower leg extension is triggered by a sudden change in muscle length, as occurs when a reflex hammer is applied to the patellar tendon.(26–30) When the patellar tendon is stretched, that level of stretch is detected by peripheral receptors, which stimulate sensory neurons to send a message to the spinal cord.(29, 30) Within the L2-L4 segments of the spinal cord, sensory neurons synapse with motor neurons that regulate contraction of the quadriceps muscle.(29, 30) This neural communication effectively produces movement of the lower leg through contraction of the quadriceps muscle.(29, 30) The lower leg kicks forward and up.(29, 30)

The ability to demonstrate a patellar reflex doesn't require forethought. It doesn't require conscious integration within the cerebrum. It just happens.

The same can be said of grief.

Grief evokes reactions inside of us that we cannot always explain and that we cannot always regulate.(9, 31–34)

Grief is, in a sense, a biological stimulus.(33) A biological stimulus causes a detectable change in our environment. For example, one stimulus for plant growth is sunlight. Plants grow in the direction in which the sun shines. The sunlight can be said to foster plant growth.

Sunlight, in this example, represents a positive stimulus. Biological stimuli can be negative, too. When an external threat is perceived by an organism, its behavioral inhibition system (BIS) is activated.(35) Much like an automatic brake, the BIS kicks in to mediate threat reactivity and to avoid the potential threat.(35)

In both examples of biological stimuli, reactions are triggered by an external event. Grief is also a reaction to an external change.(34)

In considering the many ways in which grief is impactful, there are several primary reactions to grief:(9, 31, 32, 34)

- physical
- cognitive
- social
- emotional
- spiritual.

3.4 Physical Manifestations of Grief

Physical manifestations of grief are commonly described by the bereaved and have been affirmed in the grief literature.(9, 31, 32, 34, 36) Parkes' 1970 longitudinal study was one of the first of its kind to track the first year of bereavement in widows in London, England.(37) As part of this study, Parkes documented the immediate and delayed reactions in 22 women following the deaths of their spouses.

The immediate physical reaction to death was described by ten widows as numbness. Numbness lasted for up to seven days in five cases and was protracted for more than a month in two.(37) One respondent explained that:(37)

"'I felt numb and solid for a week. It's a blessing ... Everything goes hard inside you ... like a heavy weight.' She felt that the numbness enabled her to cope without weeping."

The numbness that is associated with grief is thought to be protective. It shields the body from becoming overwhelmed in the initial period following the death of a loved one.(36, 38)

As the numbness subsides, it may give way to other physical manifestations of grief. The widows in Parkes' study displayed symptoms and actions that included:(37)

- episodes of vomiting
- waves of anxiety
- panic attacks
- headaches
- changes in appetite and associated changes in weight (loss or gain)

- insomnia or other sleep disturbances
- restlessness: one widow described it as "restless busyness"
- phantom sensations: one widow shared that "I can almost feel his skin or touch his hands"
- conscious physical displacement from the home environment: one widow sought refuge at a neighboring flat
- physically holding treasured possessions.

One widow in Parkes' study articulately captures the perception that she was on the verge of physically fracturing. She described herself as being fragile and stated that "if somebody gave me a good tap, I'd shatter into a thousand pieces."(37)

Physical pain associated with grief is commonly reported. So-called grief pangs vary in terms of descriptor and intensity, but have been described by some as "spiky" or "stabbing."(36)

For others, grief elicits a "physical feeling of sickness in my stomach, a griping sort of feeling."(36)

A widow in Pearce's 2022 study described the physical pain of grief in vivid imagery:(36)

> *I've explained about the physical pain and I always thought that was a metaphor; it's not, it's physical. My whole body cavity just screamed in pain, and even now when I'm stressed my sternum feels like all my tendons are pulling off it physically. I just had this view of the inside of my body being this black and splattered cavity where my heart and soul had just splattered into a million soggy pieces.*

This portrait of grief's impact is one of violence as painted by the widow's word choice: *screamed, pulling off,* and *splattered.*(36) These real-to-life sensations gnawed at her in the same way that a physical injury might.

In his published journal, *A Grief Observed*, C.S. Lewis chronicled his journey through grief after the untimely death of his wife. Through his grief, Lewis became acutely aware of human frailty and the impact that bereavement had on his body.

Lewis compares the death of his wife to an "amputation."(39) In other words, death has taken from him a body part that he can never get back, and he will forever know that a part of him is missing.

Lewis also acknowledges other physical manifestations of grief that he endured:(39) "At other times it feels like being mildly drunk, or concussed. There is a sort of invisible blanket between the world and me. I find it hard to take in what anyone says. Or perhaps, hard to want to take it in. It is so uninteresting."

Lewis compares grief to physical pain that kept him up at night:(39)

I once read the sentence "I lay awake all night with a toothache, thinking about the toothache and about lying awake." That's true to life. Part of every misery is, so to speak, the misery's shadow or reflection: the fact that you don't merely suffer but have to keep on thinking about the fact that you suffer. I not only live each endless day in grief, but live each day thinking about living each day in grief.

Lewis captures the seemingly endless quality of grief in this excerpt. Grief draws itself out exponentially and the bereaved are acutely aware of the sluggishness of the passage of time, hour by hour, minute by minute, second by second.

Grieving is painful and does not abate. Lewis shares that:(39) "It doesn't really matter whether you grip the arms of the dentist's chair or let your hands lie in your lap. The drill drills on." In this respect, the pain is inescapable. It will occur whether you accept it or not, whether you like it or not, and you will experience its pulsations in your utmost core whether you resist it or not.

C.S. Lewis' imagery is clear. Pain will happen, period. The bereaved lack a say in the matter. They have no choice but to endure.

In addition to physical pain, those who experience grief may report additional sensations, including, but not limited to:(34, 38, 40)

- dizziness
- lethargy
- muscle weakness
- muscle tenderness
- joint inflammation
- joint pain
- immobilization
- fatigue
- upset stomach
- nausea
- food aversion
- heaviness of the chest
- breathlessness
- heart racing
- abdominal emptiness
- abdominal tightness
- whole body tension
- difficulty falling asleep

- difficulty maintaining uninterrupted sleep
- early-morning awakening
- light or noise sensitivity
- dry mouth
- tightness in the throat
- trouble swallowing.

Recent research demonstrates that there is an evidence-based association between a wide range of physical conditions and bereavement, including, but not limited to:(40)

- tachycardia(41, 42)
- hypertension(41, 43, 44)
- increased platelet activation and circulating levels of von Willebrand factor (vWF), which may precipitate myocardial infarction (MI) (45)
- major acute cardiovascular events, such as MI or stroke(46)
- impaired immunity
  - o weaker antibody response to two different influenza strains(47, 48)
  - o decreased lymphocyte response(49)
  - o down-regulated B cell immunity genes(50)
  - o impaired natural killer (NK) cell activity(51)
- increased adrenocortical activity(34)
  - o increased blood cortisol(40, 52, 53)
- reduced quality of life(40, 54, 55)
- increased risk of mortality.(46, 56–63)

This growing body of evidence supports that grief has a very real impact on the physical self of one who is grieving.

The bereaved are often tired. They may describe themselves as "spent." Grief may make them feel as though they have run a marathon. Because of this metaphor, some have called grief "the mourning run."

Someone who is grief-stricken may feel that their entire body aches. Their muscles may tense. They may feel sore, weak, and fatigued.

Altered sleep/wake cycles create a vicious cycle of exhaustion. They may lay awake in bed for hours. Even if the bereaved do manage to sleep, they may awake without feeling rested. They may go to bed and not feel that they have the strength to get up.

Sometimes those who are grieving lack the energy to do anything. They may be unmotivated to participate in daily activities. Taking a shower or getting dressed may take significant effort. Preparing for yet another day may seem like a chore.

Others who are grieving may want to occupy their days with something other than loss. They may increase their activity patterns to stay busy. A widow in Parkes' study described herself as "'geared to a tremendous tempo' and driving herself to avoid depression."(37)

Parkes relayed another widow's comment that:(37)

"'I think if I didn't work all the time I'd have a nervous breakdown.' Interviews [with Parkes] were carried out 'on the trot' as she passed from one household chore to another."

Staying active may release pent-up emotion and serves as a pressure release valve. It may help those who are grieving to blow off steam.

At the same time, the bereaved may overdo. They may over-exert, over-commit, and burn out.

Doing too much and doing too little are common extremes among those who are grieving. It is hard to strike a balance.

The stress of grieving may cause one's heart rate and blood pressure to climb.

The bereaved may eat more; they may eat less. Weight is likely to fluctuate during this time, impacting the way in which they see themselves.

3.5 Cognitive and Social Manifestations of Grief

Weight fluctuations may also alter how the bereaved think that they are perceived by others. In this respect, the bereaved tend to get inside of their heads. They may create their own inner dialogue that they believe to be true, when in fact, that dialogue is – at least externally – non-existent.

Grief has significant cognitive and social impacts. In the words of Lewis:(39) "Grief … gives life a permanently provisional feeling. It doesn't seem worth starting anything."

Indeed, grieving takes a toll on our minds as well as our hearts. The bereaved may feel disoriented at times and detach from their surroundings.

Sometimes grief makes the bereaved go into hiding. They may experience social withdrawal. Those who are introverted may become even more so. The bereaved may distance themselves from those they care about and activities that they used to take pleasure in. They may separate themselves from a world that has moved on.

It is also common for the bereaved to lose the ability to concentrate. They may have trouble focusing or putting thoughts together. They may have trouble following others' logic. They may fail to complete their own sentences.

The bereaved may become preoccupied with thoughts that center around the deceased.(64) They may be intent on detecting any environmental cues that suggest that the deceased is still among them.(64) In their search for the deceased, they may become distressed, not unlike non-human animals that engage in frantic searching behavior when they are forcibly separated.(64) According to White, "in the context of separation short of death, searching is adaptive."(64) When a loved one dies, it is as if the grieving brain forgets that a reunion is an impossibility.(64) The bereaved may fight tooth and nail for a reunion that is futile.(64) This has been termed *vigilance in grief*.(64)

Within the first few months of bereavement, it is common to "interpret sights and sounds as having been caused by the deceased – generally followed immediately by the realization that the loved one is dead."(64) White and Fessler refer to these moments as false recognitions.

The bereaved may swear that they hear their loved one's voice or the sound of their shoes climbing the stairs.(65) In these instances, the bereaved may be tricked by their own minds into believing that the deceased are once again alive.

The bereaved are not hallucinating the deceased into being. They are reacting to real-life, external, relevant stimuli and misinterpreting them as coming from their loved one.(64)

False recognitions are common across cultures and seem more likely to occur to those who have lost a spouse or to children grieving the loss of a parent.(64, 66–72) False recognitions are not always sightings of people. (67) Grieving owners often report mistaking sights and sounds for their pets.(67, 73)

These mistaken sightings may elicit comfort or fear, depending upon the individual who is experiencing them.(64, 65, 72, 74) The individual may feel reassurance in the moment, or they may feel that they are going crazy.

It is important for those companioning the bereaved to acknowledge that false recognitions are part of the grieving process and not a sign of mental instability.

White and Fessler explain the phenomena as follows:(64)

From a cognitive perspective, false recognitions can be understood as a product of a low baseline threshold for detecting the target person in the environment, and, relatedly, indicate that the grief process is incomplete. On our account, cognitive mechanisms responsible for quick-and-dirty interpretation of stimuli, the so-called low-road aspects of perception, continue to represent the deceased as an agent capable of producing sights and sounds that impinge on the observer. At the same time, cognitive mechanisms responsible for slower, more reflective processing, the so-called high-road components of perception, no longer represent the agent in this manner— hence the disquieting conflict between the initial interpretation of sights or sounds as caused by the loved one, followed by the subsequent recollection that the loved one is dead, and realization that the initial interpretation must be erroneous.

As time passes, the bereaved recalibrate their perceptions of the world around them.(64) Sights and sounds are no longer mistaken as having originated from the deceased.(64) False recognitions are gradually extinguished until they fade away completely.(64)

In addition to searching for their loved one, the bereaved may ruminate over past events.(75) Sometimes the bereaved must tell their story repeatedly to make sense of their loss. Rumination, in this respect, is a coping strategy. Companions of the bereaved may be tempted to interrupt, truncate, or hasten story-telling. Yet, short-circuiting this process is counterproductive. Reliving the event repeatedly is one way for the bereaved to process the grief.

Sometimes the mind continues to process grief when the body is asleep. The bereaved may relive the events of a loved one's passing by dreaming about the deceased.(38) It is as though the brain is trying to fill in the gaps and make sense of the loss.

Vivid dreams are common.(38) Dreams about the loved one may transition into pleasant memories or the bereaved may experience nightmares. (37)

3.6 Emotional Manifestations of Grief

In addition to its cognitive and social impacts, grief bombards our emotional state. In a study by Gerber, one participant shared that after his partner died, he was "unprepared for the depth of my feelings ... [and had] never been through anything like this before."(76)

Indeed, grieving takes a toll on our hearts. Grief is an emotional rollercoaster.(77, 78) Memories of our loved one may trigger outbursts of emotion, sometimes when we least expect it.

Intense emotions can come on unexpectedly and persist.

As the bereaved move through the stages of grief, they may experience one or more of the following emotional reactions:(9, 31, 32, 36, 37, 39)

- shock
- numbness
- disorientation
- disbelief
- denial
- sadness

- isolation
- despair
- anxiety
- feeling overwhelmed
- feeling disconnected
- helplessness
- fear
- panic
- terror
- irritability
- anger
- hurt
- rage
- hate
- blame
- disorganization
- frustration
- confusion
- searching
- yearning
- resentment
- jealousy
- envy
- guilt
- regret
- emptiness
- hopelessness.

Lewis likened grief to fear. He shared that:(39) "No one ever told me that grief felt so like fear. I am not afraid, but the sensation is like being afraid. The same fluttering in the stomach, the same restlessness, the yawning. I keep on swallowing."

We may feel disillusioned or disappointed by life. We may feel that life has let us down. We may feel let down by loved ones, too.

Apathy is a common reaction to grief.

- Who cares?
- Why care?
- Why care about life?
- Why care about the future?
- Why invest in living?

Living mattered to us when we had our loved ones by our side. Without these individuals to ground us, we may lose our connection to the present.

Emotions are likely to fluctuate over time, even within a given day.

In some circumstances, we may feel emotions that are confusing or contradictory to one another.(31) For example, following a prolonged death, the survivors may feel at peace or even relieved.(31) In addition to relief, they may feel joy, hope, or gratitude.(31)

Feeling these emotions during a time of grief is normal. It is normal to be relieved that a loved one's suffering has ended.(31)

It is important to provide the bereaved with a safe harbor that welcomes emotions as they arise.

It is important for the bereaved, in turn, to recognize that such feelings are normal and an appropriate way to process the death of someone they loved.

3.7 Spiritual Manifestations of Grief

Sometimes our grief causes us to search for greater meaning in life or question a higher power.

Bento explains that:(79)

*The word "spirit" means "breath" in Latin, ancient Hebrew and Greek (*spiritus, ruah *and* pneuma*). When the "breath of life" is no longer in the body of a person we love, we are hurled by grief, this "tearing open of the heart"(80), into a desperate quest to explain where that breath came from, and where it is now.*

Bento adds that:(79)

This spiritual quest for the ultimate meaning of existence is no longer an intellectual exercise; we depend on the answers, whatever they are, to define how we ourselves can go on living. Working through our grief, we are transformed from homo sapiens *into* homo poeta: *man, the meaning maker.(81)*

For some, death may reinforce or strengthen faith. Faith may provide perspective that helps to make death bearable. For example, belief in life after death may be of comfort to those who feel that their loved one lives on or that they will one day be reunited again. In this respect, spirituality may offer a sense of security and comfort to some of the bereaved.(82)

Some may find solace in scripture, prayer, meditation, ceremony, and rites of passage.(82) Religious observances, customs, and rituals may also alleviate isolation and establish a sense of community at a time when so much is uncertain.(82)

Others may experience a strikingly different grief journey within the spiritual realm. For those who considered themselves to be spiritual before a loved one's passing, death may call into question their belief system.(31) They may ask themselves if what they believed before still holds true now.(31)

The bereaved may exhibit anger towards a higher power. They may blame a higher power for depriving them of their earthly love. They may interpret the death of a loved one as punishment for a sin that must be atoned. They may feel that they were chosen by a higher power to be punished. They may feel that a higher power is angry at them.

Those who feel cast aside or abandoned by a higher power during their time of need may question, if not turn away from, the faith. Losing faith has significant implications in that it also severs connection with their spiritual community and religious practices.(83) This disruption in religious practice may perpetuate ongoing insecurity with a higher power.(83) The more one questions how a good deity can allow bad things to happen to good people, the less one may be willing to reach out during times of need.

Those who companion the bereaved may unknowingly contribute to spiritual distress. The following statements by companions may have the unintentional consequences of activating or reinforcing someone's spiritual struggle.

- "It's God's will."
- "God has a will in this."
- "There is a reason for everything."
- "God has a plan."
- "God would want you to be strong."
- "God only gives us what we can handle."
- "God needed them more than you did."
- "God called them back home."
- "God didn't want them to suffer."
- "God knew that it was their time to go."
- "Heaven needed another angel."
- "Heaven gained another set of wings."
- "If your faith is strong, then you would trust in God's plan."
- "Don't cry, they are in a better place."
- "God gave them a good, long life."

The implication of these statements is that death was desired by a higher power, so we should accept and even embrace our loss. Although this may be comforting to some, the belief that a higher power caused death to occur may incite anger and rejection of faith.

A bereaved friend of mine once said something to the effect of, "It's easy for you to say that God needed another angel because he didn't ask for yours."

3.8 "Moving With" Rather than "Moving On"

Grief forever changes us.

The journey that we walk through grief changes who we are and how we perceive the world around us.

Those who are unfamiliar or uncomfortable with grief may prompt us to move on. When they try to get us to move on, we often plant our heels into the ground and resist. This may come as a surprise to them.

I have had someone in my life ask me, following the death of a grandparent, why wouldn't I want to be happy again.

What those who are unfamiliar or uncomfortable with grief do not grasp is that their version of moving on means forgetting.

Someone who has loved and lost never forgets.

You never forget your loved one's name. Speaking their name aloud often brings comfort.

You never forget how your loved one made you feel. Sharing stories of their presence in your life may one day bring peace.

Your loved ones are engraved in your memory. And though you may fear forgetting the sound of their voice, the way they laughed, or how they smiled, there is internally-driven reassurance in knowing they are forever a part of you.

You carry them with you, always.

Because the deceased are a part of you, you never truly "move on" from grieving their deaths.

You learn to "move with" grief – or rather, grief "moves" with you. Grief "moves" with you because it has woven itself into the very fabric of your being.

Life without the deceased is never going to be "normal" again. So, it's not about getting back to what's "normal." It's about finding the "new normal."

In that respect, it's not about leading an *either/or* life – meaning that you either grieve or choose to move on.

It's about leading a *both/and* life – meaning that you can both grieve and live. Living your best life does not mean that you wall off grief or confine it to a timetable that someone else prescribed for you.

Living your best life means that you get to define what your "new normal" looks like.

It's not about timelines, it's about you.

References

1. Wolfelt A. Eleven tenets of companioning the bereaved: center for loss and life transition; 2019. Available from: https://www.centerforloss.com/2019/12/elev en-tenets-of-companioning/.
2. Tyrrell P, Harberger S, Schoo C, Siddiqui W. Kubler-Ross stages of dying and subsequent models of grief. Treasure Island, FL: StatPearls; 2022.
3. Bruce CA. Helping patients, families, caregivers, and physicians, in the grieving process. J Am Osteopath Assoc. 2007;107(12);Suppl 7:ES33-40. PMID 18165376.
4. Schuelke T, Crawford C, Kentor R, Eppelheimer H, Chipriano C, Springmeyer K, et al. Current grief support in pediatric palliative care. Children (Basel). 2021;8(4). https://doi.org/10.3390/children8040278, PMID 33916583.
5. Longfellow HW. Oliver Wendell Holmes collection. 1st ed. Boston: Houghton. Library of Congress. Ultima Thule. Mifflin and Company; 1880.
6. Friedman R, James C, James JW. The grief recovery handbook for pet loss. Vol. xi. Lanham, MD: Taylor Trade Publishing; 2014.
7. Howarth R. Concepts and controversies in grief and loss. J Ment Health Couns. 2011;33(1):4–10. https://doi.org/10.17744/mehc.33.1.900m56162888u737.
8. Humphrey KM. Counseling strategies for loss and grief. Vol. xv. Alexandria, VA: American Counseling Association; 2009.
9. Wolfelt A. Understanding grief: helping yourself heal. Vol. xvi. Muncie, IN: Accelerated Development Inc; 1992.
10. Margolis OS. Acute grief: counseling the bereaved. Vol. xiii. New York: Columbia University Press; 1981.
11. Neimeyer RA, Burke LA. Loss, grief, and spiritual struggle: the quest for meaning in bereavement. In: Paloutzian RF, Park CL, editors. Handbook of the psychology of religion and spirituality. 2nd ed. New York: Guilford Press; 2013. p. 131–8.
12. Lichtenthal WG, Neimeyer RA, Currier JM, Roberts K, Jordan N. Cause of death and the quest for meaning after the loss of a child. Death Stud. 2013;37(4):311–42. https://doi.org/10.1080/07481187.2012.673533, PMID 24520890.
13. Viegas J. Kinetic and potential energy: understanding changes within physical systems. New York: The Rosen Publishing Group Inc; 2004.
14. Huang M. Vehicle crash mechanics. Vol. xvi. Boca Raton, FL: CRC Press; 2002.
15. Hewitt PG, Wolf PR. Conceptual physics fundamentals. Vol. xvii. San Francisco: Pearson Addison Wesley; 2008.
16. Halliday D, Resnick R, Walker J. Fundamentals of physics. 7th ed. Hoboken, NJ: Wiley; 2005.
17. Safri SNA. Sultan MtH, Yidris N, Mustapha F. Low velocity and high velocity impact test on composite. Int J Eng Sci. 2014;3(9):50–60.
18. Huelke DF, Buege LJ, Harger JH. Bone fractures produced by high velocity impacts. Am J Anat. 1967;120(1):123–31. https://doi.org/10.1002/aja.1001200110.

19. Wilson DM, Rodríguez-Prat A, Low G. The potential impact of bereavement grief on workers, work, careers, and the workplace. Soc Work Health Care. 2020;59(6): 335–50. https://doi.org/10.1080/00981389.2020.1769247, PMID 32510280.

20. Wilson DM, MacLeod R, Houttekier D. Examining linkages between bereavement grief intensity and perceived death quality: qualitative findings. Omega (Westport). 2016;74(2):260–74. https://doi.org/10.1177/0030222815598442.

21. Mallon B. Dying, death and grief: working with adult bereavement. Thousand Oaks, CA: SAGE; 2008.

22. Machin L. Working with loss and grief: a new model for practitioners. London: SAGE; 2009.

23. Maille A, Schradin C. Survival is linked with reaction time and spatial memory in African striped mice. Biol Lett. 2016;12(8). https://doi.org/10.1098/rsbl.2016.0346, PMID 27484646.

24. Dimberg U, Thunberg M, Elmehed K. Unconscious facial reactions to emotional facial expressions. Psychol Sci. 2000;11(1):86–9. https://doi.org/10.1111/1467-9280.00221, PMID 11228851.

25. Jung CG. Instinct and the unconscious. III. Br J Psychol. 1919;10(1):15–22.

26. Fearing F. The history of the experimental study of the knee-jerk. Am J Psychol. 1928;40(1):92–111. https://doi.org/10.2307/1415312.

27. Bowditch HP, Warren JW. The knee-jerk and its physiological modifications. J Physiol. 1890;11(1–2):25–64. https://doi.org/10.1113/jphysiol.1890.sp000318, PMID 16991942.

28. Lombard WP. The variations of the normal knee-jerk, and their relation to the activity of the central nervous system. Am J Psychol. 1887;1(1): 5–17. https://doi.org/10.2307/1411231.

29. Reece WO, Erickson HH, Goff JP, Uemura EE. Dukes' physiology of domestic animals. Chichester: John Wiley & Sons Inc; 2015.

30. Hall JE. Guyton and hall textbook of medical physiology. 14th ed. Philadelphia: Elsevier; 2020.

31. Wolfelt A. Grief feelings. Center for Loss and Life Transition. Available from: https://www.centerforloss.com/grief/im-seeking-help/.

32. Wolfelt A. The journey through grief: reflections on healing. Fort Collins, CO: Companion Press; 1997.

33. Osterweis M, Solomon F, Green M. Toward a biology of grieving. In: Osterweis M, Solomon F, Green M, editors. Bereavement: reactions, consequences, and care. Washington, DC: National Academies Press; 1984. p. 143–76.

34. Mughal S, Azhar Y, Mahon MM, Siddiqui WJ. Grief reaction. Treasure Island, FL: StatPearls; 2022.

35. Levita L, Bois C, Healey A, Smyllie E, Papakonstantinou E, Hartley T, et al. The Behavioural Inhibition System, anxiety and hippocampal volume in a non-clinical population. Biol Mood Anxiety Disord. 2014;4(1):4. https://doi.org/10.1186/2045-5380-4-4, PMID 24607258.

36. Pearce C, Komaromy C. Recovering the body in grief: physical absence and embodied presence. Health (London). 2022;26(4):393–410. https://doi.org/10.1177/1363459320931914, PMID 32506960.

37. Parkes CM. The first year of bereavement. A longitudinal study of the reaction of London widows to the death of their husbands. Psychiatry. 1970;33(4):444–67. https://doi.org/10.1080/00332747.1970.11023644, PMID 5275840.

38. Brown JT, Stoudemire GA. Normal and pathological grief. JAMA. 1983;250(3): 378–82. https://doi.org/10.1001/jama.1983.03340030038025, PMID 6854902.

39. Lewis CS. A grief observed. San Francisco: Harper & Row; 1989.

40. Buckley T, Sunari D, Marshall A, Bartrop R, McKinley S, Tofler G. Physiological correlates of bereavement and the impact of bereavement interventions. Dialogues Clin Neurosci. 2012;14(2):129–39. https://doi.org/10.31887/DCNS.2012.14.2/tbuckley, PMID 22754285.

41. Buckley T, Mihailidou AS, Bartrop R, McKinley S, Ward C, Morel-Kopp MC, et al. Haemodynamic changes during early bereavement: potential contribution to increased cardiovascular risk. Heart Lung Circ. 2011;20(2):91–8. https://doi.org/10.1016/j.hlc.2010.10.073, PMID 21147029.

42. O'Connor MF, Allen JJ, Kaszniak AW. Autonomic and emotion regulation in bereavement and depression. J Psychosom Res. 2002;52(4):183–5. https://doi.org/10.1016/s0022-3999(02)00292-1, PMID 11943236.

43. Prigerson HG, Bierhals AJ, Kasl SV, Reynolds CF, Shear MK, Day N, et al. Traumatic grief as a risk factor for mental and physical morbidity. Am J Psychiatry. 1997;154(5):616–23. https://doi.org/10.1176/ajp.154.5.616, PMID 9137115.

44. Santić Z, Lukić A, Sesar D, Milicević S, Ilakovac V. Long-term follow-up of blood pressure in family members of soldiers killed during the war in Bosnia and Herzegovina. Croat Med J. 2006;47(3):416–23. PMID 16758520.

45. Buckley T, Morel-Kopp MC, Ward C, Bartrop R, McKinley S, Mihailidou AS, et al. Inflammatory and thrombotic changes in early bereavement: a prospective evaluation. Eur J Prev Cardiol. 2012;19(5):1145–52. https://doi.org/10.1177/1741826711421686, PMID 21900365.

46. Carey IM, Shah SM, DeWilde S, Harris T, Victor CR, Cook DG. Increased risk of acute cardiovascular events after partner bereavement: a matched cohort study. JAMA Intern Med. 2014;174(4):598–605. https://doi.org/10.1001/jamainternmed.2013.14558, PMID 24566983.

47. Vitlic A, Khanfer R, Lord JM, Carroll D, Phillips AC. Bereavement reduces neutrophil oxidative burst only in older adults: role of the HPA axis and immunesenescence. Immun Ageing. 2014;11(13): 1–6. https://doi.org/10.1186/1742-4933-11-13, PMID 25191511.

48. Phillips AC, Carroll D, Burns VE, Ring C, Macleod J, Drayson M. Bereavement and marriage are associated with antibody response to influenza vaccination in the elderly. Brain Behav Immun. 2006;20(3):279–89. https://doi.org/10.1016/j.bbi.2005.08.003, PMID 16198083.

49. Bartrop RW, Luckhurst E, Lazarus L, Kiloh LG, Penny R. Depressed lymphocyte function after bereavement. Lancet. 1977;1(8016):834–6. https://doi.org/10.1016/s0140-6736(77)92780-5, PMID 67339.

50. O'Connor MF, Schultze-Florey CR, Irwin MR, Arevalo JMG, Cole SW. Divergent gene expression responses to complicated grief and non-complicated grief. Brain Behav Immun. 2014;37:78–83. https://doi.org/10.1016/j.bbi.2013.12.017, PMID 24380850.

51. Irwin M, Daniels M, Smith TL, Bloom E, Weiner H. Impaired natural killer cell activity during bereavement. Brain Behav Immun. 1987;1(1):98–104. https://doi.org/10.1016/0889-1591(87)90011-0, PMID 3451784.

52. Buckley T, Bartrop R, McKinley S, Ward C, Bramwell M, Roche D, et al. Prospective study of early bereavement on psychological and behavioural cardiac risk factors.

Intern Med J. 2009;39(6):370–8. https://doi.org/10.1111/j.1445-5994.2009.018 79.x, PMID 19460057.

53. Gerra G, Monti D, Panerai AE, Sacerdote P, Anderlini R, Avanzini P, et al. Long-term immune-endocrine effects of bereavement: relationships with anxiety levels and mood. Psychiatry Res. 2003;121(2):145–58. https://doi.org/10.1016/s0165-1781(03)00255-5, PMID 14656449.

54. Breier AAE. A.E. Bennett award paper. Experimental approaches to human stress research: assessment of neurobiological mechanisms of stress in volunteers and psychiatric patients. Biol Psychiatry. 1989;26(5):438–62. https://doi.org/10.1016/0006-3223(89)90066-8, PMID 2551397.

55. Nicolson NA. Childhood parental loss and cortisol levels in adult men. Psychoneuroendocrinology. 2004;29(8):1012–8. https://doi.org/10.1016/j.psyneu en.2003.09.005, PMID 15219652.

56. Moon JR, Kondo N, Glymour MM, Subramanian SV. Widowhood and mortality: a meta-analysis. PLOS ONE. 2011;6(8):e23465. https://doi.org/10.1371/journal. pone.0023465, PMID 21858130.

57. Shor E, Roelfs DJ, Curreli M, Clemow L, Burg MM, Schwartz JE. Widowhood and mortality: a meta-analysis and meta-regression. Demography. 2012;49(2):575–606. https://doi.org/10.1007/s13524-012-0096-x, PMID 22427278.

58. Acharya D, Haas G. Bereavement and mortality in heart failure. JACC Heart Fail. 2022;10(10):765–7. https://doi.org/10.1016/j.jchf.2022.06.007, PMID 36175062.

59. Shah SM, Carey IM, Harris T, Dewilde S, Victor CR, Cook DG. The effect of unexpected bereavement on mortality in older couples. Am J Public Health. 2013;103(6):1140–5. https://doi.org/10.2105/AJPH.2012.301050, PMID 23597341.

60. Lichtenstein P, Gatz M, Berg S. A twin study of mortality after spousal bereavement. Psychol Med. 1998;28(3):635–43. https://doi.org/10.1017/s0033291798006692, PMID 9626719.

61. Stahl ST, Arnold AM, Chen JY, Anderson S, Schulz R. Mortality after bereavement: the role of cardiovascular disease and depression. Psychosom Med. 2016;78(6): 697–703. https://doi.org/10.1097/PSY.0000000000000317, PMID 26894326.

62. Martikainen P, Valkonen T. Mortality after death of spouse in relation to duration of bereavement in Finland. J Epidemiol Community Health. 1996;50(3):264–8. https:// doi.org/10.1136/jech.50.3.264, PMID 8935456.

63. Simeonova E. Marriage, Bereavement and mortality: the role of health care utilization. J Health Econ. 2013;32(1):33–50. https://doi.org/10.1016/j.jhealeco.2012.10.010, PMID 23202255.

64. White C, Fessler DMT. An evolutionary account of vigilance in grief. Evol Med Public Health. 2018;2018(1):34–42. https://doi.org/10.1093/emph/eox018, PMID 29492265.

65. Parkes CM. Bereavement: studies of grief in adult life. Vol. xiii. New York: International Universities Press; 1972.

66. Maciejewski PK, Zhang B, Block SD, Prigerson HG. An empirical examination of the stage theory of grief. JAMA. 2007;297(7):716–23. https://doi.org/10.1001/ jama.297.7.716, PMID 17312291.

67. Archer J, Winchester G. Bereavement following death of a pet. Br J Psychol. 1994;85(2):259–71. https://doi.org/10.1111/j.2044-8295.1994.tb02522.x, PMID 8032709.

68. Glick IO, Weiss RS, Parkes CM. The first year of bereavement. Vol. xvii. New York: Wiley; 1974.

69. Olson PR, Suddeth JA, Peterson PJ, Egelhoff C. Hallucinations of widowhood. J Am Geriatr Soc. 1985;33(8):543–7. https://doi.org/10.1111/j.1532-5415.1985. tb04619.x, PMID 4020000.

70. Dewi Rees W. The hallucinations of widowhood. Br Med J. 1971;4(5778):37–41. https://doi.org/10.1136/bmj.4.5778.37, PMID 5096884.

71. Castelnovo A, Cavallotti S, Gambini O, D'Agostino A. Post-bereavement hallucinatory experiences: a critical overview of population and clinical studies. J Affect Disord. 2015;186:266–74. https://doi.org/10.1016/j.jad.2015.07.032, PMID 26254619.

72. Silverman PS, Worden JW. Children's reactions to the death of a parent. In: Stroebe MS, Stroehe W, Hansson RO, editors. Handbook of bereavement: theory, research, and intervention. Cambridge: Cambridge University Press; 1993. p. 300–29.

73. Carmack BJ. The effects on family members and functioning after the death of a pet. Marriage Fam Rev. 1985;8(3–4):149–61. https://doi.org/10.1300/J002v08n03_11.

74. Grimby A. Bereavement among elderly people: grief reactions, post-bereavement hallucinations and quality of life. Acta Psychiatr Scand. 1993;87(1):72–80. https://doi.org/10.1111/j.1600-0447.1993.tb03332.x, PMID 8424323.

75. Nolen-Hoeksema S, McBride A, Larson J. Rumination and psychological distress among bereaved partners. J Pers Soc Psychol. 1997;72(4):855–62. https://doi.org/10.1037//0022-3514.72.4.855, PMID 9108698.

76. Gerber K, Brijnath B, Lock K, Bryant C, Hills D, Hjorth L. "Unprepared for the depth of my feelings" – Capturing grief in older people through research poetry. Age Ageing. 2022;51(3). https://doi.org/10.1093/ageing/afac030, PMID 35284925.

77. McGahan K. Only gone from your sight: Jack McAfghan's little guide to pet loss and grief: McGahan, K; 2018.

78. Gould JB. "A picture is worth a thousand words": a strategy for grief education. Death Stud. 1994;18(1):65–74. https://doi.org/10.1080/07481189408252643.

79. Bento RF. When the show must go on: disenfranchised grief in organizations. J Manag Psychol. 1994;9(6):35–44. https://doi.org/10.1108/02683949410070197.

80. Levine S. Who dies? An investigation of conscious living and conscious dying. Vol. xiv. Garden City, NY: Anchor Press. Doubleday Publishing; 1982.

81. Becker E. The structure of evil; an essay on the unification of the science of man. Vol. xviii. New York: G Braziller; 1968.

82. Pargament KI, Koenig HG, Perez LM. The many methods of religious coping: development and initial validation of the RCOPE. J Clin Psychol. 2000;56(4):519–43. https://doi.org/10.1002/(sici)1097-4679(200004)56:4<519::aid-jclp6>3.0.co;2-1, PMID 10775045.

83. Burke LA, Neimeyer RA. Inventory of complicated spiritual grief (ICSG). In: Neimeyer RA, editor. Techniques of grief therapy: assessment and intervention. New York: Routledge; 2016. p. 76–80.

CHAPTER 4

Children, Adolescence, and Grief

The preceding chapter emphasized the uniqueness of grief among the bereaved. Although grief-associated physical, cognitive, social, emotional, and spiritual manifestations have been described, we all experience grief in our own way, on our own timeline. Yet, until this point in the text, we have only considered the grieving process through the lens of an adult.

Children experience grief and grieving, death and dying, too.(1–4)

4.1 Prevalence of Bereavement Among Children

It was estimated in 1979 that 5% of children in the United States mourned the death of one or both of their parents by age 15.(5) Estimates are infrequently updated with respect to the population of pediatric mourners; however, in more recent years, the numbers of those affected appear to be climbing. In 2022, it was reported that nearly 8% of children (1 in 13) experience parental or sibling death by age 18.(6) Eight percent may not seem significant; however, that amounts to an estimated 5.6 million bereaved children and teens.(6)

This increase in childhood bereavement is thought to be multifactorial. (7) One contributing factor is that people are delaying parenthood until older ages (8). Other factors are increased deaths by suicide(9) and overdose.(10)

A 2017 Bereavement Survey by the New York Life Foundation reported that seven out of every ten teachers was at that time instructing one or more pupils who were experiencing grief.(11)

Four percent of single parents were reported to have been widowed, according to the 2000 U.S. Census, and nearly 14% of these family units included children less than 12 years old.(12)

The Childhood Bereavement Estimation Model (CBEM) was developed in 2020 as an epidemiological tool to approximate the prevalence of childhood bereavement.(7) According to this approximation, one out of every 14 children in the U.S. will lose a parent or sibling to death prior to their 18th birthday.(7) Estimates double if statisticians extend the timeline for bereavement to include any loss up to age 25.(7)

There appears to be geographical variance in the rate at which children experience significant loss. Within the U.S., California is among the states with the lowest rates of childhood bereavement (5.9%) as compared with West Virginia, a state with one of the highest (12.4%).(6)

Race also appears to influence the prevalence of childhood loss. Black children within the U.S. experience loss at a higher rate.(6)

4.2 The Primary and Secondary Impacts of Bereavement on Children

Grief is significant to all who mourn. Childhood bereavement carries additional impact in that loss at such an influential age has the capacity to disrupt developmental competence.(3, 7, 13) Those who grieve at young ages may be at greater risk of experiencing relationship, academic and career dysfunction.(7) In addition, this subset of the bereaved is more likely to be challenged by mental health and substance abuse.(7) Risks of suicide and early mortality are also increased among those who grieve during childhood.(7, 14–21)

Additional disruptions that are associated with loss of a parent or other caregiver include the possibility that the bereaved child may have to transition to a new home and/or school.(3, 7, 18, 22) These changes become secondary stressors(22) and are additional sources of grief that may not always be acknowledged or even recognized by those companioning the bereaved through the grieving process.

The bereaved child may also grieve intangible losses, too.(4) A family unit that has experienced death is never again the same. The death of a loved one may shatter hopes for unity and togetherness.(4) Hopes and dreams for the future must be recalibrated. That is not an easy task for an adult mourner, let alone a child.(4)

The bereaved child may also be made aware of and/or experience financial insecurity in the aftermath of a loved one's death.(3, 7, 18, 22) Such shifts in lifestyle are not always openly discussed in households, but the child may perceive that the family can no longer afford 'x' without loved one 'y.'

Childhood bereavement is not limited to grieving the loss of a parent or caregiver. Children may also grieve children. Over 50,000 children died in the U.S. in the year 2000.(23) Of these deaths, 19,582 were children under the age of one, and sudden infant death syndrome (SIDS) was the number one cause of infant mortality.(24) These numbers are impactful for surviving parents. We must consider surviving siblings, too.(13)

The longest-lasting family tie is the sibling relationship.(23) Family heritage and, in some cases, genetic background, is shared by siblings.(23) Siblings are influencers in each other's lives, not only during childhood development but also throughout life.(13, 23, 25–29) Irrespective of whether these influences are positive or negative, they are long-lasting. Nearly 8% of the population experience a sibling death before age 25.(23) It is as common to lose a sibling during childhood as it is to experience maternal death.(23, 30) In some ways, the death of a sibling is even more disruptive to the child's worldview because children are not supposed to die before their parents.(13, 31, 32)

Childhood bereavement is critical to acknowledge and address because it impacts so many in so many ways, and because the ways in which our children cope with loss carry forward into adulthood.(1) Osterweis explains that:(1) "Individuals continue to grow and develop throughout life, but during no other period beyond childhood and adolescence are specific reactions as likely to be influenced by the level of development." Osterweis adds that:(1)

Repercussions and meanings of major object loss will be colored by the individual child's level of development. Psychiatrists and others have generally been struck by how often major childhood loss seems to result in psychopathology. Studies of adults with various mental disorders, especially depression, frequently reveal childhood bereavement, suggesting that such loss may precipitate or contribute to the development of a variety of psychiatric disorders and that this experience can render a person emotionally vulnerable for life. This special vulnerability of children is attributed to developmental immaturity and insufficiently developed coping capacities.

4.3 Unique Aspects of Childhood Bereavement

Because children are especially vulnerable, we must tailor our approach to their respective journeys through bereavement.(1) Historically, there has been a tendency to impose the adult model of grieving onto the child, yet research has consistently demonstrated that children's responses to grief do not always mirror adults.(1)

Osterweis provides several examples as a means to highlight key distinctions in childhood bereavement:(1)

Often what seems glib and unemotional in the small child—such as telling every visitor or stranger on the street, "my sister died"—is the child's way of seeking support and observing others to gauge how he or she should feel. Children may be observed playing games in which the death or funeral activities are reenacted in an effort to master the loss. A child may ask the same questions about the death over and over again, not so much for the factual value of the information as for reassurance that the story has not changed. A four- or five-year-old might resume playing following a death as if nothing distressing had happened. Such behavior reflects the cognitive and emotional capacity of the child and does not mean that the death had no impact.

Adults who are unfamiliar with childhood grief might call out the child's behavior as being inappropriate.(33)

Adults often misinterpret grief-related reactions in children as episodes of misbehavior.(1) Acting out may be the only way the child knows how to express depth of emotion.(1)

Adults may also misinterpret the brevity of children's emotional bursts as signs that they are "done" grieving. It is important to recognize that children frequently fluctuate between approaching and avoiding their emotions.(1)

Young children do experience strong emotions (e.g., anger, fear, and sadness), yet they do not consistently sustain these emotions for the duration that adults do.(1, 4) Doing so might run the risk of overwhelming them.(1)

Instead, young children seem to float in and out of emotions (4) like a light switch – they're either "on" or "off." That doesn't mean during "off" times that they have forgotten about their loss. They are still aware of it. They have simply shifted their approach.

Some might say that just like the physical feature of height, children grieve in spurts.(33)

Because young children tend to prioritize their needs as being immediate, they may shift quickly from expressing grief to searching for a replacement. This replacement may be another person, a non-human animal, or an object. This action on the part of the child does not mean that they are unfeeling or that they have "gotten over it."(34) It is often an age-appropriate means by which the child copes with their own needs in the absence of a loved one.(1)

Another age-appropriate mechanism by which children cope with grief involves symbolic play.(4) When emotions overwhelm them and/or they do not know how to articulate what it is that they are feeling, they may play out their emotions.(4) This may occur on their own or they may engage siblings and/or friends in the experience.(4) They may recreate a funeral, coffin, or burial using props to work through and assimilate their feelings about their recent experiences with loss.(4)

Crenshaw writes, as an example, that:(4) "When dealing with a devastating loss, for example, a child may repetitively play out with puppets a turtle looking for its mother. The turtle is sad. After these futile searches, the turtle is exhausted but won't give up looking." According to Crenshaw:(4)

> *Self-initiated symbolic play "allows graded and safe exposure … Since the child can break off the play at any moment, the child remains in control of the process, the timing, and the pacing. The child also determines the degree to which the symbolic representation is distant from the actual experience(s)."*

Symbolic play is one way that children try to make sense of a changed world in which they find themselves.(13) In the words of Crenshaw:(4)

> *Children externalize compelling facets of their inner world when they play out a drama with puppets, make a picture in a sand tray, draw or paint a picture, create a figure out of clay, or create a play scene in a family play house. What gets externalized is experienced as more manageable than that which remains internalized.*

Play therapy also offers the opportunities for children to navigate "big problems" that overwhelm them through miniaturization. It is thought that working with puppets literally and figuratively "shrinks" obstacles in question down to a level that is more easily managed and processed by children.(4)

In the same way that we might "shrink" a sizeable problem into a bearable one through puppetry, adults might adjust their vocabulary and conceptualization of death to match the child's age and developmental capacity.

Age-appropriateness is an important starting point so that we begin to understand child bereavement in terms of comprehension level and coping strategies.(13, 35–37) This chapter is not intended to be comprehensive or a substitute for human physicians, mental health consultants, or bereavement counselors. What the authors hope to accomplish is to paint a portrait of what the grieving child understands as they age so that you, the adult, can tailor your conversations accordingly and recognize when additional interventions are indicated.

According to Osterweis:(1)

> *In order for complete "mourning" to occur in the true psychoanalytic sense of detaching memories and hopes from the dead person(38, 39), the child must have some understanding of the concept of death, be capable of forming a real attachment bond, and have a mental representation of the attachment figure.*

In order for children to fully process death, they must be able to wrap their heads around four main concepts.(13)

- Universality: death happens to everyone; at some point in everyone's lifetime, life ceases to exist.
- Irreversibility: when death happens, it is permanent.
- Nonfunctionality: when death occurs, all body function ceases to exist.
- Causality: understanding what causes death and what does not.

What "complete mourning" entails and at what age children fully comprehend death continue to be active areas of research.(1, 13, 40–51)

4.4 Children Under the Age of Three Years Old

Prior to age three, it is thought that children lack the ability to conceptualize death.(1) In those early years, they are building a mental database of significant figures in their lives and the growing expectation that those to whom they have attached will be constant.(1)

Infants and toddlers do not know what death means, even if it is explained to them.(13) Their reactions to life's events are not based on an understanding of loss.(13) They know only whether a significant person is present. If that person is absent, they do not comprehend why that might be, although they may experience signs of insecurity or abandonment upon separation.(13, 52)

Rather than process that their significant figure is absent because they died, infants and toddlers react to changes in their immediate surroundings.(13, 34, 52) Specifically, they may react to distress in one of the following ways:(13)

- increased "irritability"
- crying more
- sleeping more or sleeping less
- changes in elimination
- increased "clinginess" – they may need to be held more
- increased anxiety around strangers
- possible withdrawal from play or food.

Babies and toddlers are perceptive of others' emotions.(34) If those around them are anxious, then they are likely to feel anxious, too.(34)

Infants may need to be held more during times of loss and to spend more time with caregivers.(13) If time with immediate caregivers is reduced, infants are more likely to experience social withdrawal.(13) It is thought that mistrust develops.(13) The infant may ultimately reject being held or cuddling.(13, 53)

Toddlers do not understand the passage of time. Separation for any amount of time precipitates insecurity.(13)

Toddlers may ask for the missing person by name. They often search for them. They are waiting for them to return. It is separation from their significant figure that they are grieving, not death. They do not know why the person is missing. They just know that their loved one is absent but must be coming back.

Infants and toddlers whose families are experiencing grief may be supported by maintaining routines and safe spaces. Maintaining a sense of calm when holding them or speaking to them in a calm voice may provide reassurance. Making favorite attachment objects available, such as blankets and stuffed toys, may also reduce anxiety by maintaining some semblance of what is familiar.

4.5 Nagy's Three-Stage Model of Childhood Bereavement

In 1948, Nagy proposed a conceptualized view of the stages in which children aged three years and older perceive death.(54) This three-stage model is based upon her trauma research working with Hungarian children, and is still widely referenced today:(54)

- Stage 1: children between the ages of three and five years old
- Stage 2: children between the ages of five and nine years old
- Stage 3: children who are ten years old and up.

4.6 Children Between the Ages of Three and Five (Stage 1)

Children between the ages of three and five do not see death as having permanence.(1, 47, 49, 54–56) Children of this age are wrestling with the biological concept of what it means to be alive. They have reached a surface level of understanding that dead is "not alive," but they have not quite figured out yet what the distinction is between the two states.

Death can be confused with sleeping in that both states seem to be "less alive."(1, 13, 54, 57) In comparing the two – dead to alive – the former may appear to resemble "prolonged sleep."(58)

Preschoolers may be curious about death. They may have encountered dead insects and non-human animals. They may have wanted to touch them, pick them up, or carry them. They may ask what happened to make the animal die. They may ask how death happens or even why.

This is normal.

Before children even experience loss, it is okay to engage them in conversation about death, particularly if they are already fascinated by it. Help them to explore the life cycle with you by their side. Teach them what the circle of life is, in age-appropriate ways. They will not understand in the moment that death is permanent, but talk plants an initial seed of understanding that you can draw upon during times of need.

After children of this age group experience loss, they may recall this memory. You may recall it for them and use it as a starting point for a new conversation about the death of a loved one.

Be prepared to accept that children between the ages of three and five do not understand that death is forever. They see it as transient in the same way that water can be one of many phases (e.g., liquid, solid, or gas).

Because death is seen as temporary, preschoolers often believe that the deceased can come back to life.(34, 59) Such "magical thinking"(60) is reinforced by cartoons. In *Tom and Jerry* and *Looney Tunes,* primary characters die, yet death is reversible. In every episode, Coyote comes back to life in order for Roadrunner to try to end Coyote's life once more.

"Magical thinking" also extends to the perception by children that they are in control of all life events.(13) Children of this age group are egocentric.(13, 34) As such, they may respond to the death of a loved one by taking on the belief that something they did caused the person to die. (13) They may believe that if they had just done "x," then their loved one would never have left, or that if they just did "x" now, then their loved one would return. They may try to reverse death through their actions, not fully understanding that doing so is impossible. This apparent failure may confuse them and perpetuate guilt or shame.

Children who are three to five years old are very literal when it comes to language.

"Lost" means "lost," not "dead." Saying that you "lost" someone implies that they are "missing" and can be "found."

Expressions such as "passed away" have no meaning.

Saying that a loved one went to a "better place" is not, to a child, what we think it means. "Went" implies that their loved one left to go somewhere but can come back. A "better place" could mean Disney World.

If as the adult your core belief is in an afterlife and you believe that the deceased is now in "Heaven," then use that word in conversations with the bereaved child and explain what your perception of "Heaven" is.

Death must be explained to this age group in a direct manner, using the actual words that we mean rather than euphemisms.(3)

When navigating pet loss, adults should avoid saying that the dog or cat was "put to sleep." Children of this age group may subsequently fear bedtime thinking that they can be "put to sleep," too.

Likewise, avoid saying that a loved one is "sleeping" or "resting."(3, 61) That may precipitate fear that if they sleep or rest, then they, too, will die.

Be cautious of linking sickness and death in a way that implies that everyone who is ill dies.(34) Reassure this age group that they cannot "catch" death like they can the common cold, in language that they can understand.(34)

Preschoolers are often perceptive of changes in their immediate environment and may react with feelings of fear or insecurity. They may exhibit the following symptoms:

- irritability
- tantrums
- increased tears
- increased tantrums(13)
- increased clinginess
- searching for the person who has died
- asking (repeatedly) when the person who has died will "come back"(34)
- asking if the person died because of them
- talking to the person who has died as if they are still there
- changes in appetite
- sleep disturbances
- changes in sociability
- temporary regression(13)
    - bedwetting
    - a child that was walking may default to crawling
    - a child that was toilet-trained may ask to wear diapers
    - asking for a bottle.

Children who are between the ages of three to five may be supported by:

- asking if they have any questions
- clarifying their questions: understand what the child is asking before you answer

- answering questions simply, but honestly; follow the child's lead
- explaining that death is a part of life and providing examples that are found in nature (e.g., plants or non-human animals)
- helping them to understand what "dead" means:
  - "dead" means not alive
  - when someone dies, their body has stopped living
  - they do not breathe
  - they do not walk or talk
  - they do not eat or sleep
  - they do not go to the bathroom
  - they do not need to do any of these activities because they are not alive
- reading children's books together on grief and grieving, death and dying [refer to *Appendix: Bereavement Resources*]
- maintaining routines(34)
- reassuring them through touch (with permission): e.g., "It looks like you could use a hug; would that be okay?"
- reassuring them that they are looked out for
- reassuring them that they are loved
- reassuring them that they are safe
- reassuring them that they did not cause their loved one to die
- reassuring them that death is not their fault
- asking what they want to talk about
- encouraging them to use words that describe what they are feeling
- acknowledging and affirming their feelings (e.g., "it's okay to cry.")
- encouraging creative outlets to express themselves through words, art, music, dance, theatre, and sports
- inviting them to participate in family rituals that are associated with grieving, for example:(34)
  - sitting shiva
  - attending funerals
  - visiting the cemetery
  - lighting candles
  - saying prayers
  - reading eulogies
- inviting them to participate in less formal memorialization, for example:(62)
  - planting trees
  - drawing pictures
  - writing poems
- giving them the choice to participate rather than forcing them to
- inviting them to share memories of the deceased(62)

- inviting them to gather mementos of the one who died; these so-called "linking objects" make them feel connected to the deceased(62)
- inviting them to create a memory book.(62)

4.7 Children Between the Ages of Five and Nine (Stage 2)

Children who are between the ages of five and nine are beginning to accept death as permanent but detach themselves from it. They do not see death as universal; they see it as something that only happens to other people.(1, 54)

Although they do not yet make the connection that death could one day happen to them, they may become concerned that it could happen to someone they know and love. This may precipitate fear of additional loss.

Because this subset of children is still wrapping their heads around the permanence of death, they may "forget" at times that death is not temporary. There may be times when they expect the person to return.

When they realize that the person is not coming back, they may still ascribe characteristics that are associated with the living to them. For instance, they may worry that the person who died might get cold or hungry.(13) A common fear among this age group, after burying the dead, is that the deceased will be afraid of the dark. Children may ask how it feels to be buried.(13, 63)

These children may begin to contemplate what happens after death as they wrestle to make sense of what death means to them. They may ask about body aftercare. They may ask what happens to the body after death. They may ask where their loved one is now that they have died.

Questions about life after death tend to be direct. Children who are raised with religious beliefs may call those beliefs into question. Gaps in understanding that they were unaware of prior to experiencing loss may now come to the surface. Recognize that these questions are being asked to gather information rather than question the belief. The intention is to clarify what isn't crystal clear in the moment.

Be direct in your answers. Exhibit transparency with your responses. If you do not know the answer to something, feel comfortable enough to say, "I don't know."

It's also okay to say, "I believe this because … but I'm not sure. This is what I think … ."

Ask children of this age group if they need additional explanations. Follow their lead. Sometimes what you think they're asking is not at all what they meant to ask. Clarify their questions before you answer to make sure that you're getting it right.

After you answer their initial question, ask if what you shared makes sense. You might ask them to explain to you in their own words what they heard you say. Check for mutual understanding before you provide additional layers of information that they may or may not be ready for.

At the same time, give them enough to work with. If you err too much on the side of caution and are intentionally vague or unclear, then children of this age group are likely to fill in any gaps with their own imagination.

This age group may also blame themselves for their loved one's death. They may take on a tremendous sense of guilt. Blame may give them a sense of control, which death has otherwise taken from them.

This age group can be supported through many of the same activities as children ages three through five. This age group may need to receive explanations again and again in response to their questions about what happened and why. Their questions may feel repetitive. They may need to ask the same question repeatedly to make sense of what happened.

This age group may benefit from asking where it hurts. You might initiate conversation by asking them if they ever feel sick or have pains when they are sad. Ask them how they feel and where. They may point out their grief "pangs" on themselves. They may feel more comfortable referencing pain points using the game of *Operation*.

4.8 Pre-teens (Stage 3)

Children who are ten or older recognize both the permanence and the universality of death. They understand that death happens to everyone and that death is inevitable.(1, 54)

Because they recognize the irreversibility of death, pre-teens see death as the ultimate separation from those they love and may fear being left behind.(3) They may worry "what if," as in "what if something bad happens to someone else I love?"

Pre-teens may ask higher level questions about death and dying that grieving adults often ask of themselves, too. These questions include:

- "Did I cause this to happen?"(1)
- "Will it happen to me?"(1)

By asking these questions and by processing the answers that they receive, pre-teens start to piece together causality.(3) They begin to wrap their heads around what causes death and what does not.(3)

Pre-teens may also focus on the impact that death has on the family unit. They want to know how death will affect them. It is normal for them to question, "Who will take care of me now (or if something happens to my surviving caretaker)?"(1)

Death is a disruption of routine. If the deceased was intimately tied to routine (e.g., "Dad took me to baseball games every Friday night"), then a secondary grief becomes the loss of routine. Pre-teens may ask, "Who will take me now?" or "Am I still able to go?" Pre-teens may focus on the logistics because these are tangible, concrete aspects of day-to-day life. They may emphasize events not necessarily because the event itself is significant but because the event is tied to someone who was.

It is normal for pre-teens to oscillate between journeying through grief and reengaging in activities of the living. Likewise, they may oscillate between wanting to be with others and wanting to be alone. Denial may become heavily entrenched, and they may cope by acting as though nothing has happened.

The Wendt Center for Loss and Healing suggests that you "invite expression."(64) Examples that the center provides on their website include:

- "Create: Draw the color of your heart, use lines, shapes, and color to express your emotions."(64)
- "Music: Find a song that matches your mood/energy or facilitates a mood-shift, or create a playlist about your grief."(64)
- "Movement: Use movement to release the energy, make your body as big as your grief."(64)

You can help this age group by making yourself available to engage in dialogue. Allow them to share what they feel ready to share with you and help them to identify what they are feeling in healthy ways.

When they aren't willing or wanting to talk, accept that as their current path. Give them space. Respect their need to process in their own way.

Connect with other adults (e.g., neighbors, parents of friends, teachers, coaches) that your pre-teen trusts and broaden their net of resources.

Let your pre-teen know that they have others looking out for them who are there and want to help. Sometimes just knowing that they have multiple people to turn to can be of help.

Consider reaching out to licensed professionals if your pre-teen would like to talk to someone neutral. They may not be comfortable sharing their innermost thoughts with you during their time of grief, but they may be open to the possibility of talking with someone else.

4.9 Staging Childhood Grief as Being Descriptive Rather than Prescriptive

Recognize that these stages, as first outlined by Nagy, are intended to provide a guide to age-appropriate conceptions of death among children.(1, 54) However, there is considerable individual variation between one child's response to death and another's.(1, 54)

How an individual child grieves is just as unique as the grief journey for an adult.

Grief is unique, period.

A child's grief journey is influenced by age and developmental stage as well as by:

- their temperament(35, 62)
  - the child's grief is likely to reflect their temperament
    - introverted children are more likely to exhibit introspective grief
- their relationship with the person who has died(65)
- how the person died
  - specifically the nature of the death(65) and whether the child was present(35)
- whether the child was present immediately before or immediately after the death(35)
- whether the child was prepared for the death and, if so, how(35)
- whether the child experienced anticipatory grief(35)
- their relationships with those who are still living
- what the child has been told about grief and grieving, death and dying
- prior experiences with grief and grieving, death and dying
- how others around them are grieving
- coping strategies that they have witnessed(35)
  - strategies that are effective
  - strategies that are ineffective
- culture(65)
  - what roles do culture and community play in the family's grief journey?
    - children have a tendency to be protected from conceptualizations of death in European-American culture(65)
    - children are routinely exposed to and participate openly in death rituals in Mexican culture:(65, 66)

       □ "Cultural practices like *dia de los muertos* provide socialization opportunities that influence youths' cognitive and affective understanding of death."(65)

- rituals and beliefs(35)
  - what roles do family traditions and/or religion play in the family's grieving?
  - what role, if any, did the child play in the funeral?
  - did the child attend the funeral?
  - what has the child been taught to believe surrounding what happens after death?
  - what does the child believe happens after death?
- their support networks
- concurrent stresses(35, 62), such as financial, housing, or food insecurity; poverty; mental health or addiction issues(67–69)
  - simultaneous stressors may intensify grief
  - simultaneous stressors may delay grief.

How someone dies is significant to a child. When death is unexpected, sudden, and/or traumatic, there is no time to prepare just as there is no time to say goodbye.(35)

The child may feel as if the ground dropped out from beneath them, leaving them suspended mid-air.

If the deceased died on the operating table, then the child may fear hospitals or surgery. They may consciously or unconsciously link death to healthcare.

The child may feel as though they are wading through unfinished business. There may be things left unsaid that they wished they had spoken aloud when the deceased were still alive. They may struggle with regret, particularly if they wish they could amend their last living memory of the deceased. Maybe their last words to the deceased were said in anger. Maybe they quarreled.

Maybe they had made plans and were supposed to go out, but never got the chance to.

They may feel frustrated because they are missing out on all the activities that they had planned together. They may feel angry that there will never be another time to do "x."

Even when death is "expected," as following a protracted terminal condition, death can still come as a shock. Sometimes the adults are aware of the trajectory of illness yet choose to shield children from the reality of the situation. In these circumstances, children may find themselves surprised that death came "so soon," thinking that they had more time with their loved one. When death comes, it may be shocking and launch them into denial because, simply put, "it can't be!"

There are so many variables when it comes to bereavement and its multifaceted impact on the child. Stages of childhood bereavement are intended to be descriptive rather than prescriptive because we cannot predict for certain how an individual will react to loss.

What is essential is to recognize that what is "normal" for this child may be out of character for another. When out of character behavior arises, acknowledge it and take measures to address the underlying "why." It is important to find out why it is happening because "acting out" is a common manifestation of grief in children. Explore grief and grieving, death and dying in age-appropriate conversations that allow for shared understanding. Find ways to support one another, without expecting the child to take on the weight of your grief. They carry a weight that is all their own. They cannot carry yours to the finish line just as you cannot carry theirs. Grief is individual, even when shared.

4.10 Delayed Impacts of Childhood Bereavement

Until now, our discussion about grief has focused on the immediate aftermath of loss. What is essential to note about children is that they often exhibit delayed effects of grief.(13)

Several studies set out to investigate this delay in the emotional impact of grief in school-aged children prior to 1996. However, results were inconsistent and inconclusive due to low sample size and methodological limitations.(70)

The Child Bereavement Study, published in 1996 by Worden and Silverman, expanded the data set to include 70 families with 125 bereaved children who resided in the greater Boston area.(70) Participants were interviewed at four months, one year, and two years after their loss. A child from each of the grieving families was randomly selected for matching by school personnel with a child who was not grieving, so as to make comparisons between age, gender, grade of education, and socioeconomic background.(70) These so-called controls were evaluated at the same one- and two-year mark as the bereaved child.(70)

Results of the Child Bereavement Study demonstrate that there can be significant changes to the bereaved child's perception of self-worth and self-efficacy at the one- and two-year anniversaries of their loss.(70)

Worden and Silverman document these changes as follows:(70)

At one year bereaved children, as compared to controls, saw themselves as performing less well scholastically … and as less well-behaved … than their peers. By the second anniversary the bereaved saw themselves as performing less well socially … and being less well-behaved … than their peers when compared to the responses of the control children. Two years after the death of their parent, bereaved children also had significantly lower scores on overall self-worth than controls … .

Worden and Silverman also evaluated the ability to which the bereaved and non-bereaved children felt that they could control their environment and the course of their lives. Worden and Silverman defined this as the "Locus of Control."(70) Historically, younger children feel less empowered than older children to change their surroundings; they are more likely to feel helpless.(70) What Worden and Silverman found was that the bereaved, irrespective of age, mirrored typical findings of younger children. At both one- and two-year anniversaries of their loved one's death, the bereaved children scored lower in terms of their sense of empowerment than the controls.(70) The bereaved were less likely than the non-bereaved to feel that they could effectively control life events.(70)

These results confirm others' suspicions that bereaved children may postpone grief and/or experience grief on an expanded timeline.(70) Significant figures in children's lives may believe that at one and two years post-death, the bereaved are "okay." In fact, bereaved children may feel significantly different about themselves, their lives, their self-esteem, and sense of self-worth.(70)

Bereaved children are also more likely to experience and report anxiety that may not emerge until one or two years after the loss.(70) Anxiety may reflect their own underlying concerns about safety of self or they may find that they are anxious to protect the surviving parent.(70)

Bereaved children are also likely to exhibit physical manifestations of grief.(70) They do not necessarily take ill more often than the non-bereaved, but they do exhibit higher levels of headaches and stomachaches.(70)

Traditionally, hospice-affiliated programs provide up to one year of grief support for the bereaved following the death of a loved one.(70) What the Worden and Silverman study shows is that bereaved children require extended follow-up, beyond 12 months.(70) Maintaining correspondence with bereaved families is essential so that healthcare professionals can identify delayed sequelae to loss that may not arise until one or two years post-death.(70)

4.11 Grief is Not About "Fixing"

Children and the adults who care for them need to know that, especially when it comes to childhood grief, "grief doesn't have an expiration date; it's not a carton of eggs or a quart of milk."(71)

More than ever, what bereaved children need is:(71) "a 'significant adult' who brings sensitivity, honesty, a sense of inclusion and compassion, and allows children to be their own experts. We can't take away or 'fix' our children's pain, anger, or fear; but we can support them through their grief process."(71)

Just as we cannot "fix" grief in adults who mourn, adults cannot "fix" grief in bereaved children.

We may instinctually try to shield children from the physical, cognitive, social, emotional, and spiritual manifestations of grief. Our instinct is often to protect the younger generation from the harsh truths of adult living.

Sometimes, adults do not want to talk about the death, assuming that by doing so, children will be spared some of the pain and sadness. Yet, when they are ignored, children may suffer more from feeling isolated than from the actual death itself.

The truth is that we cannot predict how a child will react to a loss. What we as adults assume to be protective may in fact be counterproductive. The only thing we know for sure is that children need to be given the freedom to grieve in their own way.

We must learn to accept children where they are at in their own grief process and recognize that, in the words of Alan Wolfelt, "Anyone old enough to love is old enough to grieve."(71)

Just because they are "kids" doesn't mean that they hurt less. Grief impacts all the bereaved in different ways. It's not that grief is "more" for some and "less" for others. It is, simply put, different.

Adults who are willing to talk openly about the death help children understand that grief is a natural feeling when someone loved has died. Children need adults to affirm that it's okay to be sad and to cry, and to be reassured that the hurt they feel now will not last forever.

Openness to grief and willingness to sit with it – the ability to gain comfort with the discomfort – sets the stage for resilience. Resilience has been defined as the ability to bounce back from – in effect overcome – significant adverse experiences.(4, 72–75)

Building a resilient mindset is essential for the bereaved child so that they not only survive their loss but thrive in spite of it.(76, 77) Having resilience does not mean that one is happy to have experienced loss. Building resiliency does mean that over time, the individual is able to more effectively "bounce back from disappointments, adversity, and trauma, to develop clear and realistic goals, to solve problems, to relate comfortably with others, and to treat oneself with respect."(78)

4.12 Adolescent Grief

Adolescence is a protracted state of development in which children are coming into their own as they mature and transition into adulthood. It is not set by any one particular date so much as it refers to a broad range in time during which the adolescent experiences biological, cognitive, cultural, and societal influences.(79)

Early adolescence is said to take place between 12–18 years of age. (79) Within this time frame, puberty exerts itself and creates extensive physical change. Adolescents experience themselves physically evolving before their own eyes as they encounter growth spurts, muscle and/or breast development, change in voice, body size, and shape. (79) Advancements in physical maturity may take place prior to other developmental changes, including cognitive, social, and emotional.(79) Outwardly, a "child" may appear to be all grown up when in fact their brain is still in the process of reshaping. They are, day by day, relearning themselves, who they are, and how and where they fit into new and changing relationships.

Although identity development is a lifelong process, it plays a particularly critical role during adolescence. Adolescence is often the first time that people truly begin to explore and clarify who they are and how their unique identity affects not only their lives, but those around them.(80)

Adolescents become acutely aware of themselves and their changing identities.(80, 81) Their self-consciousness influences how they act and interact with their family units, circles of friends, academic classes, teams, and communities. They learn quickly who is accepting of them and who is not, and this often influences the way in which they elect to portray themselves to different audiences.

Who they are and who they perceive themselves to be forms the basis for self-esteem. During adolescence, how teens see themselves may experience one or more shifts as they continually respond to peer groups and families. Self-identity is inherently tied to our sense of belonging. We learn who our people are, who we want to hang out with, and who we want to be more like.

Adolescence is, in a sense, about finding oneself. In that process, teens strive for independence as they work through their own sense of inherent value and self-worth.(79) They may constantly balance what they aspire to be against what society expects them to be as they consider social norms and societal expectations while establishing their own sense of purpose.(79)

A significant challenge that faces teens who grieve is that at a time when they are striving for independence, they are made vulnerable by the death of a loved one. They may desire to express grief in the same way that adults do, yet many feel conflicted about opening themselves up to others emotionally.

Teens may be inhibited from expressing emotion if others have modeled that behavior for them. Alternatively, they may inhibit themselves from open expressions of emotion to avoid being flagged as "different" from their peer group.

Even though contemporary society is moving away from traditional gender roles, teens may still encounter and experience traditional gender role expectations that influence the way in which they grieve.(79) Gender binary roles in a non-binary world may be losing steam, yet many are still raised with the expectation that girls should nurture and boys shouldn't cry.(79)

The reality is that the word, "shouldn't," has no place in bereavement, particularly when teens must find their own way to cope. All teens grieve when a loved one dies.(82) To reconcile their loss, they must feel secure and openly accepted for the way they choose to display grief.(82)

In many ways, grieving teens seek permission to mourn.(82) They often have a preconceived notion of what it means to act "grown up" and in the process of maturing, they naturally separate themselves from authority and other attachment figures.(82) Often what they need to hear from us is that it is okay to feel. It is okay to talk about feelings. It is okay not to talk about feelings.

The most critical piece of support that we can provide to them during their time of need is that it is okay to be true to themselves – feeling what they need to feel, sharing what they need to share, with whom they want to share, at a time of their choosing, in a space where they feel safe.(82)

Teens have an adult understanding of what death means, but they rely on us to model coping skills. They do not have the experiences or the behavior of an adult. Teens may also experience a wide range of emotions that they are not certain how to handle. Accordingly, they may look to us consciously or unconsciously to demonstrate appropriate paths for moving forward.

Note that grief is not about "moving on."(62) Grief is about "moving with." The loss will always be there. It's about the teen learning to come to terms with it, on their own timetable.

You can support teens best by giving them the space they need.

Avoid pushing them to be who they used to be. Give them the time to figure out their "new normal." Be accepting of this "new normal" as the bereaved grieve at their own pace.

Help the bereaved to remember their loved one, in their own time, in their own way. Don't be afraid to ask them what they would like in terms of discussing the loved one. Don't assume that they would rather not talk about the loved one, if bringing up the loved one's name causes tears. The bereaved may appreciate hearing that the loved one is remembered, even if by experiencing the memory, emotions resurface.

Understand that the bereaved are forever changed. It does not mean that they will never be themselves again, it means they need to find themselves again.

In the process of finding themselves, it is normal for teens to exhibit one or more of the following as they grieve:

- testing the limits
- acting moody, impulsive, egocentric, or rebellious
- turning to peers for support more so than family.

Red flags that suggest you may need additional support for your teen include if they:

- get into fights or legal trouble
- isolate from family and friends
- take on a dramatic change in personality or attitude
- engage in substance use/abuse
- engage in inappropriate sexual behaviors
- develop the symptoms of clinical depression(62) or chronic depressive disorders:(35)
  - "Depressed mood most of the day, nearly every day, as indicated by subjective report (e.g., feels sad or empty) or observation by others (e.g., appears tearful)."(83)
  - "Markedly diminished interest or pleasure in all, or almost all, activities most of the day, nearly every day."(83)
  - "Significant weight loss when not dieting or weight gain, or decrease or increase in appetite nearly every day."(83)
  - "Insomnia or hypersomnia nearly every day."(83)
  - "Psychomotor agitation or retardation nearly every day (observable by others, not merely subjective feelings or restlessness or being slowed down)."(83)
  - "Fatigue or loss of energy nearly every day."(83)
  - Feelings of worthlessness or excessive or inappropriate guilt nearly every day (not merely self-reproach or guilt about being sick)."(83)

- o "Diminished ability to think or concentrate, or indecisiveness, nearly every day (either by subjective account or as observed by others)."(83)
- o "Recurrent thoughts of death (not just fear of dying), recurrent suicidal ideation without a specific plan, or a suicide attempt or specific plan for committing suicide."(83)

Depressive symptoms may include:(35)

- dysphoria
- social withdrawal
- sleep disturbances
- changes in eating habits
- poor academic performance.

Know your limits and encourage the bereaved to seek help when or if you become concerned about the duration or course of their grief journey. Let them know you are concerned because you care, not because you are judging their progress.

4.13 Avoiding Clichés When Navigating Adolescent and Adult Grief

Clichés are what we default to when we do not know what else to say. Unfortunately, what we mean to say and what the bereaved hear us say are two very different things.

The intent is lost in translation and there can be adverse impact, particularly among teens and adults who are grieving.

Consider, for example, the following clichés.

- When you say: "Everything happens for a reason."
  - o *What they hear: "There is a reason my loved one died."*
- When you say: "This is a test to make you stronger."
  - o *What they hear: "My loved one had to die to make me strong."*
- When you say: "They had a long life."
  - o *What they hear: "I don't have the right to complain about this death because they got to live longer than some."*
  - o How they feel: "It wasn't long enough."
- When you say: "At least they didn't suffer."
  - o *What they hear: "Stop complaining. Their death could have been worse."*
  - o How they feel: "I am suffering."

- When you say: "Time will heal."
  - *What they hear: "Stop complaining. You'll get over this."*
  - How they feel: "I'll never get over this."
- When you say: "You're holding up so well."
  - *What they hear: "We like when you appear put together so that we aren't made to feel uncomfortable."*
  - How they feel: "Inside, I am cracking."
- When you say: "You are never given more than you can handle."
  - *What they hear: "Stop complaining: you can handle this."*
  - How they feel: "I don't know how to handle this."

It is best to think before you speak and consider how your words might be received. Ask yourself how you might feel if the roles were reversed.

4.14 Don't Say "You Know" When You Don't

In addition to clichés, avoid the following phraseology when speaking with teens and adults about their grief:

- "I get it."
- "I know what you're going through."
- "I understand how you feel."

Although it may be true that you have experienced something similar – for example, perhaps you, too, experienced the death of a parent – you are forgetting that your experience was still unique to you.

You experienced loss your way.

Your teen's experience may be distinct for any number of reasons, some of which you may be aware of, others you may not.

To validate the uniqueness of loss, it would be preferred to make use of the following statements instead:

- "I can only imagine what you're going through."
- "I can't begin to understand how you feel."
- "I can imagine how I'd feel, but I'm not you. Tell me what you are experiencing. Tell me about you."

4.15 Be Honest and Be Present

When you are uncomfortable, it is okay to be upfront with the teen as long as you don't cross the line and ask them to comfort you instead of the other way around.

If you are at a loss for words, it is okay to say:

- "I'm sorry. I don't know what to say."
- "I'm sorry. There are no words for a time such as this."

If you cannot think of anything helpful to say, a silent presence may effectively demonstrate that you care and that you are willing to be there for the other person, no matter what.

It is worth noting that in order to be present, you must mean it both in words and actions. If you ask, "How are you?", then you need to be willing to stick around to hear the answer.

Active listening is a skill. Listen to hear and to comprehend fully rather than listening to respond.

References

1. Osterweis M, Solomon F, Green M. Bereavement during childhood and adolescence. In: Osterweis M, Solomon F, Green M, editors. Bereavement: reactions, consequences, and care. Washington, DC: National Academies Press; 1984.
2. Lieberman AF. Losing a parent to death in the early years: guidelines for the treatment of traumatic bereavement in infancy and early childhood. 1st ed. Vol. xvi. Washington, DC: Zero To Three Press; 2003.
3. Jones AM, Deane C, Keegan O. The development of a framework to support bereaved children and young people: the Irish Childhood Bereavement Care Pyramid. Bereavement Care. 2015;34(2):43–51. https://doi.org/10.1080/0268262 1.2015.1063857.
4. Crenshaw DA, Kelly JE. "Dear Mr. Leprechaun": nurturing resilience in children facing loss and grief. In: Crenshaw DA, Brooks RB, Goldstein S, editors. Play therapy interventions to enhance resilience. New York: The Guilford Press; 2015. p. 82–106.
5. Kliman G. Childhood mourning: a taboo within a taboo. In: Gerber I, Wiener A, Kutscher A, Battin D, Arkin A, Goldberg I, editors. Perspectives on bereavement. New York: Arno Press; 1979.
6. Delaney K. Childhood grief: elevating awareness of prevalence and the need for requisite support. J Child Adolesc Psychiatr Nurs. 2022;35(4):299–300. https://doi.org/10.1111/jcap.12398, PMID 36308395.
7. Burns M, Griese B, King S, Talmi A. Childhood bereavement: understanding prevalence and related adversity in the United States. Am J Orthopsychiatry. 2020;90(4):391–405. https://doi.org/10.1037/ort0000442, PMID 31999137.

8. Khandwala YS, Zhang CA, Lu Y, Eisenberg ML. The age of fathers in the USA is rising: an analysis of 168 867 480 births from 1972 to 2015. Hum Reprod. 2017;32(10):2110–6. https://doi.org/10.1093/humrep/dex267, PMID 28938735.

9. Curtin SC, Warner M, Hedegaard H. Increase in suicide in the United States, 1999–2014. NCHS Data Brief. 2016;(241):1–8. PMID 27111185.

10. Seth P, Scholl L, Rudd RA, Bacon S. Overdose deaths involving opioids, cocaine, and psychostimulants – United States, 2015–2016. MMWR Morb Mortal Wkly Rep. 2018;67(12):349–58. https://doi.org/10.15585/mmwr.mm6712a1, PMID 29596405.

11. The New York Life. Foundation's 2017 bereavement survey: key findings. The New York Life Foundation; 2017. Available from: https://www.newyorklife.com/assets/newsroom/docs/pdfs/NYLF_2017_Bereavement_Survey.pdf.

12. One-parent family groups with own children under 18, by marital status, and race and Hispanic origin of the reference person. Washington, DC: United States Census Bureau; 2001.

13. Machajewski V, Kronk R. Childhood grief related to the death of a sibling. J Nurse Pract. 2013;9(7):443–8. https://doi.org/10.1016/j.nurpra.2013.03.020.

14. Brent D, Melhem N, Donohoe MB, Walker M. The incidence and course of depression in bereaved youth 21 months after the loss of a parent to suicide, accident, or sudden natural death. Am J Psychiatry. 2009;166(7):786–94. https://doi.org/10.1176/appi.ajp.2009.08081244, PMID 19411367.

15. Brent DA, Melhem NM, Masten AS, Porta G, Payne MW. Longitudinal effects of parental bereavement on adolescent developmental competence. J Clin Child Adolesc Psychol. 2012;41(6):778–91. https://doi.org/10.1080/15374416.2012.717 871, PMID 23009724.

16. Cerel J, Fristad MA, Verducci J, Weller RA, Weller EB. Childhood bereavement: psychopathology in the 2 years postparental death. J Am Acad Child Adolesc Psychiatry. 2006;45(6):681–90. https://doi.org/10.1097/01.chi.0000215327.58799.05, PMID 16721318.

17. Guldin MB, Li J, Pedersen HS, Obel C, Agerbo E, Gissler M, et al. Incidence of suicide among persons who had a parent who died during their childhood: a population-based cohort study. JAMA Psychiatry. 2015;72(12):1227–34. https://doi.org/10.1001/jamapsychiatry.2015.2094, PMID 26558351.

18. Kaplow JB, Saunders J, Angold A, Costello EJ. Psychiatric symptoms in bereaved versus nonbereaved youth and young adults: a longitudinal epidemiological study. J Am Acad Child Adolesc Psychiatry. 2010;49(11):1145–54. https://doi.org/10.1016/j.jaac.2010.08.004, PMID 20970702.

19. Keyes KM, Pratt C, Galea S, McLaughlin KA, Koenen KC, Shear MK. The burden of loss: unexpected death of a loved one and psychiatric disorders across the life course in a national study. Am J Psychiatry. 2014;171(8):864–71. https://doi.org/10.1176/appi.ajp.2014.13081132, PMID 24832609.

20. Li J, Vestergaard M, Cnattingius S, Gissler M, Bech BH, Obel C, et al. Mortality after parental death in childhood: a nationwide cohort study from three Nordic countries. PLOS Med. 2014;11(7):e1001679. https://doi.org/10.1371/journal.pmed.1001679, PMID 25051501.

21. Yu Y, Liew Z, Cnattingius S, Olsen J, Vestergaard M, Fu B, et al. Association of mortality with the death of a sibling in childhood. JAMA Pediatr. 2017;171(6):538–45. https://doi.org/10.1001/jamapediatrics.2017.0197, PMID 28437534.

22. Thompson MP, Kaslow NJ, Price AW, Williams K, Kingree JB. Role of secondary stressors in the parental death-child distress relation. J Abnorm Child Psychol. 1998;26(5):357–66. https://doi.org/10.1023/a:1021951806281, PMID 9826294.

23. Fletcher J, Mailick M, Song J, Wolfe B. A sibling death in the family: common and consequential. Demography. 2013;50(3):803–26. https://doi.org/10.1007/s13524-012-0162-4, PMID 23073753.

24. Murphy SL, Kochanek KD, Xu J, Arias E. Mortality in the United States, 2020. NCHS Data Brief. 2021;(427):1–8. PMID 34978528.

25. Kramer L, Kowal AK. Sibling relationship quality from birth to adolescence: the enduring contributions of friends. J Fam Psychol. 2005;19(4):503–11. https://doi.org/10.1037/0893-3200.19.4.503, PMID 16402865.

26. Schultheiss DEP, Palma TV, Predragovich KS, Glasscock JMJ. Relational influences on career paths: siblings in context. J Couns Psychol. 2002;49(3):302–10. https://doi.org/10.1037/0022-0167.49.3.302.

27. Whiteman SD, McHale SM, Crouter AC. Explaining sibling similarities: perceptions of sibling influences. J Youth Adolescence. 2007;36(7):963–72. https://doi.org/10.1007/s10964-006-9135-5.

28. Rende R, Slomkowski C, Lloyd-Richardson E, Niaura R. Sibling effects on substance use in adolescence: social contagion and genetic relatedness. J Fam Psychol. 2005;19(4):611–8. https://doi.org/10.1037/0893-3200.19.4.611, PMID 16402876.

29. East PL, Khoo ST. Longitudinal pathways linking family factors and sibling relationship qualities to adolescent substance use and sexual risk behaviors. J Fam Psychol. 2005;19(4):571–80. https://doi.org/10.1037/0893-3200.19.4.571, PMID 16402872.

30. Jacobs JR, Bovasso GB. Re-examining the long-term effects of experiencing parental death in childhood on adult psychopathology. J Nerv Ment Dis. 2009;197(1):24–7. https://doi.org/10.1097/NMD.0b013e3181927723, PMID 19155806.

31. Crehan G. The surviving sibling: the effects of sibling death in childhood. Psychoanal Psychother. 2004;18(2):202–19. https://doi.org/10.1080/14749730410001700723.

32. Worden JW, Davies B, McCown D. Comparing parent loss with sibling loss. Death Stud. 1999;23(1):1–15. https://doi.org/10.1080/074811899201163, PMID 10346731.

33. Lawrence ST. The grieving child in the classroom: a guide for school-based professionals. 1st ed. New York; London: Routledge/Taylor & Francis Group. Vol. xii; 2020.

34. Stuber ML, Mesrkhani VH. "What do we tell the children?": understanding childhood grief. West J Med. 2001;174(3):187–91. https://doi.org/10.1136/ewjm.174.3.187, PMID 11238354.

35. Pearlman MY, Schwalbe KDA. Cloitre Mn. Grief in childhood: fundamentals of treatment in clinical practice. 1st ed. Vol. vii. Washington, DC: American Psychological Association; 2010.

36. Lehmann L, Jimerson SR, Gaasch A. Mourning child grief support group curriculum: early childhood edition: kindergarten—grade 2. Vol. vii. Philadelphia: Brunner-Routledge; 2000.

37. Lehmann L, Jimerson SR, Gaasch A. Mourning child grief support group curriculum: middle childhood edition: grades 3–6. Vol. vii. Philadelphia: Brunner-Routledge; 2000.

38. Freud S. Totem and taboo. In: Strachey J, editor. The standard edition of the complete psychological works of Sigmund Freud. 13. London: Hogarth Press and Institute for Psychoanalysis; 1955. p. 1–161.

39. Freud S. Mourning and melancholia. In: Strachey J, editor. The standard edition of the complete psychological works of Sigmund Freud. 14. London: Hogarth Press and Institute for Psychoanalysis; 1955. p. 237–60.

40. Anthony HS. The child's discovery of death; a study in child psychology. London: K. Paul, Trench, Trubner & Co.; 1940.

41. Bluebond-Langner M. The private worlds of dying children. Vol. xv. Princeton, NJ: Princeton University Press; 1978.

42. Silverman PR, Kelly M. A parent's guide to raising grieving children: rebuilding your family after the death of a loved one. Oxford: Oxford University Press; 2009.

43. Gibney H. What death means to children. Parent's Mag. 1965 (March).

44. Betz CL, Poster EC. Children's concepts of death. Implications for pediatric practice. Nurs Clin North Am. 1984;19(2):341–9. https://doi.org/10.1016/S0029-6465(22)01836-9, PMID 6563585.

45. Sodoy CC. Children's concepts of death. Bull Am Protestant Hosp Assoc. 1978;42(2):129–32. PMID 10240982.

46. Kane B. Children's concepts of death. J Genet Psychol. 1979;134(1):141–53. https://doi.org/10.1080/00221325.1979.10533406.

47. Koocher GP. Childhood, death, and cognitive development. Dev Psychol. 1973;9(3):369–75. https://doi.org/10.1037/h0034917.

48. Menig-Peterson C, McCabe A. Children talk about death. Omega (Westport). 1978;8(4):305–17. https://doi.org/10.2190/JKJ4-UTB3-HKG0-47M9.

49. Piaget J, Tomlinson J, Tomlinson A. The child's conception of the world. London. New York: Routledge; 2011.

50. Spinetta JJ. The dying child's awareness of death: a review. Psychol Bull. 1974;81(4):256–60. https://doi.org/10.1037/h0036229, PMID 4594964.

51. Tallmer M, Formanek R, Tallmer J. Factors influencing children's concepts of death. J Clin Child Psychol. 1974;3(2)(Summer):17–9. https://doi.org/10.1080/15374417409532564.

52. Hames CC. Helping infants and toddlers when a family member dies. J Hosp Palliat Nurs. 2003;5(2):103–10. https://doi.org/10.1097/00129191-200304000-00016.

53. Murray JS. Understanding sibling adaptation to childhood cancer. Issues Compr Pediatr Nurs. 2000;23(1):39–47. https://doi.org/10.1080/014608600265200, PMID 11011662.

54. Nagy M. The child's theories concerning death. J Genet Psychol. 1948;73(First Half):3–27. https://doi.org/10.1080/08856559.1948.10533458, PMID 18893204.

55. Koocher G. Children's conception of death. In: Bibare R, Walsh M, editors. New directions for child development: children's conceptions of health, illness, and bodily functions. San Francisco: Jossey-Bass; 1981.

56. Lonetto R. Children's conceptions of death. New York: Springer; 1980.

57. Busch T, Kimble CS. Grieving children: are we meeting the challenge? Pediatr Nurs. 2001;27(4):414–8. PMID 12025282.

58. Melson GF. Children's experiences of pet loss and separation: a child development framework. In: Kogan L, Erdman P, editors. Pet loss, grief, and therapeutic interventions: practitioners navigating the human-animal bond. New York: Routledge; 2020. p. 21–34.

59. Furman E. A child's parent dies: studies in childhood bereavement. Vol. xi. New Haven, NY: Yale University Press; 1974.

60. Piaget J. The origins of intelligence in children. New York: International Universities Press; 1952.

61. Mahon MM. Death of a sibling: primary care interventions. Pediatr Nurs. 1994;20(3):293–5, 328. PMID 8008481.

62. Wolfelt A. When your pet dies: a guide to mourning, remembering, and healing. Fort Collins, CO: Companion Press; 2004.

63. Reynolds LA, Miller DL, Jelalian E, Spirito A. Anticipatory grief and bereavement. In: Roberts MC, editor. Handbook of pediatric psychology. 2nd ed. New York: Guilford Press; 1995. p. 142–64.

64. Talking to kids about grief: Wendt center for loss and healing; 2021. Available from: https://www.wendtcenter.org/talking-to-kids-about-grief/.

65. Alvis L, Zhang N, Sandler IN, Kaplow JB. Developmental manifestations of grief in children and adolescents: caregivers as key grief facilitators. J Child Adolesc Trauma. 2022:1–11. https://doi.org/10.1007/s40653-021-00435-0, PMID 35106114.

66. Gutiérrez IT, Menendez D, Jiang MJ, Hernandez IG, Miller P, Rosengren KS. Embracing death: Mexican parent and child perspectives on death. Child Dev. 2020;91(2):e491–511. https://doi.org/10.1111/cdev.13263, PMID 31140591.

67. Penny A, Stubbs D. Bereavement in Childhood – what do we know in 2014. U.K.; 2014.

68. Stephen AI, Macduff C, Petrie DJ, Tseng FM, Schut H, Skår S, et al. The economic cost of bereavement in Scotland. Death Stud. 2015;39(1–5):151–7. https://doi.org/1 0.1080/07481187.2014.920435, PMID 25255790.

69. Harper M, O'Connor R, Dickson A, O'Carroll R. Mothers continuing bonds and ambivalence to personal mortality after the death of their child–an interpretative phenomenological analysis. Psychol Health Med. 2011;16(2):203–14. https://doi. org/10.1080/13548506.2010.532558, PMID 21328148.

70. Worden JW, Silverman PR. Parental death and the adjustment of school-age children. Omega (Westport). 1996;33(2):91–102. https://doi.org/10.2190/ P77L-F6F6-5W06-NHBX.

71. Olin R. A child's grief. Brain, child magazine. 2016. Available from: https://02f 0a56ef46d93f03c90-22ac5f107621879d5667e0d7ed595bdb.ssl.cf2.rackcdn.com/ sites/14962/uploads/24215/Harvard_Child_Bereavement_Study20180706-20166- 3e6sod.pdf.

72. Rutter M. Implications of resilience concepts for scientific understanding. Ann N Y Acad Sci. 2006;1094:1–12. https://doi.org/10.1196/annals.1376.002, PMID 17347337.

73. Wolin SJ, Wolin S. The resilient self: how survivors of troubled families rise above adversity. 1st ed. Vol. xiv. New York: Villard Books; 1993.

74. Wolin S, Wolin SJ. The challenge model: working with strengths in children of substance-abusing parents. Child Adolesc Psychiatr Clin N Am. 1996;5(1):243–56. https://doi.org/10.1016/S1056-4993(18)30396-1.

75. Wolin SJ, Wolin S. The challenge model: how children rise above adversity. Fam Dyn Addict Q. 1992;2(2):10–22.

76. Brooks RB, Goldstein S. Raising resilient children: fostering strength, hope, and optimism in your child. Lincolnwood. IL: Contemporary Books; 2001.

77. Brooks RB, Goldstein S. Nurturing resilience in our children: answers to the most important parenting questions. Vol. xiv. Chicago: Contemporary Books; 2003.

78. Goldstein S, Brooks RB. Why study resilience? In: Goldstein S, Brooks RB, editors. Handbook of resilience in children. 2nd ed. New York: Springer; 2013. p. 3–14.

79. Uttley CM. Adolescence, pet loss, grief, and therapeutic intervention. In: Kogan L, Erdman P, editors. Pet loss, grief, and therapeutic interventions: practitioners navigating the human-animal bond. New York: Routledge; 2020. p. 35–54.

80. Steinberg LD. Adolescence. 8th ed. New York: McGraw-Hill Higher Education; 2008.
81. Erikson EH. Identity, youth, and crisis. 1st ed. New York: W W Norton; 1968.
82. Wolfelt A. Healing your grieving heart for teens: 100 practical ideas. Fort Collins, CO: Companion Press; 2001.
83. Moore R, Garland A. Cognitive therapy for chronic and persistent depression. Vol. xvi. Chichester, West Sussex: Wiley; 2003.

CHAPTER 5

Complicated Grief

"You can clutch the past so tightly to your chest that it leaves your arms too full to embrace the present."—*Jan Glidwell*

Chapters 2, 3, and 4 emphasized the uniqueness of grief as a journey through which the bereaved individual navigates.(1, 2) Although the one who is grieving may be companioned by friends and family through the process, ultimately it is the bereaved who must commit to rebuilding life and healing from their loss.(3)

5.1 Grief as an Adaptive Process

In this respect, grief is an adaptive process(4) and the timeline for the bereaved varies.(3) The bereaved must establish for themselves a "new normal" with a renewed self of identity that has been influenced by their grief and their decision to "move with" grief into their next chapter of living.(5)

"Moving with" grief is about accepting reality – the reality of loss as well as the reality that there is a very real distinction between that which we do and do not have control over.(4)

"Moving with" grief is about rebuilding autonomy(4), that is, taking the reins back from the grieving process and stepping back into control over those life aspects that are within one's reach (6)

"Moving with" grief is about the many ways that the bereaved find to "turn the light on in the world again."(6)

"Moving with" grief is about learning to desire life again and seek out new experiences – not because the deceased have been forgotten, but rather because their memories have become an intangible yet very real part of who we are.(6)

In the words of Shear:(6) "A successful mourning process entails effective emotional regulation and assimilation of new learning in long-term memory." Shear explains:(6)

Our loved ones exist in long-term memory, but there are different kinds of memory. Episodic, semantic, and implicit memory(7–11) are inter-related but serve different functions, entail different brain systems, and have different properties. Close attachments are mapped in each of these systems, so each must be updated when a loved one dies.

Updating memory is a bit like rebooting a hard-wired system and navigating glitches in the coding:(6)

To update explicit memory means learning new stories and facts. To update semantic memory means learning new meanings and rules, and to update implicit memory means extinguishing conditioned reward responses and learning new motor patterns and other procedural responses that are permanently out of awareness.

The process is lengthy by intentional design. Our body needs time to update the internal wiring. The time it takes to rewire our thoughts is the time it takes for us to process our grief. According to Shear:(6)

Given this multifaceted goal, it makes sense that mourning is a complex process that is often lengthy and arduous. We must repeatedly engage with information about the death and its myriad consequences in order to adequately assimilate it and amend existing information about the deceased in each memory system.

As we navigate our own respective journeys through grief, we learn to embrace that our loved ones live on inside of us through memories.(6) In many ways, these memories drive us forward. They remind us of what used to be. They remind us of what can be. Therein is hope.

It is hope that the bereaved often cling to during difficult days.

It is often that same hope that the bereaved may credit with helping them to come through the fog of grief to the other side.

Grief is for many the most empty place that we can go to inside of ourselves and it's there that we become most in tune with what we need to coax ourselves out.

That journey to understand ourselves and our needs is a significant part of the grieving process.(4) A better understanding of self provides clarity as we learn what we must hold on to tightly and what we can let go of in order to effectively and successfully make it through.(4)

Author Suzanne Collins alludes to this journey of self-discovery when, in the novel, *Mockingjay*, she documented Katniss the protagonist's thoughts as follows:(12)

> *… what I need to survive is not Gale's fire, kindled with rage and hatred. I have plenty of fire myself. What I need is the dandelion in the spring. The bright yellow that means rebirth instead of destruction. The promise that life can go on, no matter how bad our losses. That it can be good again.*

The bereaved want to believe that life can be good again. The mourning process is about learning how to "feel deeply connected to deceased loved ones while also able to imagine a satisfying future without them."(6)

As we adapt to our "new normal," the symptoms of grief should improve over time, that is, they should lessen. That does not mean that we no longer feel our losses. Some days we may feel those losses more deeply than others.

Special occasions, such as birthdays, holidays, and anniversaries are more likely to reignite the blaze of grief inside of us as these moments emphasize who is *not* present to celebrate with us, more often than those who are.

However, as we mourn the absence of those we love over time, we are, in essence, learning how to sit with our loss. We ultimately make the choice to integrate loss into our lives. Grief becomes one manifestation of our identity. In this way, we are able to restore meaning and value to the lives we choose to lead.(6, 13)

5.2 Becoming "Stuck" in Grief

Unfortunately, a minority of the bereaved become "stuck" in their grief. (6, 14–16) Estimates appear to vary regionally and by country as reported below:(17)

- 2.4% in Japan(18)
- 3.7% in Germany(14)
- 4.2% in Switzerland(19)

For the estimated 7%–10% of the global grieving population(14, 15, 17, 20, 21), mourning goes awry and coping strategies are not achieved.(6, 14) Instead, the affected individuals become trapped within the pain of grief, and grief is said to be "complicated."(6, 14, 22–32) It is as if the vehicle in which the bereaved is travelling has stalled or as if one's tires have gotten entrenched in mud, and no further forward progress can be made.

When someone becomes "stuck" in their grief, their grief is "prolonged."(17, 33) Prolonged grief disorder (**PGD**) or complicated grief (**CG**) is a syndrome in which acute grief is protracted and interferes with healing.(6, 14, 16, 33) "Traumatic grief" has historically been referenced as a synonym(17, 34–38); however, complicated grief is not always related to post-traumatic stress syndrome (**PTSD**).(37)

It may be that the affected mourner has become "stuck" in one of the phases of grieving. It may mean that their symptoms are worsening rather than reducing.

According to Shear:(6)

We use the term "complicated" in the medical sense to refer to a superimposed process that alters grief and modifies its course for the worse. Think about a physical wound that produces an inflammatory response as part of the healing process. A wound complication, for example an infection, increases the inflammation and delays healing.

You can think of bereavement as analogous to an injury and grief as analogous to the painful inflammatory response and complicated grief as analogous to a superimposed infection. The result is delayed healing and increased pain which occurs because aspects of a person's response to the circumstances or consequences of the death derail the mourning process, interfering with learning, and preventing the natural healing process from progressing.

The authors have previously shared that there is no definitive timeline for grief. Grief takes as long as it takes.

Complicated grief is said to occur when someone who is grieving has made little to no progress in their grief journey within the first six months following a loved one's death.(4, 6, 17)

5.3 Symptoms Associated with Complicated Grief

Those who experience complicated grief exhibit one or more of the following symptoms for the *duration* of their protracted grief:(4, 6, 17, 21, 30, 39–41)

- persistent yearning for the deceased
- intense loneliness
- static emptiness
- ongoing perception that life is meaningless

- preoccupation with thoughts of the deceased
  - thoughts are intrusive
    - they constantly interrupt one's ability to function
    - they interfere with activities
    - they interfere with relationships with other survivors
- recurrent desire to join the deceased
  - this may be reflective of "magical thinking," as though the bereaved can bring the dead back to life "if only"…
  - this may be reflective of suicidal ideation and should be explored by those who are companioning the bereaved through grief.

The syndrome of complicated grief as outlined above causes significant disturbance in the individual's ability to connect to others.(17) Social, domestic, and/or occupational functions are impaired.(17) In this way, complicated grief sets the stage for dysfunctional relationships.(17) These are perpetuated by the mourner's inability to trust since their loss.(17) The less they trust, the less they reach out. The less they reach out, the more they lose connection to their surroundings and shut people out. Isolation breeds isolation. It is increasingly more difficult to get the affected individual out of their shell because they have essentially cocooned themselves to block out the possibility that they could experience additional loss. It may be perceived as more beneficial to never experience connection again than to risk the chance that someone else they let in might abandon them.

Although complicated grief typically affects a small subset of the grieving population six months into bereavement, it may manifest itself earlier in the mourning process, particularly when two or more of the following symptoms last for one or more months.(4, 6, 17, 21, 39)

- Incessant questioning.
  - How did the death occur?
  - Why did the death occur?
  - Could the death have been prevented?
  - Why wasn't the death prevented?
- Persistent bargaining as though the bereaved was in complete control over the death and could have either prevented the loss or could now reverse it.
  - "If onlys."
  - "What ifs."
- Tendencies to catastrophize about the future.
  - Only bad things will happen now that their loved one has died.
    - "It's all over."
    - "This is the beginning of the end."

- Persistent numbness or shock.
  - "This didn't happen!"
  - "This couldn't have happened!"
- Difficulty accepting the death.
- Recurrent dreams of the deceased.(42)
  - It is rare for the nonbereaved to dream of a deceased person: it is said to occur in 1% of dreams reported by women, <1% of dreams reported by men, and in 2% of college students.(42)
  - Those who experience complicated grief dream about the deceased more frequently, particularly if the dreamer identifies as female.(42)
- Inability to trust others following the death of a loved one.
- Anger towards others who had nothing to do with the death, as if they are responsible for having caused it.
- Anger towards others outside of the circle of grief for not having experienced the death of a loved one.
- Bitterness towards the death itself.
- Making death into an enemy.
- Hating death as though it were a person.
- Altering behavior.
  - Excessive avoidance:(41)
    - e.g., avoiding places, people, or things that the mourner has linked to the deceased.
  - Excessive proximity-seeking:
    - e.g., seeking visual, auditory, olfactory, and tactile reminders of the deceased.
  - Note that both avoidance and proximity-seeking behaviors may be observed.
- Intense reactions to memories of the deceased or to reminders of the loss.
  - Memories of the deceased may not bring comfort.
  - Memories of the deceased may reignite the blaze of anger, blame, resentment, envy, and/or frustration.
- Intense activation of negative valence emotions (e.g., anger, bitterness, resentment).
- Lack of respite from negative valence emotions with positive emotions, or guilt that clouds over any positive emotions.
- Lack of forward planning and future thinking.(43)
- Difficulty imagining future events that are positive.(43)
- Ease of imagining future events relating to the loss.(43)
- Sensations that they are feeling what it was that the deceased person felt when they were still alive (e.g., pain).
- Visual or auditory hallucinations: seeing or hearing the deceased.

Note that hallucinations are distinct from false recognitions.

Recall from Chapter 3 that false recognitions are common across cultures and occur with greater frequency among those who have lost either a spouse or a parent.(44–51) False recognitions are a normal part of the grieving process. In false recognitions, the bereaved are not hallucinating the deceased into being. They are reacting to real-life, external, relevant stimuli and misinterpreting them as coming from their loved one.(44) For instance, the bereaved actually hear the sound of a someone coming up the staircase. For that split second, the sound of shoes upon the stairs prompts them to believe that the deceased is coming home from work. The bereaved didn't invent the sound in their mind. They heard a sound that in the past was linked to an action of the deceased and they are momentarily mistaken. They ultimately recognize their mistake and reconcile with the fact that the deceased is truly physically absent. By contrast, those who hallucinate truly believe that the deceased is present and cannot be convinced otherwise.

5.4 Similarities and Distinctions Between Acute Grief and Complicated Grief

Many of the symptoms of complicated grief overlap with those of normal acute grief.(41, 42) However, individuals who experience complicated grief are essentially reliving a heightened sense of mourning each day, every day.(6) By contrast, the symptoms for normal acute grief reduce in intensity and frequency over time. In other words, symptoms of acute grief abate, whereas symptoms of complicated grief perpetuate, if not intensify.

5.5 Similarities and Distinctions Between Complicated Grief and Depression

Many of the symptoms of complicated grief overlap with those for clinical depression(15, 17, 21, 41–43), but can be differentiated as follows:(6)

[Complicated grief] symptoms are strongly centered on the loss. For example, guilt is specifically related to letting the deceased down, whereas guilt in depression is pervasive and multifaceted. A grieving person maintains a sense of self-esteem and self-worth, whereas depressed people have lost faith in themselves. Additionally, grief symptoms not seen in major depression include intense yearning or longing for the deceased, strong wishes to be reunited with the lost loved one, a desire to feel close to

the deceased, intrusive or preoccupying thoughts of the deceased, and efforts to avoid reminders of the loss. People with [complicated grief] feel the world could be made right instantly by the reappearance of the deceased, whereas those with depression have no such illusions.

That being said, one can experience both complicated grief and depression, and concurrent depression will exacerbate symptoms of complicated grief.(6, 15)

5.6 The Health-Related Impacts of Complicated Grief on the Bereaved

Complicated grief is important to recognize by companions and professionals alike because the state of being puts the mourner at increased risk for:(15, 33, 52)

- sleep disorders(53)
- immune dysfunction
- hypertension
  - o older widows who experience complicated grief are ten times as likely to develop high blood pressure(35)
- social impairment
- occupational impairment
- cardiac events
- hospitalization
- neoplasia.

Complicated grief strains existing relationships between the bereaved and others that they love, further isolating them from their surroundings. This is just one of the many ways in which complicated grief is said to reduce quality of life.(25, 28, 33, 35, 54–56)

Individuals who experience complicated grief may lapse into destructive behavior.(33) They are at increased risk of substance abuse.(33) This risk is intensified if there is a family history of substance abuse.

5.7 Complicated Grief, Maladaptive Thoughts, and Risk of Death by Suicide

Individuals who experience complicated grief may also have maladaptive thoughts(15), including suicidal ideation.(33) They may share that there is no point in living without the deceased. They may openly express that they would be better off joining their loved one in death.

Although feeling hopeless and wanting their loved one back is normal for the bereaved to express in the early stages of acute grief, these feelings should not persist. There is a difference between saying, "I wish [name of loved one] were here" and "I wish that I could die to be with [name of loved one]." When conversations take the latter approach and consistently so, it is concerning.

Those who are experiencing acute grief do not actually want to die. What they are desiring and in fact hoping for is to be able to hit the imaginary "pause" button on life. It is "magical thinking" in the sense that they want life to "stop" – not forever, but momentarily, so they can catch a break, catch a breath, and adjust to the whirlwind changes that have overtaken their lives.

By contrast, those who are experiencing complicated grief may mean what they say, that they want to die. Companions of the bereaved and professionals alike must be prepared to ask follow-up questions to clarify meaning and intent.

It is important to be direct and not shy away from asking life-saving questions.

- "When you say that you want to die, what do you mean by that? Tell me more."
- "Are you thinking about hurting yourself?"
  - "How?"
  - "In what way?"
  - "Do you have a plan?"
- "Are you thinking about killing yourself?"(57)
- "Does it ever get so tough that you think about ending your life?"(57)
- "How often are you having these thoughts?"(57)
- "When it gets really bad, what do you do?"(57)
  - "What scares you about these thoughts?"(57)
  - "What do you need to do to feel safe?"(57)

Reflect aloud what you hear them say. Check for understanding.
Reassure them that they are heard.
Let them know that they are supported.
Consider sharing with them: "The fact that you're having these thoughts tells me something significant is going on for you right now. The good news is, help is out there. I want to help you get connected to resources that can help."(57)

Those who are experiencing complicated grief can feel as though they have been swallowed up by a huge hole.

They may be aware that they are sinking deeper and deeper into a hole from which they want to get out. They may not know how to articulate that or even where to begin. They may struggle with getting out of the hole on their own. They may struggle to ask for help.

Many who experience complicated grief know that something is wrong, but aren't aware of what until they are diagnosed.(58)

Sometimes those who experience complicated grief may not see themselves as needing help or being in crisis.

It is important that companions of the bereaved assess each situation individually and seek professional help for those in mourning as early as the need arises.

5.8 Risk Factors for Complicated Grief

Knowing the risk factors for complicated grief can be of assistance in terms of knowing when professional assistance is most often indicated.

Risk factors for complicated grief include:(6, 30, 33)

- age
  - adults aged 60 and older are at increased risk of experiencing spousal loss as well as the deaths of friends or non-spousal relatives(59–61)
  - one study reported that over a 2.5 year period, 70% of older participants experience bereavement(60)
- gender
  - those who identify as females are more likely than those who identify as males to experience complicated grief(21)
  - women who are 61 years of age or older experience complicated grief more than three times as often as younger adults(14)
- low level of education(21)
- low socioeconomic status(21)
- pre-existing mental health condition
- insomnia(37)
- pre-existing history of substance abuse
- history of abuse or betrayal by the deceased
- lack of a support system(21)
- multiple losses in a short period of time
- survivors of those who have died by suicide(37, 62)
- survivors of those who have died by homicide(63)

- survivors of those who have experienced accidental death(64)
- survivors of those who died in a natural disaster(16)
- those who have witnessed violent or traumatic death(64)
- those who have discovered the body in a case of traumatic death(65)
- those who have experienced the loss of a child
- childhood separation anxiety(37, 66)
- controlling parents(67)
- parental abuse or death(37, 68)
- a close kinship relationship to the deceased(62, 65, 69)
- insecure attachment styles(70)
- the death of a partner(39)
- marital supportiveness and dependency(37, 70, 71)
- extreme emotional dependency upon the deceased(21, 37, 72)
- lack of preparation for the death(73, 74).

Pre-existing spirituality prior to experiencing loss may be protective against developing complicated grief.(21, 75–77)

5.9 Supporting Those Who Experience Complicated Grief

Complicated grief is best addressed by seeking professional help. There is no shame in seeking assistance from those who have the training and expertise to companion those who are "stuck" and get them back on course.

Support for complicated grief begins with acknowledgment. In the words of Shear:(4) "We consider grief to be the form love takes when someone we love dies and we honor its myriad forms and waxing and waning intensity as it seeks its rightful place in a bereaved person's life."

To understand and work through complicated grief, one must put judgment aside. It is easy for an outsider looking in to presume to know where someone else should be in their respective grief journey.

It is the role of the trained professional to meet the bereaved where they are at and provide them with the tools that they need to accept their new reality.(4) Reality can be an enormously steep mountain to climb. To quote a widow who experienced the sudden death of her 71-year-old husband and companion of 40 years:(78)

Grief turns out to be a place none of us know until we reach it … Nor can we know ahead of the fact … the unending absence that follows, the void, the very opposite of meaning, the relentless succession of moments during which we will confront the experience of meaninglessness itself.

Grief is, to paraphrase this survivor's description, isolating and unfathomable. Those who experience complicated grief often feel alone.(4) It is a confusing experience that can exhaust the bereaved, who may already be overwhelmed by emotional dysregulation.(4)

The trained professional plays a supportive role in allowing the survivor to share their unique story of love and grief.(4) Their story, as only they can tell it, holds the key to them reimagining the future.(4)

References

1.   Humphrey KM. Counseling strategies for loss and grief. Vol. xv. Alexandria, VA: American Counseling Association; 2009.

2.   Wolfelt A. Understanding grief: helping yourself heal. Vol. xvi. Muncie, IN: Accelerated Development Inc; 1992.

3.   Parkes CM. The first year of bereavement. A longitudinal study of the reaction of London widows to the death of their husbands. Psychiatry. 1970;33(4):444–67. https://doi.org/10.1080/00332747.1970.11023644, PMID 5275840.

4.   Shear MK, Gribbin Bloom C. Complicated grief treatment: an evidence-based approach to grief therapy. J Rat-Emo Cognitive-Behav Ther. 2017;35(1):6–25. https://doi.org/10.1007/s10942-016-0242-2.

5.   Tyrrell P, Harberger S, Schoo C, Siddiqui W. Kubler-Ross stages of dying and subsequent models of grief. Treasure Island, FL: StatPearls; 2022.

6.   Shear MK. Grief and mourning gone awry: pathway and course of complicated grief. Dial Clin Neurosci. 2012;14(2):119–28. https://doi.org/10.31887/DCNS.2012.14.2/mshear, PMID 22754284.

7.   Fujiwara E, Levine B, Anderson AK. Intact implicit and reduced explicit memory for negative self-related information in repressive coping. Cogn Affect Behav Neurosci. 2008;8(3):254–63. https://doi.org/10.3758/cabn.8.3.254, PMID 18814462.

8.   Dillon DG, Ritchey M, Johnson BD, LaBar KS. Dissociable effects of conscious emotion regulation strategies on explicit and implicit memory. Emotion. 2007;7(2):354–65. https://doi.org/10.1037/1528-3542.7.2.354, PMID 1751 6813.

9.   Menon V, Boyett-Anderson JM, Schatzberg AF, Reiss AL. Relating semantic and episodic memory systems. Brain Res Cogn Brain Res. 2002;13(2):261–5. https://doi.org/10.1016/s0926-6410(01)00120-3, PMID 11958970.

10. Sakaki M, Gorlick MA, Mather M. Differential interference effects of negative emotional states on subsequent semantic and perceptual processing. Emotion. 2011;11(6):1263–78. https://doi.org/10.1037/a0026329, PMID 22142207.

11. Sakaki M. Semantic self-knowledge and episodic self-knowledge: independent or interrelated representations? Memory. 2007;15(1):1–16. https://doi.org/10.1080/09658210601055750, PMID 17479921.

12. Collins S. Mockingjay. New York: Scholastic Press; 2010.
13. Bonanno GA, Moskowitz JT, Papa A, Folkman S. Resilience to loss in bereaved spouses, bereaved parents, and bereaved gay men. J Pers Soc Psychol. 2005;88(5): 827–43. https://doi.org/10.1037/0022-3514.88.5.827, PMID 15898878.
14. Kersting A, Brähler E, Glaesmer H, Wagner B. Prevalence of complicated grief in a representative population-based sample. J Affect Disord. 2011;131(1–3):339–43. https://doi.org/10.1016/j.jad.2010.11.032, PMID 21216470.
15. Shear MK, Reynolds CF, 3rd, Simon NM, Zisook S, Wang Y, Mauro C, et al. Optimizing treatment of complicated grief: A randomized clinical trial. JAMA Psychiatry. 2016;73(7):685–94. https://doi.org/10.1001/jamapsychiatry.2016.0892, PMID 27276373.
16. Gesi C, Carmassi C, Cerveri G, Carpita B, Cremone IM, Dell'Osso L. Complicated grief: what to expect after the coronavirus pandemic. Front Psychiatry. 2020;11:489. https://doi.org/10.3389/fpsyt.2020.00489, PMID 32574243.
17. Rosner R, Pfoh G, Kotoučová M. Treatment of complicated grief. Eur J Psychotraumatol. 2011;2. https://doi.org/10.3402/ejpt.v2i0.7995, PMID 22893810.
18. Fujisawa D, Miyashita M, Nakajima S, Ito M, Kato M, Kim Y. Prevalence and determinants of complicated grief in general population. J Affect Disord. 2010; 127(1–3):352–8. https://doi.org/10.1016/j.jad.2010.06.008, PMID 20580096.
19. Maercker A, Znoj H. The younger sibling of PTSD: similarities and differences between complicated grief and posttraumatic stress disorder. Eur J Psychotraumatol. 2010;1. https://doi.org/10.3402/ejpt.v1i0.5558, PMID 22893801.
20. He L, Tang S, Yu W, Xu W, Xie Q, Wang J. The prevalence, comorbidity and risks of prolonged grief disorder among bereaved Chinese adults. Psychiatry Res. 2014;219(2):347–52. https://doi.org/10.1016/j.psychres.2014.05.022, PMID 24924526.
21. Shear MK, Ghesquiere A, Glickman K. Bereavement and complicated grief. Curr Psychiatry Rep. 2013;15(11):1–13. https://doi.org/10.1007/s11920-013-0406-z, PMID 24068457.
22. Prigerson HG, Maciejewski PK, Reynolds CF, 3rd, Bierhals AJ, Newsom JT, Fasiczka A, et al. Inventory of complicated grief: a scale to measure maladaptive symptoms of loss. Psychiatry Res. 1995;59(1–2):65–79. https://doi.org/10.1016/0165-1781(95)02757-2, PMID 8771222.
23. Dillen L, Fontaine JR, Verhofstadt-Denève L. Are normal and complicated grief different constructs? a confirmatory factor analytic test. Clin Psychol Psychother. 2008;15(6):386–95. https://doi.org/10.1002/cpp.590, PMID 19115457.
24. Boelen PA, van den Bout J. Complicated grief and uncomplicated grief are distinguishable constructs. Psychiatry Res. 2008;157(1–3):311–4. https://doi.org/10.1016/j. psychres.2007.05.013, PMID 17916387.
25. Prigerson HG, Frank E, Kasl SV, Reynolds CF, 3rd, Anderson B, Zubenko GS, et al. Complicated grief and bereavement-related depression as distinct disorders: preliminary empirical validation in elderly bereaved spouses. Am J Psychiatry. 1995;152(1):22–30. https://doi.org/10.1176/ajp.152.1.22, PMID 7802116.
26. Prigerson HG, Bierhals AJ, Kasl SV, Reynolds CF, 3rd, Shear MK, Newsom JT, et al. Complicated grief as a disorder distinct from bereavement-related depression and anxiety: a replication study. Am J Psychiatry. 1996;153(11):1484–6. https://doi. org/10.1176/ajp.153.11.1484, PMID 8890686.
27. Horowitz MJ, Siegel B, Holen A, Bonanno GA, Milbrath C, Stinson CH. Diagnostic criteria for complicated grief disorder. Am J Psychiatry. 1997;154(7):904–10. https:// doi.org/10.1176/ajp.154.7.904, PMID 9210739.

28. Latham AE, Prigerson HG. Suicidality and bereavement: complicated grief as psychiatric disorder presenting greatest risk for suicidality. Suicide Life Threat Behav. 2004;34(4):350–62. https://doi.org/10.1521/suli.34.4.350.53737, PMID 15585457.

29. Ogrodniczuk JS, Piper WE, Joyce AS, Weideman R, McCallum M, Azim HF, et al. Differentiating symptoms of complicated grief and depression among psychiatric outpatients. Can J Psychiatry. 2003;48(2):87–93. https://doi.org/10.1177/070674370304800204, PMID 12655905.

30. Simon NM. Treating complicated grief. JAMA. 2013;310(4):416–23. https://doi.org/10.1001/jama.2013.8614, PMID 23917292.

31. Simon NM, Pollack MH, Fischmann D, Perlman CA, Muriel AC, Moore CW, et al. Complicated grief and its correlates in patients with bipolar disorder. J Clin Psychiatry. 2005;66(9):1105–10. https://doi.org/10.4088/jcp.v66n0903, PMID 16187766.

32. Boelen PA, van den Bout J. Complicated grief, depression, and anxiety as distinct post-loss syndromes: a confirmatory factor analysis study. Am J Psychiatry. 2005;162(11):2175–7. https://doi.org/10.1176/appi.ajp.162.11.2175, PMID 16263861.

33. Prigerson HG, Horowitz MJ, Jacobs SC, Parkes CM, Aslan M, Goodkin K, et al. Prolonged grief disorder: psychometric validation of criteria proposed for DSM-V and ICD-11. PLOS Med. 2009;6(8):e1000121. https://doi.org/10.1371/journal.pmed.1000121, PMID 19652695.

34. Jacobs S. Traumatic grief: diagnosis, treatment, and prevention. Philadelphia: Taylor & Francis Group; 1999.

35. Prigerson HG, Bierhals AJ, Kasl SV, Reynolds CF, Shear MK, Day N et al. Traumatic grief as a risk factor for mental and physical morbidity. Am J Psychiatry. 1997;154(5):616–23. https://doi.org/10.1176/ajp.154.5.616, PMID 9137115.

36. Shear MK, Frank E, Foa E, Cherry C, Reynolds CF, 3rd, Vander Bilt J, et al. Traumatic grief treatment: a pilot study. Am J Psychiatry. 2001;158(9):1506–8. https://doi.org/10.1176/appi.ajp.158.9.1506, PMID 11532739.

37. Lobb EA, Kristjanson LJ, Aoun SM, Monterosso L, Halkett GK, Davies A. Predictors of complicated grief: a systematic review of empirical studies. Death Stud. 2010;34(8):673–98. https://doi.org/10.1080/07481187.2010.496686, PMID 24482845.

38. Lichtenthal WG, Cruess DG, Prigerson HG. A case for establishing complicated grief as a distinct mental disorder in DSM-V. Clin Psychol Rev. 2004;24(6):637–62. https://doi.org/10.1016/j.cpr.2004.07.002, PMID 15385092.

39. Shear MK. Clinical practice. Complicated grief. N Engl J Med. 2015;372(2):153–60. https://doi.org/10.1056/NEJMcp1315618, PMID 25564898.

40. Germain A, Caroff K, Buysse DJ, Shear MK. Sleep quality in complicated grief. J Trauma Stress. 2005;18(4):343–6. https://doi.org/10.1002/jts.20035, PMID 16281231.

41. Shear K, Shair H. Attachment, loss, and complicated grief. Dev Psychobiol. 2005;47(3):253–67. https://doi.org/10.1002/dev.20091, PMID 16252293.

42. Germain A, Shear KM, Walsh C, Buysse DJ, Monk TH, Reynolds CF, 3rd, et al. Dream content in complicated grief: a window into loss-related cognitive schemas. Death Stud. 2013;37(3):269–84. https://doi.org/10.1080/07481187.2011.641138, PMID 24524436.

43. Maccallum F, Bryant RA. Imaging the future in complicated grief. Depress Anxiety. 2011;28(8):658–65. https://doi.org/10.1002/da.20866, PMID 21796741.

44. White C, Fessler DMT. An evolutionary account of vigilance in grief. Evol Med Public Health. 2018;2018(1):34–42. https://doi.org/10.1093/emph/eox018, PMID 29492265.

45. Maciejewski PK, Zhang B, Block SD, Prigerson HG. An empirical examination of the stage theory of grief. JAMA. 2007;297(7):716–23. https://doi.org/10.1001/jama.297.7.716, PMID 17312291.

46. Archer J, Winchester G. Bereavement following death of a pet. Br J Psychol. 1994;85(2):259–71. https://doi.org/10.1111/j.2044-8295.1994.tb02522.x, PMID 8032709.

47. Glick IO, Weiss RS, Parkes CM. The first year of bereavement. Vol. xvii. New York: Wiley; 1974.

48. Olson PR, Suddeth JA, Peterson PJ, Egelhoff C. Hallucinations of widowhood. J Am Geriatr Soc. 1985;33(8):543–7. https://doi.org/10.1111/j.1532-5415.1985. tb04619.x, PMID 4020000.

49. Dewi Rees W. The hallucinations of widowhood. Br Med J. 1971;4(5778):37–41. https://doi.org/10.1136/bmj.4.5778.37, PMID 5096884.

50. Castelnovo A, Cavallotti S, Gambini O, D'Agostino A. Post-bereavement hallucinatory experiences: A critical overview of population and clinical studies. J Affect Disord. 2015;186:266–74. https://doi.org/10.1016/j.jad.2015.07.032, PMID 26254619.

51. Silverman PS, Worden JW. Children's reactions to the death of a parent. In: Stroebe MS, Stroehe W, Hansson RO, editors. Handbook of bereavement: theory, research, and intervention. Cambridge University Press; 1993. p. 300–29.

52. Wittouck C, Van Autreve S, De Jaegere E, Portzky G, van Heeringen K. The prevention and treatment of complicated grief: a meta-analysis. Clin Psychol Rev. 2011;31(1):69–78. https://doi.org/10.1016/j.cpr.2010.09.005, PMID 21130937.

53. Szanto K, Prigerson H, Houck P, Ehrenpreis L, Reynolds CF, 3rd. Suicidal ideation in elderly bereaved: the role of complicated grief. Suicide Life Threat Behav. 1997;27(2):194–207. PMID 9260302.

54. Prigerson HG, Bridge J, Maciejewski PK, Beery LC, Rosenheck RA, Jacobs SC, et al. Influence of traumatic grief on suicidal ideation among young adults. Am J Psychiatry. 1999;156(12):1994–5. https://doi.org/10.1176/ajp.156.12.1994, PMID 10588419.

55. Jacobsen J, Vanderwerker L, Block SD, Friedlander R, Maciejewski PK, Prigerson H. Depression and demoralization as distinct syndromes: preliminary data from a cohort of advanced cancer patients. Indian J Palliat Care. 2006;12(1):8–15. https://doi.org/10.4103/0973-1075.25913.

56. Silverman GK, Jacobs SC, Kasl SV, Shear MK, Maciejewski PK, Noaghiul FS, et al. Quality of life impairments associated with diagnostic criteria for traumatic grief. Psychol Med. 2000;30(4):857–62. https://doi.org/10.1017/s0033291799002524, PMID 11037094.

57. I'm right here with you. American Foundation for Suicide Prevention (AFSP); 2022. Available from: https://afsp.org/story/if-someone-tells-you-they-re-thinking-about-sui cide-a-realconvo-guide-from-afsp.

58. Johnson JG, First MB, Block S, Vanderwerker LC, Zivin K, Zhang B, et al. Stigmatization and receptivity to mental health services among recently bereaved adults. Death Stud. 2009;33(8):691–711. https://doi.org/10.1080/07481180903070392, PMID 19697482.

59. Williams BR, Baker PS, Allman RM. Nonspousal family loss among community-dwelling older adults. Omega (Westport). 2005;51(2):125–42. https://doi.org/10.2190/BUBQ-J0VP-EVPW-V95V.

60. Williams BR, Sawyer Baker P, Allman RM, Roseman JM. Bereavement among African American and White older adults. J Aging Health. 2007;19(2):313–33. https://doi.org/10.1177/0898264307299301, PMID 17413138.

61. Newson RS, Boelen PA, Hek K, Hofman A, Tiemeier H. The prevalence and characteristics of complicated grief in older adults. J Affect Disord. 2011;132(1–2):231–8. https://doi.org/10.1016/j.jad.2011.02.021, PMID 21397336.

62. Mitchell AM, Kim Y, Prigerson HG, Mortimer-Stephens M. Complicated grief in survivors of suicide. Crisis. 2004;25(1):12–18. https://doi.org/10.1027/0227-5910.25.1.12, PMID 15384652.

63. van Denderen M, de Keijser J, Kleen M, Boelen PA. Psychopathology among homicidally bereaved individuals: a systematic review. Trauma Violence Abuse. 2015;16(1):70–80. https://doi.org/10.1177/1524838013515757. PMID 24346707.

64. Nakajima S, Ito M, Shirai A, Konishi T. Complicated grief in those bereaved by violent death: the effects of post-traumatic stress disorder on complicated grief. Dialogues Clin Neurosci. 2012;14(2):210–4. https://doi.org/10.31887/DCNS.2012.14.2/snakajima, PMID 22754294.

65. Crunk AE, Burke LA, Robinson EHM. Complicated grief: an evolving theoretical landscape. J Couns Dev. 2017;95(2):226–33. https://doi.org/10.1002/jcad.12134.

66. Vanderwerker LC, Jacobs SC, Parkes CM, Prigerson HG. An exploration of associations between separation anxiety in childhood and complicated grief in later life. J Nerv Ment Dis. 2006;194(2):121–3. https://doi.org/10.1097/01.nmd.0000198146.28182.d5, PMID 16477190.

67. Johnson JG, Zhang B, Greer JA, Prigerson HG. Parental control, partner dependency, and complicated grief among widowed adults in the community. J Nerv Ment Dis. 2007;195(1):26–30. https://doi.org/10.1097/01.nmd.0000252009.45915.b2, PMID 17220736.

68. Silverman GK, Johnson JG, Prigerson HG. Preliminary explorations of the effects of prior trauma and loss on risk for psychiatric disorders in recently widowed people. Isr J Psychiatry Relat Sci. 2001;38(3–4):202–15. PMID 11725418.

69. Cleiren M, Diekstra RF, Kerkhof AJ, van der Wal J. Mode of death and kinship in bereavement: focusing on "who" rather than "how". Crisis. 1994;15(1):22–36. PMID 8062585.

70. van Doorn C, Kasl SV, Beery LC, Jacobs SC, Prigerson HG. The influence of marital quality and attachment styles on traumatic grief and depressive symptoms. J Nerv Ment Dis. 1998;186(9):566–73. https://doi.org/10.1097/00005053-199809000-00008, PMID 9741563.

71. Johnson JG, Vanderwerker LC, Bornstein RF, Zhang B, Prigerson HG. Development and validation of an instrument for the assessment of dependency among bereaved persons. J Psychopathol Behav Assess. 2006;28(1):1–8.

72. Denckla CA, Mancini AD, Bornstein RF, Bonanno GA. Adaptive and maladaptive dependency in bereavement: distinguishing prolonged and resolved grief trajectories. Pers Individ Dif. 2011;51(8):1012–7. https://doi.org/10.1016/j.paid.2011.08.014, PMID 21984858.

73. Barry LC, Kasl SV, Prigerson HG. Psychiatric disorders among bereaved persons: the role of perceived circumstances of death and preparedness for death. Am J Geriatr

Psychiatry. 2002;10(4):447–57. https://doi.org/10.1097/00019442-200207000-00011, PMID 12095904.

74. Hebert RS, Dang Q, Schulz R. Preparedness for the death of a loved one and mental health in bereaved caregivers of patients with dementia: findings from the REACH study. J Palliat Med. 2006;9(3):683–93. https://doi.org/10.1089/jpm.2006.9.683, PMID 16752974.

75. Schaal S, Jacob N, Dusingizemungu JP, Elbert T. Rates and risks for prolonged grief disorder in a sample of orphaned and widowed genocide survivors. BMC Psychiatry. 2010;10:55. https://doi.org/10.1186/1471-244X-10-55, PMID 20604936.

76. Seirmarco G, Neria Y, Insel B, Kiper D, Doruk A, Gross R et al. Religiosity and mental health: changes in religious beliefs, complicated grief, posttraumatic stress disorder, and major depression following the September 11, 2001 attacks. Psychology of Religion and Spirituality;4(1):10–8. https://doi.org/10.1037/a0023479.

77. Chiu YW, Huang CT, Yin SM, Huang YC, Chien CH, Chuang HY. Determinants of complicated grief in caregivers who cared for terminal cancer patients. Support Care Cancer. 2010;18(10):1321–7. https://doi.org/10.1007/s00520-009-0756-6, PMID 19816716.

78. Didion J. The year of magical thinking. 1st ed. New York: A. A. Knopf; 2005.

CHAPTER 6

Disenfranchised Grief

The Invisible Wound

"There is no grief like the grief that does not speak."
—*Henry Wadsworth Longfellow*

Twelve weeks before writing this textbook, I unexpectedly sustained significant orthopedic trauma to my right knee. The inciting event had in fact occurred months prior, with the degree of damage unbeknownst to me. That single domino set into motion a chain reaction for which there could be only one end to the story: my right knee fell apart during a basic backstep action in foxtrot, and I collapsed into my dance instructor's frame.

There was nothing that anyone could have done to have prevented it.

I didn't trip or slip. No one saw it coming. My knee just gave out beneath me. And in the blink of an eye, the world as I knew it changed.

The weeks that followed were a blur of doctor's appointments and a constellation of diagnostic imaging tests that culminated in the telephone conversation that no competitive dancer wants to hear: "you need surgery."

Surgery meant that I was effectively benched. *Indefinitely.*

Surgery meant appreciable time away from the sport that I was passionate about outside of the office.

We weren't talking about an absence on the order of days or weeks. We were talking months, if not years. And, at a time in my life when dance was the only thing outside of my profession that defined me, months felt like a lifetime.

The irony is that dance had not always been a part of my life. As a child, I practically kicked myself out of ballet.

I hadn't known then that performing arts would change the lens through which I saw myself.

I hadn't known then that I would dream of tango in the middle of the night.

I hadn't known then that I would practice my dance routines in the hallway on the way to teach class; that I would spend the better part of a decade training in the art of ballroom; and that I would develop sufficient skill to qualify for finals in the Pro-Am division of my sport.

I hadn't known then that I would fall in love with something other than medicine.

When my instructor, Lowell Fox, joined Arrowhead Arthur Murray and became my permanent instructor in July 2014, he built me as a dancer from the ground up. He accepted me for who I was and, in an uncanny sort of way, knew who I would become.

Under Lowell's tutelage, I grew immensely. I learned that dance wasn't just about the steps, I had to feel the music, and develop trust.

There was surprising peace in surrendering, that is, learning how to close my eyes and listen to the rhythmic language of body movement rather than words.

I learned that I could be good at something other than science, and that work ethic mattered more than raw talent. If I wanted something badly enough and if I worked at something hard enough, I could achieve it.

In those early years, dance was a constant opportunity to face my fears. I was insecure and worried … about *everything*. I worried that I wasn't "good enough," "athletic enough," or "strong enough." I worried about body image. I didn't look like what I thought a dancer was supposed to look like. I was curvy, not slender. I had thick legs. I worried that I wasn't "small enough."

Nail by nail, board by board, dance rebuilt my foundation with a sturdier base of growing confidence that I needed to take flight. I learned to believe in me, through my dance, because – for starters – Lowell did.

He taught me that it was okay to try and fail, as long as you gave it your all and tried again.

I learned that it was okay to fall and that everyone does. The problem was that this time I couldn't get back up. I didn't know how.

Overnight, I went from competing to watching from the sidelines.

I went from refining our open choreography to learning a bench routine.

I went from making the two-and-a-half-hour commute from home base Tucson to the Peoria studio, and back again, every Saturday, to not being able to drive at all.

I went from being a 39-year-old single, independent, professional woman to someone who, post-operatively, couldn't even put on socks.

I was surrounded by the love of family during this critical transitional period in my life and by my determined coach, Lowell, who never gave up on me. I enrolled in physical therapy and established a strong connection to an entire healthcare team that was committed to my recovery, meaning my re-entry into everyday living.

Despite this forward push, I felt frustrated in those early weeks after surgery.

I didn't know how to articulate the losses that I was experiencing so acutely.

I just knew that there were many:

- loss of independence
- loss of the use of and sensation of a limb
- loss of mobility
- loss of exercise as an outlet
- loss of the competitive nature of the sport
- loss of my dance "team"
- loss of how I defined myself.

And even though those losses were said to be transient, there was a gnawing sensation inside of me: *what if they weren't?*

When I tried to be open about my feelings and express those fears to anyone outside of my immediate circle, I was met with resistance. I was told that I should be "grateful" because:

- "It could have been a lot worse."
- "You still have two legs."
- "You didn't lose your leg."
- "At least it is operable."
- "At least you'll be able to walk again."

Several friends shared that their dog had endured the "same surgery" and they were "just fine."

When I expressed my fear of never being able to dance again, to anyone other than Lowell, I was told by most that I should be "happy" because I had gotten "eight good years in."

I allowed those words to sink into my core. They made me feel greedy or selfish to ask for more.

When I expressed my fear of not being able to visit the distant studio until spring of the following year, to anyone other than Lowell, I was told that "next year isn't that far away" and "not to push" myself, because there will always be "some other event" to spectate.

My concept of time did not align with theirs. Next year felt like a lifetime for someone who had not even stepped away from dance during the height of the COVID pandemic.

As for the concept of "some other event," I couldn't track that far ahead. All I could see was what I was missing out on *now*.

What I was expressing in my brief exchanges with others was grief. Based upon Worden's definition, change equals loss, and loss equals grief.(1)

My acute grief was not recognized as such. In fact, it was discounted by others because my grief did not fit the classic mold. What I experienced nonetheless was a type of grief, what bereavement experts refer to as being *disenfranchised* grief.

6.1 Introducing the Concept of Disenfranchised Grief

Disenfranchised grief refers to loss that is not "openly acknowledged, socially validated or publically [sic] mourned."(1)

Every culture, religion, community, and society frames grief in accordance with a set of norms that dictate who and what we grieve.(2) Societal norms dictate which losses are significant and which are not.(2)

Grieving the death of family members is universally acceptable.(1) Yet, not all deaths involve family members, and not all losses involve death.(1, 3)

One may grieve secondary losses, for instance, losses that are associated with transitional periods in one's life:(1, 4)

- moving out of state
- moving to a new school
- the end of childhood
- the end of a relationship
- the end of college
- the end of an internship
- the end of a residency
- the end of employment.

One may grieve the loss of a place and the meaning that we have ascribed to it. Alex Gitterman explains that:(4)

Akin to developing emotional bonds with people, we develop attachments towards places that are significant to us. We interact with places; we develop identification with places; we often describe ourselves as "belonging" to these places.(5) An attachment to a meaningful place "is a universal affective tie that fulfills fundamental human needs".(6) The attachment to a place helps us develop and maintain our self-identity and sense of well-being.

What Gitterman highlights is likely one of the primary reasons that Miranda Lambert's "The House That Built Me" was her fastest-rising single at that time in her career. Lambert's lyrics remind us how intimately our childhood home is tied to sense of self. On the outside, it may be just a residence, but on the inside, it provided the earliest foundation for our identity to develop and blossom. It's where we once belonged. It's where we came to know ourselves best.

Lambert sings that:(7)

I know they say you can't go home again.
I just had to come back one last time.
Ma'am, I know you don't know me from Adam,
But these hand prints on the front steps are mine.

Up those stairs in that little back bedroom
Is where I did my homework and I learned to play guitar,
And I bet you didn't know under that live oak
My favorite dog is buried in the yard.

I thought if I could touch this place or feel it
This brokenness inside me might start healing.
Out here, it's like I'm someone else.
I thought that maybe I could find myself.

If I could just come in, I swear I'll leave,
Won't take nothin' but a memory
From the house that built me.

Through these lyrics, Lambert expresses the innate desire to find herself again within her childhood home. It is as though the home's memory is self-sustaining and will give her back what she is searching for, but cannot find, in the grown-up world.

Gitterman shares that it is not unusual to bond with a safe space:(4)

Children's developmental task of learning to trust, for example, is based on the
security of stable physical arrangements, as well as on secure relationships.
Children refer to my toys, my clothes, my room, my house, my playground, and my
neighborhood and view these as extensions of themselves.(8)

Gitterman adds that:(4)

We develop and become embedded in the physical as well as social connections that
accrue from living in the same place over time. Therefore, the absence of familiar and

cherished places and structures that comforted us and has been part of our individual and group identities leaves us with feelings of grief associated with being uprooted and adrift.

In addition to grieving for the loss of place and the comfort that such a place has afforded, we may grieve in anticipation of the loss of something or someone.(1) For example, caregivers of those with terminal disease grieve that the death of someone they love is impending, even if that day is weeks, months, or years away.(1)

As a second example, owners of geriatric pets may experience anticipatory grief because they are increasingly aware, acutely so, that their loved one will not live forever. I felt this way myself, having never owned a cat that lived beyond the age of 15 until champagne mink Tonkinese cat Bailey came into my world.

There are cats, and then there are *cats*.

Bailey was *mine* in a way that is simultaneously indescribable and irreplaceable. Every birthday that passed (her 16th, her penultimate 17th, and her finale year, the 18th), I held my breath because I knew that it could be her last.

As she aged, I grew acutely aware that time was not on our side. In advance of her passing, I anticipated what life would be like without her at my side. I mourned the loss before it hit because I knew that it was coming.

The aforementioned losses – losses associated with transitions, spaces, places, and anticipatory grief – are outside of the typical lens through which societies view grief and grieving, death and dying.(2) Because of this, such losses may not be acknowledged, discussed, affirmed, or validated.(2)

Losses often go unvoiced and/or unheard. Expressions of loss may even be actively silenced by people and communities that cannot accept or even relate to these unique experiences of the bereaved.

When one's grief is not embraced or even acknowledged by others as being valid, that grief becomes internalized.(2) Internalized grief is a risk factor for the development of complicated grief.(2, 9) When grief becomes complicated, it is not resolved(10) and bereavement intensifies rather than abates.(2)

6.2 Examples of Disenfranchised Grief

There are many types of disenfranchised grief.(2) Disenfranchised grief occurs when:(2, 11–13)

- the loss is not recognized
  - death of a pet(14, 15)
  - a pet runs away and is never found
  - relinquishment of a pet to a shelter
  - estrangement from family
  - estrangement from friends
  - orphan status (as an adult), meaning that the grown-up child has experienced the loss of their parent(s)
  - loss of lifestyle
  - loss of home; housing insecurity(16)
  - loss of culture(17)
  - being on the "losing" side in a war
  - loss of homeland(18)
  - chronic illness(19)
  - transplant failure(20)
  - traumatic brain injury(19)
    - diminished cognitive processing
    - communication barriers
    - personality changes
  - loss of memory(19)
  - loss of sight
  - loss of hearing
  - loss of mobility
  - loss of independence
  - unintended childlessness
    - e.g., "women who are 'contingently childless'; that is women who have always seen themselves as having children but find themselves at the end of their natural fertility without having done so for social rather than (at least initially) biological reasons."(21)
  - loss of desired birth plan(22)
    - e.g., having to flex from natural childbirth to caesarean section
  - loss of relationship(19, 23, 24)
  - loss of marriage(19)
  - loss of innocence, as experienced by victims of abuse(19)
  - symbolic losses(19)
    - loss of self
    - loss of identity
    - loss of hope
    - loss of aspirations
  - infertility
  - giving up a baby to adoption(25)

- o ectopic pregnancy(26)
- o miscarriage(26, 27)
- o stillbirth(28)
- o perinatal death(26, 29)
- o abortion
- either the relationship or the magnitude of the relationship is not recognized
  - o grieving someone you don't know
  - o grieving your patient(30–33)
    - grief among human and veterinary healthcare workers is often disenfranchised, particularly in the field of hospice
    - hospice workers may form emotional attachments to their patients, even though they are terminally ill(34)
    - when patients die, hospice workers' grief is often overlooked because society sees them as having just done their job when in fact workers can be grievers, too(35–37)
  - o grieving someone you haven't talked to for years
  - o grieving someone you never knew (e.g., your parent died prior to or at birth)
  - o grieving someone who died before you were born (e.g., a sibling died prior to your birth)
  - o the loss of a birth parent that you never knew
  - o the loss of a foster child
  - o the loss of a foster parent
  - o the loss of a stepchild
  - o the loss of a stepparent
  - o the loss of a co-worker
  - o death of a therapist
  - o same-sex partners(9, 38–44)
    - not having one's partner recognized at all
    - being told that one's partner was "just a friend"(45)
  - o non-binary partners(43)
  - o members of LGBTQIA+ who may or may not be "out" and may or may not feel safe expressing their grief(43, 46)
  - o polyamorous partners who still are connected to one or more living partners, but lost someone they loved that others in their lives may or may not know about(43)
  - o aromantic or asexual life partners(43)
  - o unmarried life partners
  - o partners involved in extra-marital affairs or other forms of cheating
  - o ex-partners

- o those who co-parent, but are no longer spouses
  - o casual partners ("friends with benefits")
- the griever is excluded from bereavement; society presumes that they are unable to grieve because they lack the capacity to understand death(47)
  - o children
  - o the elderly
  - o those experiencing mental health crises
  - o those with developmental disabilities
- the circumstances surrounding loss carry stigma
  - o incarceration of a loved one
  - o death by suicide
  - o death by drunk driving
  - o death by drug overdose
  - o death by AIDS(45, 48, 49)
  - o death by COVID(50)
    - misconceptions surrounding spread of infection
    - fear of contracting the disease
    - enforced social distancing and emotional isolation
    - restricted visitation to hospitals, including intensive care units
    - curtailed mourning rituals
      - □ lack of in-person funerals
      - □ transition to live streaming of funerals
  - o death by execution (51)
- the coping methods that are employed are perceived as inappropriate
  - o no expression of emotion
  - o "excessive" expression of emotion.

6.3 Hierarchy of Loss

Disenfranchised grief often exists because there is a spoken or unspoken ladder of loss within families, religions, cultures, societies, and communities. This so-called "hierarchy of loss" was studied extensively by Robson and influences the following:(52)

- Who is granted bereavement ("compassionate") leave?
  - o For whose death is it acceptable to take time off from work?
  - o For whose death is it not?
- Who is allowed to mourn and to what degree?
- Who is expected to attend the funeral?
- Who is allowed to deliver the eulogy?
- Who is allowed to design the memorial stone?

- Who is allowed to keep the belongings and/or the ashes of the deceased?

Societal norms dictate who is allowed to mourn whom and to what degree. Littlewood describes this hierarchy as follows:(53)

- chief mourners
- the lesser mourners.

Littlewood describes chief mourners as having:(53)

> *Few obligations other than to mourn ... This person ... also acted as an agent of the dead person, speaking, as it were, on their behalf [and] it was not seen to be appropriate to question this person's interpretation of the dead person's wishes. The majority of offers of support, condolences and practical help were directed towards chief mourners – presumably in the belief that this person would require the most support.*

Chief mourners – spouses and dependent children – receive their status primarily through inheritance law in Western societies.(52, 54) This is reinforced by etiquette – reserving the front rows at funerals for the immediate family of the bereaved. Chief mourners are also honored by Human Resources (HR) policies at most companies.(52, 55, 56)

Bento shares that:(57)

> *Organizations ... allow people a few days to deal with the death of loved ones, according to a sliding scale of love: so many days for a spouse, a child, a parent, a friend. Then the telegrams, cards, flowers and donations to favourite charities are over. An awkward pat on the back, and the bereaved worker is expected to "get over" it. The show must go on. And it does – but not always, or not as expected.*

In an age where traditional relationships are not necessarily the norm, and both divorce and remarriage are commonplace, the increasing complexities of family dynamics may call into question who is entitled by society to mourn more.

The bereaved may compete for "chief mourner status."(52) Littlewood shares that:(53)

> *Whilst on the surface such disputes might appear petty and ungenerous in spirit they undoubtedly reflected deeper and more central preoccupations ... i.e. that of exclusive possession of the memory of the dead person ... The position of chief mourner became vitally important in terms of the access it gave to the holder effectively to speak on*

behalf of the dead person, i.e. it gave them literally, as well as figuratively the last word.

Robson adds that:(52) "In sports games, the aim is to win; either you win, or you are one of the losers (an either/or result). In mourning, there may be competition for chief mourner status, but that does not mean all 'losers' are equal."

Spoken or unspoken, conscious or subconscious competitions between mourners set the stage for unhealthy, hurtful comparisons. If one person is presumed to be entitled to grieve more, then one person is presumed to grieve less.

Grief is in and of itself not a competition. Yet, when society sets it up to be, the only gain is that grief is honored for some while disenfranchised for others. "Lesser mourners" – stepchildren, stepparents, foster parents, ex-spouses, ex-partners, friends, work colleagues, health care professionals, nursing home staff, and pet owners – are likely to find that their losses are discounted.(1, 11, 52, 58, 59)

Today's society continues to privilege "nuclear family relationships, in life as well as in death, to the exclusion of attachments based on extended family or community."(52) In spite of this, grief remains a social construct that is bound to change with the times. Robson explains that:(52) "With the increasing importance of friendship alongside family in modern western societies, and the fluidity of friendship in contrast to the more formal structures of family relationships, it seems inevitable that there will be considerable variation in how the grief of friends is socially assessed."

Robson suspects that one day intimacy rather than traditional family-based hierarchies will determine who is "allowed" to grieve, for whom, and for how long.

Until then, mismatches continue to be perpetuated between the grief that is expected by society and the grief that is experienced.(52) Disenfranchised grief occurs when the latter exceeds the former.

6.4 The Words and Actions Underlying Disenfranchised Grief

Grief may become disenfranchised through words or actions.(13) Companions of the bereaved may actually call out those who are grieving on the grounds that their thoughts, feelings, and/or behaviors are inappropriate.(12, 13) The bereaved may be told that they are "taking too long" or that they need to "hurry up" and "move on."(12, 13)

In some cases, the bereaved may be told to truncate their period of mourning because it is "unnecessary" or "unhealthy" or their loved one would not "approve."(12, 13) They may be told to "count their blessings" or "stop crying." Not everyone is as direct in their communication; however, the bereaved will pick up on hints that they are not fitting in.

The burden is placed on the bereaved to change their ways if they want companionship. Those who disenfranchise grief act as though it is possible to "short-circuit reflexes" that accompany bereavement because, in their minds, there is not an "acceptable" reason to grieve.(12, 13) This presents a challenge because the bereaved cannot just turn off sadness and tears in the same way that one can turn off a faucet.

6.5 The Feelings Associated with Disenfranchised Grief

Those whose grief is disenfranchised often experience one or more of the following physical or emotional reactions:(15, 29, 49, 51, 60–62)

- shock
- sadness
- loneliness
- frustration
- depression
- devastation
- anger
- resentment
- generalized pain
- feeling isolated
- feeling abandoned.

Those experiencing disenfranchised grief want to be heard; they often feel misunderstood. Most of all, they desire the right to grieve.(13)

6.6 The Impact of Disenfranchised Grief

Having one's grief discounted is impactful. The bereaved may feel that they are forced to return to "normal" when they no longer know what "normal" is. Moreover, others' dismissive reactions towards their state of being perpetuates and reinforces their sense of isolation. Those who grieve may feel that they must "fake it until they make it" or play along if they are to ever fit back into the fold.

Those who companion others through grief may intentionally try to rush those who are grieving along. Some companions may feel that they are helping the bereaved to assimilate so that they no longer "stand out."

Others may not be aware of their impact. What these individuals need to recognize is that disenfranchising is "not simply a matter of indifference to the experiences and efforts of the bereaved. It is more actively negative and destructive as it involves denial of entitlement, interference, and even imposition of sanction."(13)

In the words of Attig: "Disenfranchising messages actively discount, dismiss, disapprove, discourage, invalidate, and delegitimate the experiences and efforts of grieving. And disenfranchising behaviors interfere with the exercise of the right to grieve by withholding permission, disallowing, constraining, hindering, and even prohibiting it."(13)

Disenfranchisement is, at its core, a failure of empathy.(13, 63) Those who engage in this behavior cannot even begin to perceive of a grief that they have never known. Because they themselves have never experienced it, they are unable to comprehend the depth of loss. Their struggle to relate to the mourner challenges their ability to offer support. Their default "support" is a verbal attempt or non-verbal cue to shut down grief, thinking that if they just don't talk about grief, it will go away.

6.7 Coping with Disenfranchised Grief

Rituals are one of the many ways in which survivors cope with grief.(1, 2, 11) Ceremonies such as funerals acknowledge and honor the loss. They cement the reality that loss happened and is permanent.(1, 2, 11, 12) They embrace survivors in togetherness by bringing people together in a way that inspires ongoing living.(1, 2, 11, 12)

According to Mortell:(2)

Because disenfranchised loss is often associated with secrecy and shame, a ritual surrounding such losses may be unheard of. For example, one would not ordinarily hold a ritual around losing a job, home, or marriage. Yet, the absence of the public acknowledgement and support around such events, as is felt through ritual, may add to the difficulties that individuals face as they try to process these losses.

Mourners often struggle. They may want to express their grief openly but feel that such outward displays of emotion are not construed as appropriate or welcomed by society. In those circumstances, it may be helpful for mourners to create opportunities to experience ritual their own way. Because meaning-making is at the core of these actions, they should be tailored to meet the individual mourner's needs, wants, and expectations. They must find what's "right" for them.

One or more of the following activities may be helpful in taking the first steps towards acknowledging and affirming one's grief, even when others do not:

- journaling
- letter writing
- writing poetry
- lighting a candle
- getting a memorial tattoo
- reading a meaningful quote or verse
- creating a memorial garden
- planting a tree of remembrance
- naming a star after a loved one
- creating a playlist in honor of the deceased
- creating a memory box or photo collage
- creating a memorial wreath
- commemorating a special date, anniversary, or event
- connecting with a therapist or a support group
- art, music, dance, or movement therapy(30, 49)
- letting go of a linking object as a means of therapeutic release
- creating a sanctuary where the loved one can be remembered
- cleansing a sacred space with sage, cedar, lavender, or an herb of choice.

References

1. Doka K. Disenfranchised grief: recognizing hidden sorrow. Lexington, MA: Lexingon Books; 1989.
2. Mortell S. Assisting clients with disenfranchised grief: the role of a mental health nurse. J Psychosoc Nurs Ment Health Serv. 2015;53(4):52–7. https://doi.org/10.3928/02793695-20150319-05, PMID 25856812.
3. Harris D. Non-death loss and grief: context and clinical implications. 1st ed. New York: Routledge; 2019.
4. Gitterman A, Knight C. Non-death loss: grieving for the loss of familiar place and for precious time and associated opportunities. Clin Soc Work J. 2019;47(2):147–55. https://doi.org/10.1007/s10615-018-0682-5.
5. Stedman RC. Toward a social psychology of place: predicting behavior from place-based cognitions, attitude, and identity. Environ Behav. 2002;34(5):561–81. https://doi.org/10.1177/0013916502034005001.

6. Scannell LG, Gifford R. Defining place attachment: a tripartite organizing framework. J Environ Psychol. 2010;30(1):1–10. https://doi.org/10.1016/j.jenvp.200 9.09.006.

7. Lambert M. Revolution [sound recording]. Nashville, TN; New York: Columbia Nashville; distributed in the USA by Sony Music Entertainment; 2009.

8. Nicotera N. The child's view of neighborhood: assessing a neglected element in direct social work practice. J Hum Behav Soc Environ. 2005;11(3–4):105–33. https://doi.org/10.1300/J137v11n03_06.

9. McNutt B, Yakushko O. Disenfranchised grief among lesbian and gay bereaved individuals. J LGBT Issues Couns. 2013;7(1):87–116. https://doi.org/10.1080/1553860 5.2013.758345.

10. Fujisawa D, Miyashita M, Nakajima S, Ito M, Kato M, Kim Y. Prevalence and determinants of complicated grief in general population. J Affect Disord. 2010; 127(1–3):352–8. https://doi.org/10.1016/j.jad.2010.06.008, PMID 20580096.

11. Doka KJ. Disenfranchised grief: new directions, challenges, and strategies for practice. Vol. xviii. Champaign, IL: Research Press; 2002.

12. Corr CA. Revisiting the concept of disenfranchised grief. In: Doka KJ, editor. Disenfranchised grief: new directions, challenges, and strategies for practice. Champaign, IL: Research Press; 2002. p. 39–60.

13. Attig T. Disenfranchised grief revisited: discounting hope and love. Omega. 2004;49(3):197–215. https://doi.org/10.2190/P4TT-J3BF-KFDR-5JB1.

14. Cordaro M. Pet loss and disenfranchised grief: implications for mental health counseling practice. J Ment Health Couns. 2012;34(4):283–94. https://doi.org/10.17744/mehc.34.4.41q0248450t98072.

15. Packman W, Carmack BJ, Katz R, Carlos F, Field NP, Landers C. Online survey as empathic bridging for the disenfranchised grief of pet loss. Omega. 2014;69(4): 333–56. https://doi.org/10.2190/OM.69.4.a, PMID 25304868.

16. Burns VF, Sussman T, Bourgeois-Guérin V. Later-life homelessness as disenfranchised grief. Can J Aging. 2018;37(2):171–84. https://doi.org/10.1017/S0714980818000090, PMID 29606165.

17. Ramirez S. Wailing for my cultura: disenfranchised grief among Mexican Americans navigating A bicultural identity. University of Texas at El Paso; 2021.

18. Lester JC. Strangers in their own land: culture loss, disenfranchised grief, and reentry adjustment. Antioch University; 2000.

19. Flynn A. Disenfranchised grief in response to non-death loss events. Humboldt State University; 2015.

20. Gill P, Lowes L. Renal transplant failure and disenfranchised grief: participants' experiences in the first year post-graft failure–a qualitative longitudinal study. Int J Nurs Stud. 2014;51(9):1271–80. https://doi.org/10.1016/j.ijnurstu.2014.01.012, PMID 24560891.

21. Tonkin L. Making sense of loss: the disenfranchised grief of women who are "contingently childless". J Motherhood Initiat;1(2):177–87.

22. DeGroot JM, Vik TA. Disenfranchised grief following a traumatic birth. J Loss Trauma. 2017;22(4):346–56. https://doi.org/10.1080/15325024.2017.1284519.

23. Kaczmarek MG, Backlund BA. Disenfranchised grief: the loss of an adolescent romantic relationship. Adolescence. 1991;26(102):253–9. PMID 1927658.

24. Robak RW, Weitzman SP. Grieving the loss of romantic relationships in young adults: an empirical study of disenfranchised grief. Omega. 1995;30(4):269–81. https://doi.org/10.2190/CY1W-V6RL-0L5V-G4Q2.

25. Davidson H. A review of the literature on three types of disenfranchised grief: grandparent grief, grief of Birtlunothers following adoption, and the grief of ex-spouses. The Graduate School at the University of Wisconsin – Stout; 2010.

26. Clower CE. Pregnancy loss: disenfranchised grief and other psychological reactions. University of North Texas; 2003.

27. Levitan F, Frei-Landau R, Sabar-Ben-Yehoshua N. I just needed a hug. Culturally-based disenfranchised grief of Jewish ultraorthodox women following pregnancy loss. Westport, CT: Omega. 2022:302228221133864.

28. Faro L. Monuments for stillborn children and disenfranchised grief in the Netherlands: recognition, protest and solace. Mortality. 2021;26(3):264–83. https://doi.org/10.10 80/13576275.2020.1779202.

29. Lang A, Fleiszer AR, Duhamel F, Sword W, Gilbert KR, Corsini-Munt S. S.C-M. Perinatal Loss and parental grief: the challenge of ambiguity and disenfranchised grief. Omega. 2011;63(2):183–96. https://doi.org/10.2190/OM.63.2.e, PMID 21842665.

30. Wlodarczyk N. The effect of a group music intervention for grief resolution on disenfranchised grief of hospice workers. Prog Palliat Care. 2013;21(2):97–106. https://doi.org/10.1179/1743291X13Y.0000000051.

31. Lamers WM. Disenfranchised grief in caregivers Doka KJ, editor. Champaign, IL: Research Press; 2002.

32. Tsui EK, Franzosa E, Cribbs KA, Baron S. Home care workers' experiences of client death and disenfranchised grief. Qual Health Res. 2019;29(3):382–92. https://doi.org/10.1177/1049732318800461, PMID 30264669.

33. Lathrop D. Disenfranchised grief and physician burnout. Ann Fam Med. 2017;15(4):375–8. https://doi.org/10.1370/afm.2074, PMID 28694277.

34. Mallett K, Price JH, Jurs SG, Slenker S. Relationships among burnout, death anxiety, and social support in hospice and critical care nurses. Psychol Rep. 1991;68(3 Pt 2):1347–59. https://doi.org/10.2466/pr0.1991.68.3c.1347, PMID 1924632.

35. Wakefield A. Nurses' responses to death and dying: a need for relentless self-care. Int J Palliat Nurs. 2000;6(5):245–51. https://doi.org/10.12968/ijpn.2000.6.5.8926, PMID 12419996.

36. Grove WJC. Remembering patients who die: exploring the meaning conveyed in notes to the researcher. Illn Crisis Loss. 2008;16(4):321–33. https://doi.org/10.2190/IL.16.4.d.

37. Lev E. A nurse's perspective on disenfranchised grief. In: Doka K, editor. Disenfranchised grief: recognizing hidden sorrow. Lexington, MA: Lexington Books; 1989.

38. O'Brien JM, Forrest LM, Austin AE. Death of a partner: perspectives of heterosexual and gay men. J Health Psychol. 2002;7(3):317–28. https://doi.org/10.1177/135910 5302007003224, PMID 22114253.

39. Fenge LA. Developing understanding of same-sex partner bereavement for older lesbian and gay people: implications for social work practice. J Gerontol Soc Work. 2014;57(2–4):288–304. https://doi.org/10.1080/01634372.2013.825360, PMID 24006957.

40. Bristowe K, Marshall S, Harding R. The bereavement experiences of lesbian, gay, bisexual and/or trans* people who have lost a partner: a systematic review, thematic synthesis and modelling of the literature. Palliat Med. 2016;30(8):730–44. https://doi.org/10.1177/0269216316634601, PMID 26944532.

41. Jenkins CL, Edmundson A, Averett P, Yoon I. Older lesbians and bereavement: experiencing the loss of a partner. J Gerontol Soc Work. 2014;57(2–4):273–87. https://doi.org/10.1080/01634372.2013.850583, PMID 24798053.

42. Whipple V. Lesbian widows: invisible grief. New York: Harrington Park Press; 2006.

43. Corns DL. Disenfranchised grief in queer companionship and chosen family. California State University – San Bernardino; 2022.

44. Timmins L, Pitman A, King M, Gao W, Johnson K, Yu P, et al. Does the impact of bereavement vary between same and different gender partnerships? A representative national, cross-sectional study. Psychol Med. 2022; May:1–9. https://doi.org/10.1017/S0033291722000496, PMID 35620818.

45. Curtin N, Garrison M. "She was more than a friend': clinical intervention strategies for effectively addressing disenfranchised grief issues for same-sex couples. J Gay Lesbian Soc Serv. 2018;30(3):261–81. https://doi.org/10.1080/10538720.2018.146 3885.

46. Lucas JJ, Bouchoucha SL, Afrouz R, Reed K, Brennan-Olsen SL. LGBTQ+ Loss and grief in a cis-heteronormative pandemic: a qualitative evidence synthesis of the COVID-19 literature. Qual Health Res. 2022;32(14):2102–17. https://doi.org/10.1177/10497323221138027, PMID 36342414.

47. Schwebach IA. Disenfranchised grief in mentally retarded and mentally ill populations. Indiana University of Pennsylvania; 1992.

48. Cadell S, Marshall S. The (re)construction of self after the death of a partner to HIV/ AIDS. Death Stud. 2007;31(6):537–48. https://doi.org/10.1080/0748118070135 6886, PMID 17726828.

49. Dominguez KM. Encountering disenfranchised grief: an investigation of the clinical lived experiences in dance/movement therapy. Am J Dance Ther. 2018;40(2): 254–76. https://doi.org/10.1007/s10465-018-9281-9.

50. Ramadas S, Vijayakumar S. Disenfranchised grief and Covid-19: how do we make it less painful? Indian J Med Ethics. 2021;VI(2):1–4. https://doi.org/10.20529/ IJME.2020.123, PMID 33908367.

51. Jones SJ, Beck E. Disenfranchised grief and nonfinite loss as experienced by the families of death row inmates. OMEGA J Death Dying. 2006–2007;54(4):281–99. https://doi.org/10.2190/a327-66k6-p362-6988, PMID 18186424.

52. Robson P, Walter T. Hierarchies of loss: a critique of disenfranchised grief. Omega. 2013;66(2):97–119. https://doi.org/10.2190/OM.66.2.a.

53. Littlewood J. Aspects of grief: bereavement in adult life. London; New York: Tavistock Publications/Routledge; 1992.

54. Cretney SM. Principles of family law. London: Sweet & Maxwell; 1997.

55. Charles-Edwards D, Charles-Edwards D. Handling death and bereavement at work. Rev ed. London; New York: Routledge; 2005.

56. Mosley C. Debrett's guide to bereavement. London: Headline; 1995.

57. Bento RF. When the show must go on: disenfranchised grief in organizations. J Manag Psychol. 1994;9(6):35–44. https://doi.org/10.1108/02683949410070197.

58. Fowlkes MR. The social regulation of grief. Sociol Forum. 1990;5(4):635–52. https:// doi.org/10.1007/BF01115395.

59. Hall CW, Reid RA. Adolescent bereavement over the deaths of celebrities. In: Balk DE, Corr CA, editors. Adolescent encounters with death, bereavement, and coping. Vol. xxiii. New York: Springer Publishing Co.; 2009. p. 237–252.

60. Mulvihill A, Walsh T. Pregnancy loss in rural Ireland: an experience of disenfranchised grief. Br J Soc Work. 2014;44(8):2290–306. https://doi.org/10.1093/bjsw/bct078.

61. Baum N, Negbi I. Children removed from home by court order: fathers' disenfranchised grief and reclamation of paternal functions. Child Youth Serv Rev. 2013;35(10):1679–86. https://doi.org/10.1016/j.childyouth.2013.07.003.
62. Doughty Horn EA, Crews JA, Guryan BA, Katsilometes BM. Identifying and addressing grief and loss issues in a person with aphasia: a single-case study. J Couns Dev. 2016;94(2):225–33. https://doi.org/10.1002/jcad.12078.
63. Neimeyer RA, Jordan JR. Disenfranchisement as empathic failure: grief therapy and the co-construction of meaning. In: Doka K, editor. Disenfranchised grief. Champaign, IL: Research Press; 2002. p. 95–117.

When the Loss of a Companion Animal Is not Recognized

Pet Loss as a Unique Form of Disenfranchised Grief

We who choose to surround ourselves with lives even more temporary than our own live within a fragile circle, easily and often breached. Unable to accept its awful gaps, we still would have it no other way. We cherish memory as the only certain immortality, never fully understanding the necessary plan.—Irving Townsend

In the preceding chapter (Chapter 6), we introduced the concept that change equals loss, and loss equals grief.(1) The bereaved can mourn the loss of something as well as someone. That someone does not have to be human.

As we explored in Chapter 1, the human–animal bond is an immensely powerful attachment (2–4) that is both mutually beneficial and dynamic, and contributes to the health and well-being of both parties.(5, 6)

Attachments are further strengthened by the following perceptions by pet owners:(7)

- they rescued the pet
- the pet rescued them
- the pet is their sole source of support
- the pet is a living "link" or connector to a person, animal, relationship, or lifestage (e.g., childhood) that has since moved on, passed away, or ended.

Because of the significance of the bond that owners often ascribe to their pets, companion animals are now considered to be members of the family by 85%–99% of pet owners.(7–13)

Many owners acknowledge that they relate to their pet as if they were human and openly profess familial love when considering interspecies relationships.(14) The love that often serves as a foundation for the human–animal bond emphasizes the value that the companion animal brings to "ownership." Many dog and cat owners no longer see themselves as being in possession of pets so much as they see their role as parent or guardian.

Within the family structure, veterinary clients may view themselves as "pet parents" and pets as their children.(5, 15–18) Pets may become child substitutes(19), "fur kids," "fur babies"(20), or even spousal replacements. Forty percent of companion animal owners within the United States also elevate their pets to the role of confidants, expressing that their pets listen to them more consistently than their partners.(21)

Other than surrogates, pets may function as the "symbiotic extension of self"(20, 22) or an invitation to sociability, in which the dog, for instance, facilitates interactions between others.(23, 24)

Today's world offers dog bakeries, doggie day cares, and pet spas. Jessica Greenebaum writes of so-called "biscuit bars" – pastry cases of dog treats – and of Fido's Barkery, in Hartford, Connecticut. She reports that:(20)

> *All the cookies, cakes, and pastries are made with natural, wholesome ingredients without the use of sugar, salt, animal fats, or artificial preservatives. Most of the cookies are dipped in carob (a chocolate substitute) or peanut butter. The cakes are topped with buttermilk-yogurt frosting mixed with peanut butter or carob. The treats look so delicious, that many first-time customers cannot believe the treats are made for dogs, rather than humans. Nothing is too indulgent for these pampered pets, including the high quality toys, collars, beds, and bowls that also sell for premium prices.*

Greenbaum adds that the "barkery" offers "Yappy Hour" between 6 and 8 o'clock on Thursday nights. She describes "Yappy Hour" as:(20)

> *… a social hour for dogs and their human companions. When the door closes, the leashes come off and the games begin. The dogs run back and forth from the front to the back of the store. The front of the store is where the dogs play and get attention from people. The back of the store is where the dogs get cake and the humans get wine or soda from Frank, the owner and "barktender."*

"Yappy Hour" reinforces the image that pets are the social butterflies that bring people together. Greenbaum shares that:(20)

> *Through this activity, the dog and dog owners become a team in constructing an image of a family. Similar to the image of soccer moms who drive their kids to games and social events, these parents take their fur babies to a weekly activity where they can play. The parents socialize with each other while encouraging their fur babies to play nicely. Just as children tend to have personalities similar to their parents, these fur babies also reflect the personalities of the parents. As a result, the dog becomes an extension and reflection of the self. Not only are the dogs elevated to the status*

of children, but the dogs also elevate the status of dog owners to parents. The dog becomes anthropomorphized through this leisure activity that promotes family life.

And for those who are convinced that it's all gone to the dogs, take note of the rising popularity of cat cafés, which were introduced in Taiwan at the end of the 1990s, then spread to Japan before going global.(25) The business model centers around a place of food or drink that allows cats to move freely around the premises.

As the guest, you decide what to purchase for yourself and/or for the cats. In this respect, you temporarily become the "protector/benefactor of the chosen animal."(25)

Giannitrapani shares that:(25)

Most of these places appear to be a true heterotopia where, for a limited period of time, the subject can have an extraordinary experience and put on hold his normal worldly relationships and then return to their usual spaces feeling, perhaps, transformed. The access procedure is orderly and subject to specific rituals (another element typical of heterotopic spaces): the customers, when entering, have to remove their shoes and wear slippers, wash their hands and, sometimes, disinfect them. Disinfecting human hands: a somewhat paradoxical gesture that reverses ordinary practices (it is usually considered a good hygienic rule to wash hands after touching an animal). In this case there is a clear projection of categorisations and practices typically cultural on the cat and some kind of sacralisation of the feline: the cat is no longer a potential carrier of germs, but a being that needs to preserve its purity, which must not be contaminated.

According to Giannitrapani:(25) "Spin-offs … of pet cafés [include] some with rabbits, others with reptiles, birds, etc., which in any case are an attempt to establish a blissful connection between men and animals, eager to be with each other, in a relationship of mutual complicity."

Indeed, it is this perception that people and animals are inherently linked through mutual need for affection and companionship that has led to the explosion of the human–animal bond.

Dogs, cats, and other pets have transitioned into many households as live-in members of family.(26, 27)

In 2007, the American Veterinary Medical Association (AVMA) reported that over 70% of homes with children aged six or older had at least one pet.(26)

Children and adults alike tend to view pets as significant "people."(28) Some adults even openly profess that they prefer their pets over human family members in large part because pets are perceived to love unconditionally.(15, 21)

Love without conditions and love irrespective of material goods or social status is priceless and rare. It is what makes the human–animal bond so intrinsically unique and so often sought after.

When that bond breaks, as through death, it becomes one of the most significant losses that a person may ever face.(29) In spite of this, such losses are not always recognized.(30, 31) Instead, they are more often than not disenfranchised, meaning that they are not "openly acknowledged, socially validated or publically [sic] mourned."(1)

In spite of this, anyone who has ever loved and lost never forgets.

7.1 Nina's Natural Wonder (April 21, 2004 – January 6, 2020): Part I – *The Death of a Best Friend*

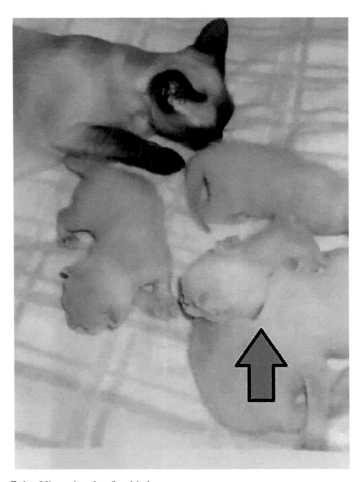

Figure 7.1   Nina, shortly after birth.

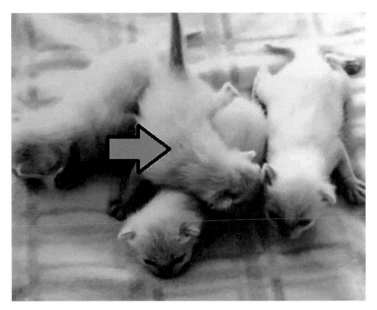

Figure 7.2 Nina at two weeks old.

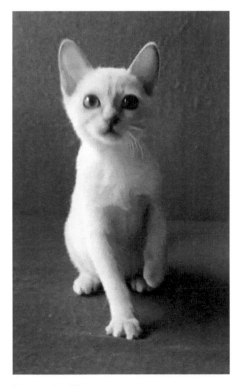

Figure 7.3 Nina at eight weeks old.

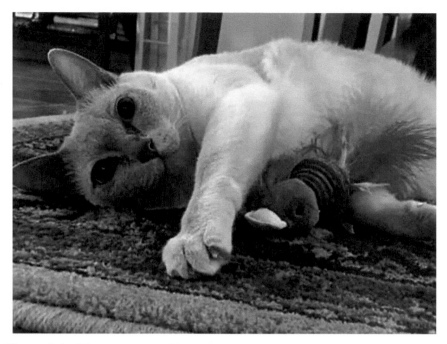

Figure 7.4   Nina at ten years old.

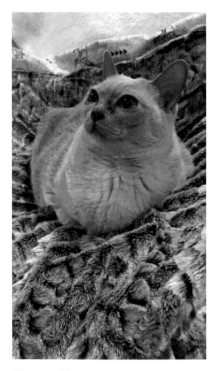

Figure 7.5   Nina at 12 years old.

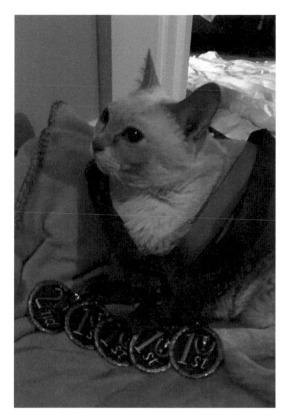

Figure 7.6 Nina at 14 years old.

January 6, 2020

Personal Facebook Post, Authored by Ryane E. Englar

> *Today, one of the brightest candles of my life was snuffed out of existence. I am heartbroken.*
>
> *Nina may have been almost 16 years old, but the truth is, she was 16 years young.*
>
> *She was born on April 21, 2004 at 9:40 AM, to mom Cara Mia and dad, Privatdancer [sic] Bobby Z of Lovnpaws ...*
>
> *Weighing in at a mere 2.4 oz, she was half of my whole world. Bailey is the other half.*
>
> *Nina spent the first four years of her life with Mom and Dad while I earned my DVM degree at Cornell. She was loved by all. My brother was her favorite.*
>
> *When I graduated in May 2008, she rejoined my household. From there, we traveled together near and far. She was with me everywhere I went. She lived my*

dreams right alongside of me. She stood by my side through thick and thin. She was there with me to celebrate my highest highs and there to commiserate with my lowest lows. She kept me going no matter what.

She was always there to greet me at the door after a long day.

She retrieved Halls cough drops.

She sat by me when I cried. She licked my tears away.

She saw me through the Dante's Inferno of early jobs and into academia.

She travelled with me from Maryland to New York, from New York to Arizona, from Arizona to Kansas, and was supposed to make the journey back home to Arizona, where I belong, just a mere 12 days from now.

We rang in 2020 together. Nina was by all accounts well on New Year's Day. She appeared as spry as ever to greet me home from the holidays. But by Saturday she'd lost the pep in her step and a mere 24 hours later, come Sunday night, I knew what I had to do.

Nina was tired. Too tired to make the journey back home with me. Too tired to write what was supposed to be her final chapter at her new retirement home in Tucson, the one I'd picked out for her and Bailey. Too tired to see us through new adventures.

In a matter of 48 hours, she spiraled downhill from happy and bouncy to icteric, hypothermic, obtunded and borderline stuporous.

As we spent our final night together last evening, I knew what she was telling me. She was ready to go, whether I was ready to accept it.

Today, I did the hardest thing I've ever had to do. I chose to end her suffering. I chose to allow her a ticket out of this world with her dignity. I chose her way out – a peaceful death, in my arms, surrounded by love.

I didn't want to let her go.

How do you say goodbye to the friend who saw you through almost half of your lifetime? On the other hand, how could I make her endure the journey, the two-day car ride back to Arizona, just for my own sake? I couldn't stomach that. Nina is and always was a free spirit. She was too wild to be confined. She was a fruit loop from the start, but she was my little fruit loop.

Tonight finds me missing her more than words can say. My heart is broken, and Bailey's is, too. We are weathering the storm the best we can, but we *hate* this "New Normal". It wasn't supposed to end this way. Nina was supposed to leave Kansas with us.

For now, I must venture on without her physical presence. And that is all too sudden and too real and too horrid of a thought to bear.

I know she will be there in spirit. But that is oh so very not the same.

Tonight finds me broken and alone and missing my very best friend.

7.2 Nina's Natural Wonder: Part II – *Three Months Later, On the Anniversary of Her Birth*

April 21, 2020

Personal Facebook Post, Authored by Ryane E. Englar

There's a certain emptiness in the Englar household today on what would have been Nina's 16th birthday. Sixteen years ago, Nina's Natural Wonder came to be.

The first time we met her, we were there to visit Bailey, who was one week her senior. Nina leaped at me from across the room like a flying squirrel, then clung to my head like a mini-koala.

She was fascinated by everything that moved.

She was a fierce hunter of insects. She pretended to be brave when it came to geckos, but one scuttle towards her sent her running for cover.

She had to be involved in everything, with everyone, all the time.

Her eyes were in a perpetual state of absorbing everything around her. They would light up like she was hyped up on amphetamine. She had big bug-eyes, and when her pupils dilated, she looked like a creature from another planet. ET. But a lovable ET.

Then she would race through the house, as if her tail were lit on fire.

In the early days, when she first joined the household, she would wait until Grandma would Swiffer. Then she'd leap onto the Swiffer handle and cling tight. It drove Grandma crazy. But Nina loved it. Every second.

Nina lived a life of reckless abandonment. She lived to enjoy. To indulge. And to live freely, not caring about the consequences.

She was in trouble more times than I can count. But she never seemed to care. No amount of loving scolding could put her in her place. Besides, she'd only curse back at you anyway with a guttural wail that would squeak into your core and curl your toes the way that chalk scrapes on a chalkboard.

Nina had the gift of life and the gift of gab. There was never a conversation that she wasn't a part of.

And as much as she at times drove me crazy, she also made me whole. Because as crazy as she was, that little ragamuffin had the most empathy of any cat I ever knew.

If you had a bad day, she was there. If you started to cry, then she stopped whatever it was she was doing and came to find you.

She loved post-competition dance bling. Unlike Bailey, who only tolerated one medal around her neck, Nina wanted them *all* … Three, four, five medals, it *didn't matter. They were hers. And she wore them proudly. And next time she expected you to bring her home even *more*.*

She was always in my way and underfoot – but I didn't realize how much I came to count on her until she was gone. Gone before we really had a chance to say goodbye. Gone before I really knew how much I would miss her.

I truly believe that Nina knew we were coming home to Arizona. She waited until I got everything in order – job interview, letter of offer, job acceptance, contract signed, old house on the market, new house purchased ... and then she went.

She left this world only after she knew that we would be okay.

Nina was my sweet pea, my flying squirrel, my snow leopard, my little peanut, my pumpkin squash, my fruit loop, my Creampuff.

She was my world in a way that I never understood ... until now.

I miss her every day, but especially today. Arizona is home, but it's not the same without my Nina.

I am absent one door greeter now.

And as much as I love my Bailey, let's face it. Bailey lives for Bailey.

Nina may have been a few Crayolas short of a box, but she lived to love. I miss that love and that selflessness. We all do.

And even though I know she would have driven me out of this world, out of my mind crazy what with the stay-at-home ordinance [due to COVID-19], a giant part of me just wants her back here again with me.

Grief is funny that way.

You manage to pull yourself back together and run on autopilot for a while . . . until you let your heart remember again ... and feel again ... and hurt all over again.

I miss you, my little warrior, tonight and forever.

7.3 Nina's Natural Wonder: Part III – *What People Said*

Three months – the period between my post about Nina's death in January 2020 and my first experience "celebrating" her birthday without her, in April 2020 – is not a significant passage of time.

In those three months, so much about my life changed, for the better.

As had been planned, I picked up my life and moved cross-country.

I became founding faculty (again). I represented a new institution (University of Arizona College of Veterinary Medicine). I was passionate about my career. I was productive and highly functional in spite of my grief journey.

Yet, I still missed Nina every day.

My new co-workers had never met Nina. She held no meaning for them, but she was everything to me.

When I reached out to my old friends about Nina, I had hoped they would understand. Instead, I was met with a surprising statement that rendered me speechless:

- *People said:* "At least you still have Bailey."
- *What I heard:* "Nina could be replaced."
- *What I felt:*
  o frustrated
  o misunderstood
  o hurt
  o resentful
  o angry.

Bailey wasn't Nina.

Nina wasn't replaceable.

Bailey's presence didn't negate Nina's death.

If you have two kids and one dies, is it okay because you still have one left?

It didn't take me long before I learned from those who "companioned" me through grief not to talk of Nina, lest someone tell me that it was time to "move on."

7.4 Bailey's Crème Brûlée: Part I – *Celebrating Her Sixteenth Birthday*

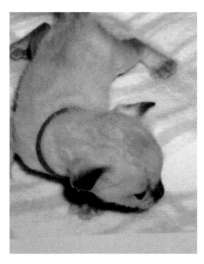

Figure 7.7   Bailey at two weeks old.

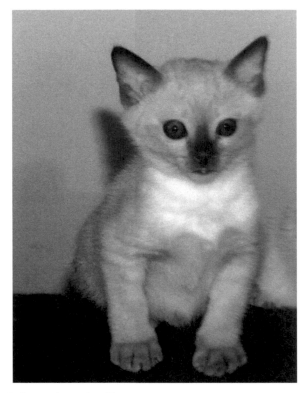

Figure 7.8   Bailey at six weeks old.

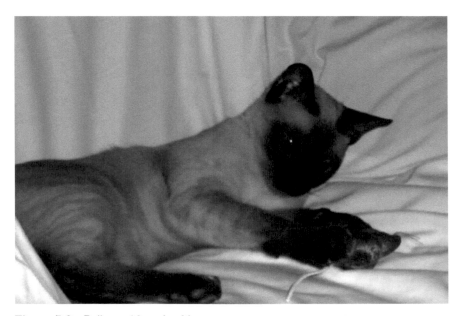

Figure 7.9   Bailey at 16 weeks old.

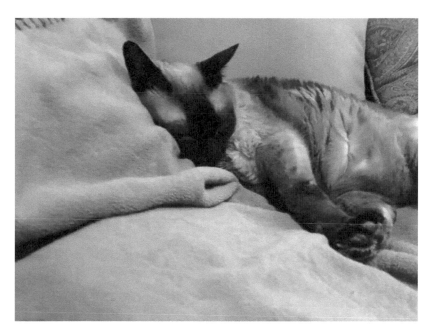

Figure 7.10   Bailey at 12 years old.

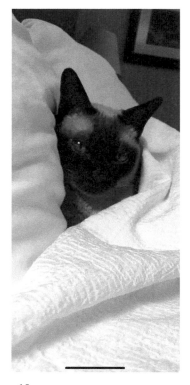

Figure 7.11   Bailey at age 15.

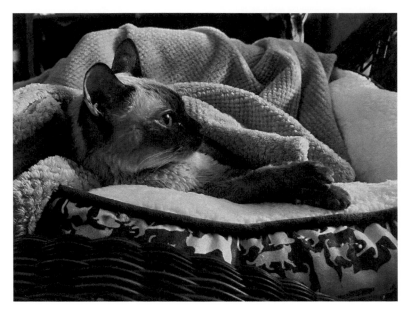

Figure 7.12 Bailey at age 18, the day before she died.

April 12, 2020

Personal Facebook Post, Authored by Ryane E. Englar

Sixteen years ago, on April 12, 2004, my beautiful Crème Brûlée came into this world at 2:30 AM.

Born to Dam Wan-Lea Sundari and Sire GC Chestnutfarm Jackson, she was all of 2.7 oz.

I loved her before I knew her. I loved her before she had even arrived.

I remember seeing her photograph on the day of her birth. She had no points at that time, which is typical of the Tonkinese breed. She was just a tiny ball of white with pink skin shining through, closed eyes and folded ears … One of a litter of two. Just her and big brother Winston.

In the moment that I saw her, I knew she had my heart … and always would. **Happy sigh …** A mother's love.

I didn't know then the extent to which she would fill my soul. I simply knew that she was meant to be and that I would love her forever.

In the days that passed, I watched her grow, first from afar, and then in person.

I remember when she was small enough to cradle in the palm of my hand.

She couldn't see me then – her eyes were still closed. But she knew I was there. And I knew she was there. And that someway, somehow, we would always have each other.

Bailey was the shyest of shy as a kitten. She was timid and cautious, ever so careful — except when coaxed by her little "sister" Nina to stir up trouble.

I remember coming home to find her "tapping" crickets — ever so gentle, never one to hurt or harm anything or anyone — just content to look at the world from afar or investigate ever so slightly with big eyes and the most gentle of "taps."

She "tapped" at my heart from the moment hers started beating.

In many ways we grew up together. Bailey entered my life the summer before vet school. She knew me before Doctor was added to my name, before my first day in clinical practice, before my debut in academia, before my first textbook …

She knew me before I found my passion in life (outside of veterinary medicine) — dance.

She's journeyed through some of my greatest chapters of my life and helped me to weather some of the most significant storms. She makes my world a better, brighter, warmer place!

Our bond is indescribable.

Bailey is not *just* a cat. She is a little person in Tonkinese clothes. And, oh my, has that "little" purrsonality grown! For those of you who don't know the Tonkinese breed, you are missing out!

Help me celebrate her today!

She's my first baby, my little panther, my grasshopper, my little princess, my diva, my gold-medalist, my champion, my heart, my everything …

PS — It is safe to say that *finally* Bailey has adapted to life in Tucson and to life as the only "child". Nina's sudden absence hit us all hard, particularly as we embarked upon this new chapter. And I was worried about the toll that it took upon my "firstborn." But Bailey has officially transitioned into life as the "only child" — and I think she's liking the fact that she now gets *all* of my attention! ☺

7.5 Bailey's Crème Brûlée (April 12, 2004 – October 17, 2022): Part II – *The Death of My Baby*

October 18, 2022

Personal Facebook Post, Authored by Ryane E. Englar

On the evening of Monday, October 17th, we helped Bailey to transition from life to death.

At 18y 6m, she was my longest relationship.

She had struggled with Chronic Kidney Disease (CKD) and Feline Orofacial Pain Syndrome (FOPS) in her final years and I knew her time with me was drawing to an end.

But I never predicted that I would have to grieve my best friend as I weathered major orthopedic reconstructive surgery and grieved my (temporary) inability to dance while rehabbing my knee.

She saw me through my best days and my worst days.

Then ✳ in the blink of an eye, she's gone.

The house is exceedingly empty.

How does one say goodbye to a friend who saw me through every adult milestone? She was my entire world. My heart is broken. I am devastated. I don't know how to do this without her.

I miss everything about her, all at once, like a torrential downpour.

Except, uncharacteristic of me, I've run out of words.

I don't know where to begin …

7.6 Bailey's Crème Brûlée: Part III – *A Significant Transitional Period in My Life*

In the final years of her life, everything outside of work revolved around Bailey, though, if I'm honest, it always had.

It had always been Bailey's way or the highway.

Now, magnify that by 255, and you can imagine life with a geriatric, 18-year-old, "only child," Tonkinese cat.

Everything had to be just so, or Bailey told you about it, in triplicate.

She had four litter boxes, split between two rooms. If one was soiled, she took it upon herself to hunt you down, wherever you were at, and demand that it be changed. It didn't matter if you were in the bathroom or in the shower. She would find you. And sit beside you. And chirp at you until you caved, threw in the towel with whatever it was you were doing, and tended to her needs.

In her final years, Bailey had gotten it down to an exact science. She would call you over to her *before* she had eliminated, just so that you would be immediately on hand to dispose of her waste.

She was the only cat I ever knew who expected you to follow her into the litter area and watch her go.

She was the only cat I ever knew who watched you scoop the litter and tracked the entire process from beginning to end. She walked you to the door, peering into the garage from the safety of indoors, as you threw out the bag of soiled litter in the trash. Then she trekked with you over to the sink to watch you wash your hands.

If you were fortunate, that was the end of chores ... for now, and she would go on her merry way, back to bed.

If you were not so fortunate, then Bailey would decide that it was time to start from square one. She would call you over just so that she could use the box again now that it was fresh.

Bailey would chirp at you as if you were Dobby, her house elf, and demand instant service. This chirp was distinct from all her other Tonkinese vocalizations. It meant *now*. Not tomorrow. Not tonight. Not in five minutes. *Now!*

Some would say that she was spoiled.

My response was always the same: you can't fault her for knowing what she likes and for refusing to settle!

As she navigated her final years, I adapted our home to meet her needs. I had often joked that my Arizona house was a retirement home ... just not mine.

Everything about the house was shifted around to make it Bailey's world. It was her home as much as it was mine, if not more so.

She was the only cat I knew who had not one bedroom, but two.

She had not one, but four orthopedic pet beds to choose from – in one bedroom alone – and she rotated among them, like royalty.

When I travelled for business, she was never alone; I hired a live-in pet sitter.

When her vision started to fade, with age, I started to leave the lights on in the house, by day and by night, to help with navigation.

When she could no longer perch on the tall cat tree, I rearranged the furniture to give her a smaller tower from which to watch the world go by.

When she wanted to lay in the sun beside the glass sliding door to the backyard, but the tile floor had become too hard for her body, I laid blankets down for her to prop herself up on.

When she could no longer jump up onto the hallway bench, I bought her kitty stairs.

The house became a clutter of steps and ramps, but I never once apologized to visitors about the mess because it was all about Bailey.

When, in her final weeks, every step seemed to be one too many – she had dropped weight and was too weary to make the trek to and from her water and feeding station – I created "rest stops" in triplicate. It gave her the autonomy to go where she wanted but trim her steps down by half.

As her functional world continued to shrink and she became less and less active, our roles reversed. I came to her, not the other way around.

I brought her food and carried her to bed at night. I held the water bowl up to her, so that she could drink, and I tucked her in.

When I underwent surgery and could temporarily not care for her myself, my mom took on that role. In the words of my mom, who had the "pleasure" of tending to her every whim during my immediate post-operative period:

> She would eat a few bites and if disgruntled by the menu would take her paw and flip her bowl upside down and then chirp as if telling me to do better next time. We opened five cans a day because she wouldn't eat the same meal twice so 3/4 of every can was wasted. I tried to trick her and got the small lids to fit over the can. She wasn't fooled and still refused the food even if I pleaded. Ryane always laughed and made excuses for her.

I did make excuses for her, always. That's what moms do!

7.7 Bailey's Crème Brûlée: Part IV – *What People Said*

Life after Bailey was the hardest "new normal" that I had ever faced.

Bailey was the last of my two babies to walk this earth. After she died, I felt a shift in my identity.

- Was I still a *cat mom* if I did not have Bailey to come home to?
- Was I still Bailey's *mom*?
- Did I still have *kids* even though my *kids* were gone?

In the immediate days that followed Bailey's death, I felt supported by close friends and family. Those who understood best had themselves known the loss of a companion animal that had spanned nearly two decades. Those my age whose own pets had seen them through most of, if not all of, their adult milestones got it.

What was most helpful in those days was hearing that her life mattered, that her life had value. What was most helpful was to hear someone else acknowledge that she meant something to someone (me), and that she would never be forgotten.

What didn't help me was the recycled variation of one of five themes:

- **Theme 1: Longevity**
  - *People said:*
    - "You were really lucky to have had her that long."

- "You gave her a good life. What cat lives to be 18?!?"
- "You knew she wouldn't live forever."
- "She lived a long life."
  o *What I heard:*
    - "You should be grateful. Not everyone's cat lives that long."
  o *How I wanted to respond:*
    - "It wasn't long enough."

- **Theme 2: "It Was Time"**
  o *People said:*
    - "She was tired."
    - "She was ready to go."
    - "She was ready to be with Nina."
    - "She saw you through major life events; she knew you would be okay."
  o *What I heard:*
    - "You didn't need her anymore."
  o *How I wanted to respond:*
    - "I needed her forever."

- **Theme 3: Relief**
  o *People said:*
    - "It must be a relief. Now, you don't have to worry about her when you travel for work."
  o *What I heard:*
    - "She was a burden that you're now relieved of."
  o *How I wanted to respond:*
    - "She was never a burden; I would gladly do it all over again."

- **Theme 4: What the Dead Would Want**
  o *People said:*
    - "Don't feel bad. Is that what Bailey would want?"
    - "Don't be sad. She wouldn't want you to be."
    - "She would want you to be strong."
  o *What I heard:*
    - "It's time to move on."
  o *How I wanted to respond:*
    - "I'm not ready to."

- **Theme 5: New Chapter**
  o *People said:*
    - "There are lots of other cats that need homes."

- "You can get a new kitten now. Do you think you'd get one or two?"
- "What are you going to do with her bedroom now that she's gone?"
- "I think you should get two new cats, so that they can bond with each other. It's too hard on you to just have the one."
- "Are you going to buy another Tonkinese cat?"
- "Maybe you should rescue a cat instead."
  o *What I heard:*
  - "Bailey was just a cat; she can be replaced."
  o *How I wanted to respond:*
  - "Bailey is not a sofa. You don't just go buy a new one."

7.8 The Significance of Pet Loss

Nina and Bailey are two examples – my examples – of the intimate attachments that can form between people and their companion animals.

As a veterinarian, I was not surprised by the depth of my grief in response to the loss of either cat because my professional identity is built around supporting the human–animal bond.

At the start of my career, I took an oath to protect animal health and welfare and benefit society.(32)

It is a lifelong obligation that I see myself fulfilling every time that I practice medicine, every time that I take another client under my wing, every time that I elicit their perspective and hear how that patient came to be.

Every patient means something to someone.

What that meaning is varies. But there is always some kind of underlying significance.

As the veterinarian, it is up to me to find out what that is, so that I can meet the needs, wants, and expectations of that partnership.

To someone, that patient may be a family member, child, or another form of significant other.

To someone, that patient may be a sibling.(33) This perspective may be reinforced among households in which children grow up with pets. In many homes, pets are ubiquitous with the childhood experience.(34) Pets are often involved in pregnancy announcements and gender-reveals. When my niece was born, my first gift to her was a onesie that said, "My siblings have tails."

To someone, that patient may be the last living link to someone else who died or to the relationship that didn't pan out.

To someone, that patient may be a companion, confidant, shoulder to lean on, or sole support.(33)

It is never just a cat.

It is never just a dog.

There is an anonymous poem that has made its rounds throughout social media that speaks to this sentiment. I read it years ago, when I was practicing in Baltimore, Maryland. When I was writing this text, the poet's words came to mind again. I found the poem online, posted by colleague Noel Fitzpatrick, a globally respected veterinary surgeon, who shared that the words resonated with him, too. I wish that I could credit the author because it's the most powerful acknowledgment of the human–animal bond that I have ever read:(35)

From time to time, people tell me, "lighten up, it's just a dog,"
or "that's a lot of money for just a dog."

They don't understand the distance travelled, the time spent,
or the costs involved for "just a dog."

Some of my proudest moments have come about with "just a dog."

Many hours have passed and my only company was "just a dog,"
but I did not once feel slighted.

Some of my saddest moments have been brought about by
"just a dog," and in those days of darkness, the gentle touch
of "just a dog" gave me comfort and reason to overcome the day.

If you, too, think it's "just a dog," then you probably understand
phrases like "just a friend," "just a sunrise," or "just a promise."

"Just a dog" brings into my life the very essence of friendship,
trust, and pure unbridled joy.

"Just a dog" brings out the compassion and patience
that make me a better person.

Because of "just a dog" I will rise early, take long walks and look
longingly to the future.

So for me and folks like me, it's not "just a dog"
but an embodiment of all the hopes and dreams of the future,
the fond memories of the past, and the pure joy of the moment.

"Just a dog" brings out what's good in me and diverts my thoughts
away from myself and the worries of the day.

I hope that someday they can understand that it's not "just a dog"
but the thing that gives me humanity and keeps me from being
"just a man" or "just a woman."

So the next time you hear the phrase "just a dog,"
just smile, because they "just don't understand." ~Unknown author

People who have never loved a dog or cat or another type of companion animal don't understand.

Maybe they never will.

They may not mean to, but their statement that incorporates *just* is disenfranchising to those who are acutely experiencing pet bereavement.

- *Just* implies sufficient. Nothing more. Nothing less.
- *Just* implies that dogs are a dime a dozen and that any animal can replace the one that is cherished.
- *Just* negates the uniqueness of the human–animal bond.
- *Just* negates the relationship and the value that relationship brought to a person's life.

The word, *just*, is ever present in today's society. It is used as a measure against which to calibrate expectations.

- It was *just* a game.
- It was *just* a joke.

The word, *just*, levels the playing field in a way that erases that which is exceptional.

Veterinary students will say to me:

- "I'm *just* a first year."
- "I'm *just* a second year."
- "I'm *just* a third year."
- "I'm *just* starting clinical year."

Doctors will say to me at conferences, "I'm *just* a baby vet."

Every time I hear the word, *just*, I think of the 2004 biographical fantasy film, *Finding Neverland*, which was based upon the 1998 play, *The Man Who Was Peter Pan*. In the movie, playwright J.M. Barrie tries to encourage four grieving brothers to use their imagination while they are on an outing at the park with their recently widowed mom. Barrie claims to make his living entertaining "princes" – the boys – with his trained "bear", Porthos. Porthos, the dog, proceeds to demonstrate tricks for the boy's entertainment. One of the boys, Peter, refuses to buy into this demonstration. He claims that *"This is absurd. It's just a dog."*(36)

Barrie responds:

Just a dog? *Just*? Porthos, don't listen! Porthos dreams of being a bear, and you want to dash those dreams by saying he's *just* a dog? What a horrible candle-snuffing word. That's like saying, 'He can't climb that mountain, he's just a man', or 'That's not a diamond, it's just a rock.' Just.(36)

I recite this quote to my students as often as is necessary. It is a reminder that the word, *just*, amends our perceptions and takes away from, rather than adds.

The significance of pet bereavement may be lost on some, but for many companion animal lovers, there are fewer more profound losses in life.(29) A human–animal relations study conducted by the University of Minnesota affirmed this, when 242 participants were asked to rate the stress level associated with all the events that they had ever endured, "including the death of a spouse, divorce, marriage, loss of children, an arrest, loss of a job, and death of a pet."(29)

According to Lagoni and her team:(29)

Researchers found that the death of a pet was the most frequently reported trauma experienced by the couples participating in the study. Survey participants said the deaths of their pets were less stressful than the deaths of human members of their immediate families but more stressful than the deaths of other relatives.

The significance of pets to human existence is multifactorial and varies between people. However, the emotional and social support that companion animals offer is an impactful driving force behind attachment.(29)

Those who underestimate the strength of the bond, including veterinarians, drive a wedge between themselves and the bereaved.(29) Yet, as far as we have come as a society in terms of recognizing the value that animals may bring us in life, not all of us are as easily able to acknowledge and affirm the value that animals brought into our lives after time of death.

For many, pet loss continues to be a type of disenfranchised grief because it is not always perceived as socially acceptable to mourn, particularly if the bereaved professes to love the pet as much as, if not more than, a human.(37)

References

1. Doka K. Disenfranchised grief: recognizing hidden sorrow. Lexington, MA: Lexington Books; 1989.
2. Johnson TP, Garrity TF, Stallones L. Psychometric evaluation of the Lexington attachment to pets scale (LAPS). Anthrozoos. 1992;5(3):160–75. https://doi.org/10.2752/089279392787011395.
3. Zilcha-Mano S, Mikulincer M, Shaver PR. An attachment perspective on human-pet relationships: conceptualization and assessment of pet attachment orientations. J Res Personal. 2011;45(4):345–57. https://doi.org/10.1016/j.jrp.2011.04.001.
4. Bowlby J. A secure base: parent–child attachment and healthy human development. Vol. xii. New York: Basic Books; 1988.
5. Applebaum JW, MacLean EL, McDonald SE. Love, fear, and the human-animal bond: on adversity and multispecies relationships. Compr Psychoneuroendocrinol. 2021;7. https://doi.org/10.1016/j.cpnec.2021.100071, PMID 34485952.
6. Human-animal bond. American Veterinary Medical Association. Available from: https://www.avma.org/one-health/human-animal-bond.
7. Lagoni L, Hetts S, Butler C. The human-animal bond. In: Lagoni L, Hetts S, Butler C, editors. The human-animal bond and grief. Philadelphia: Saunders; 1994. p. 3–28.
8. Brown JP, Silverman JD. The current and future market for veterinarians and veterinary medical services in the United States. J Am Vet Med Assoc. 1999;215(2):161–83. PMID 10416465.
9. Martin F, Ruby KL, Deking TM, Taunton AE. Factors associated with client, staff, and student satisfaction regarding small animal euthanasia procedures at a veterinary teaching hospital. J Am Vet Med Assoc. 2004;224(11):1774–9. https://doi.org/10.2460/javma.2004.224.1774, PMID 15198261.
10. Bustad LK, Hines LM, Leathers CW. The human-companion animal bond and the veterinarian. Vet Clin North Am Small Anim Pract. 1981;11(4):787–810. https://doi.org/10.1016/s0195-5616(81)50086-6, PMID 6977933.
11. Voith VL. Attachment of people to companion animals. Vet Clin North Am Small Anim Pract. 1985;15(2):289–95. https://doi.org/10.1016/s0195-5616(85)50301-0, PMID 3872510.
12. Wensley SP. Animal welfare and the human-animal bond: considerations for veterinary faculty, students, and practitioners. J Vet Med Educ. 2008;35(4):532–9. https://doi.org/10.3138/jvme.35.4.532, PMID 19228905.
13. Podberscek AL, Paul ES, Serpell J. Companion animals and us: exploring the relationships between people and pets. Cambridge, UK; New York: Cambridge University Press; 2000.
14. Bradshaw JWS, Casey RA. Anthropomorphism and anthropocentrism as influences in the quality of life of companion animals. Anim Welf. 2007;16(S1):149–54. https://doi.org/10.1017/S0962728600031869.
15. Hirschman EC. Consumers and Their Animal Companions. J Consum Res. 1994;20(4):616–632. https://doi.org/10.1086/209374.

16. Cassels MT, White N, Gee NR, Hughes C. One of the family? Measuring young adolescents' relationships with pets and siblings. J Appl Dev Psychol. 2017;49:12–20. https://doi.org/10.1016/j.appdev.2017.01.003.

17. Laurent-Simpson A. "They make me not wanna have a child": effects of companion animals on fertility intentions of the childfree. Sociol Inq. 2017;87(4):586–607. https://doi.org/10.1111/soin.12163.

18. Laurent-Simpson A. Considering alternate sources of role identity: childless parents and their animal "kids". Sociol Forum. 2017;32(3):610–34. https://doi.org/10.1111/socf.12351.

19. Guo Z, Ren X, Zhao J, Jiao L, Xu Y. Y. Can pets replace children? The interaction effect of pet attachment and subjective socioeconomic status on fertility intention. Int J Environ Res Public Health. 2021;18(16). https://doi.org/10.3390/ijerph18168610, PMID 34444359.

20. Greenebaum J. It's a dog's Life: elevating status from pet to "fur baby" at yappy hour. Soc Animals. 2004;12(2):117–35. https://doi.org/10.1163/1568530041446544.

21. Silcox D, Castillo YA, Reed BJ. The human animal bond: applications for rehabilitation professionals. J Appl Rehabil Couns. 2014;45(3):27–37. https://doi.org/10.1891/0047-2220.45.3.27.

22. Veevers JE. The Social meaning of pets: alternative roles for companion animals. Marriage Fam Rev. 1985;8(3–4):11–30. https://doi.org/10.1300/J002v08n03_03.

23. Wolch JR, I. Companions in the park: Laurel Canyon dog park. Landscape. 1992;31:16–23.

24. Robins DM, Sanders CR, Cahill SE. Dogs and their people: pet-facilitated interaction in a public setting. J Contemp Ethnogr. 1991;20(1):3–25. https://doi.org/10.1177/089124191020001001.

25. Giannitrapani A. Cat cafes and dog restaurants. In: Marrone G, editor. Semiotics of animals in culture: zoosemiotics 20. New York: Springer; 2018. p. 91–102. https://doi.org/10.1007/978-3-319-72992-3_7.

26. Mueller MK, Fine AH, O'Haire ME. Understanding the role of human-animal interaction in the family context. In: Fine AH, editor. Handbook on animal-assisted therapy: foundations and guidelines for animal-assisted interventions. 4th ed. Amsterdam; Boston: Elsevier Academic Press; 2015. p. 237–48.

27. Albert A, Bulcroft K. Pets, families, and the life course. Journal of Marriage and the Family. 1988;50(2):543–52. https://doi.org/10.2307/352019.

28. Gunter B, Furnham A. Pets and people: the psychology of pet ownership. Vol. vi. London: Whurr Publishers; 1999.

29. Lagoni L, Hetts S, Butler C. The human-animal bond and grief. Philadelphia: Saunders; 1994.

30. Cordaro M. Pet loss and disenfranchised grief: implications for mental health counseling practice. J Ment Health Couns. 2012;34(4):283–94. https://doi.org/10.17744/mehc.34.4.41q0248450t98072.

31. Packman W, Carmack BJ, Katz R, Carlos F, Field NP, Landers C. Online survey as empathic bridging for the disenfranchised grief of pet loss. Omega. 2014;69(4):333–56. https://doi.org/10.2190/OM.69.4.a, PMID 25304868.

32. Veterinarian's oath. American Veterinary Medical Association. Available from: https://www.avma.org/resources-tools/avma-policies/veterinarians-oath.

33. Barton Ross C, Baron-Sorensen J. Pet loss and human emotion: a guide to recovery. 2nd ed. Vol. xvii. New York: Routledge; 2007.

34. Kogan L. Pet loss, grief, and therapeutic interventions: practitioners navigating the human-animal bond. New York: Routledge; 2020.

35. Just a dog [cited Nov 20 2022]. Available from: https://www.noelfitzpatrick.vet/blog/just-a-dog/.

36. Forster M, Gladstein RN, Magee D, Depp J, Winslet K, Christie J, et al. Finding neverland. Miramax Films; 2004.

37. Sife W. The loss of a pet: a guide to coping with the grieving process when a pet dies. 4th ed. New York. Vol. xii. New York: Howell Book House; 2014.

CHAPTER 8

Suffering, Quality of Life, Anticipatory Grief, and Pet Loss

Preparing for the Ultimate Goodbye

The veterinary oath is a leading principle for our healthcare profession. We pledge our commitment to the "prevention and relief of animal suffering"(1) as one of the guiding principles by which we practice medicine. This requires us to draw upon our medical knowledge and skills, in concert with the ethical delivery of healthcare, to partner with clients to positively impact patient outcomes.

8.1 Shared Decision-Making

Partnership plays a vital role in both human and veterinary healthcare. Research has effectively demonstrated that human medical patients who contribute to decision-making about their own health have better clinical outcomes.(2) These include, but are not limited to the following.(3)

- Patient satisfaction is improved when patients are invited to share their perspective.(4)
- Patients are happier when their expectations have been acknowledged, affirmed, and/or addressed.(5–7)
- Patients are more satisfied when their questions are elicited and they have the opportunity to clarify their concerns.(8)
- Patients feel better connected to the healthcare team when the team's eye contact, posture, and facial expressions confirm mutual understanding; they feel heard.(9–12)
- Patient compliance with and adherence to healthcare recommendations increase when they are asked to provide insight concerning their knowledge base and core beliefs.(13–15)

- Patients report shorter durations of illness and speed through recovery periods at faster clips if they are involved in designing their own care plans.(16, 17)
- Patients are more likely to accept healthcare recommendations when they are allowed to ask clarifying questions and negotiate care. (18, 19)
- Patients are less anxious about treatment recommendations when they can collaborate on the design of their care plan.(20)

Veterinary medicine is a unique healthcare profession because its providers care for non-human patients who cannot articulate their symptoms, needs, wants, expectations, and reservations about care in the same way that a human might.(3) Veterinary practice, in many respects, resembles the delivery of pediatric human healthcare.(3, 21)

Nowhere else in medicine is there such an inherently ingrained tripartite relationship.(3, 21–23) The professional relationships, veterinarian–client–patient and the pediatrician–parent–child, are truly unique, with overlap in each caregiver's responsibilities to the patient.(3, 21, 22)

The veterinary client bears responsibility for the veterinary patient in the same way that the human parent is responsible for the child.(3, 21, 22) Both are healthcare advocates who weigh in on decisions that will directly impact the patient.(21, 22)

8.2 Advocacy for Veterinary Patients

One of the most critical decisions that a veterinary client will ever face, in partnership with the healthcare team, surrounds the concept of suffering.

As veterinarians, we often ask ourselves what it means to suffer. We question if our patient is suffering, and if so, to what degree.

We intervene in life to expedite death so that our patients don't suffer. We agonize over those final moments more than any other aspect of our patients' lives and we fear that moment in time when suffering is ever permissible.

The cases that keep us up at night are most often the ones that suffered. The ones we didn't get to quickly enough. The ones who weren't brought in to us soon enough. The ones who passed on their own, without us, in times when they needed us most.

Suffering distresses us as both veterinarians and as human beings because it jeopardizes our ability to provide compassionate care. When our hands are tied and/or we are incapable of alleviating suffering, then we question what good we were able to do, either in the course of that patient's life, or, particularly, at that patient's end.

8.3 The Subjectivity of Suffering

Suffering means different things to different people. It has been defined as "the tolerance or endurance of evil, injury, pain, or death."(24) It has also been likened to "some symptom or process (physical or otherwise) that poses a threat."(25)

Suffering may be momentary or prolonged.

Is there such a thing as bearable suffering? Is suffering for a fraction of time worth it if it facilitated the return of high-quality life?

There are no easy answers, and the information upon which we base our assessment of the degree to which a patient is suffering is largely subjective.(25)

Suffering is inferred by others looking from the outside in but is ultimately determined by the individual who is experiencing it.

Cassell explains that:(25)

> *The meanings and the fear are personal and individual, so that even if two patients have the same symptoms, their suffering would be different. The complex techniques and methods that physicians usually use to make a diagnosis, however, are aimed at the body rather than the person. The diagnosis of suffering is therefore often missed, even in severe illness and even when it stares physicians in the face.*

Doctors may struggle to identify suffering because, in the words of Cassell:(25)

> *The language that describes and defines the patient's suffering is different from the language of medicine ... Physicians are trained primarily to find out what is wrong with the body ... in terms of diseases or pathophysiology; they do not examine what is wrong with persons. It would seem, from looking at training programs and physicians' actions, that people, with all their ideas, conceptions and misconceptions, fears and fancies, and misleading behaviors, are too often seen as something a physician has to get out of the way in order to diagnose and treat diseases and their manifestations. When physicians attend to the body rather than to the person, they fail to diagnose suffering.*

Veterinarians are challenged even further by their inability to hear directly from the patient what it is that the patient is experiencing, from their own perspective. This requires us to partner with the client to dissect each clinical case from the empathic lens through which they relate to the patient, make our best guess, and err on the side of caution when faced with uncertainty.

It is a constant struggle to do right by the patient and right by the client. Mark Oyama et al. add another layer to the struggle when he and his research team share that:(24)

> *It would appear that veterinarians are dedicated to improving the quality (e.g., alleviating injury and pain) as well as the quantity (e.g., preventing death) of their patients' lives. This dual mission is deeply ingrained into everyday veterinary practice, and it is tempting to assume that these goals are equally important to all veterinarians and pet owners. In ideal circumstances, each veterinary treatment would ensure high quality of life and increase longevity; however, in many instances treatment may fail to achieve one or even both of these goals.*

The classic case example in companion animal medicine that Oyama's research team references involves the canine patient with heart disease. They collectively share that:(24)

> *Dogs with advanced heart disease are perceived to have a reduced quality of life because of respiratory distress, poor appetite, and reduced activity. Most causes of heart disease in dogs, such as mitral valve disease and cardiomyopathy, are progressive and reduce the life span of severely affected patients. When dealing with heart disease–affected dogs, veterinarians commonly prescribe medications that diminish clinical signs and improve survival time (e.g., diuretics, angiotensin-converting enzyme inhibitors, and pimobendan). Yet, among dogs receiving such standard treatments, there is a wide degree of variation with respect to adverse effects, development of refractory clinical signs, and financial burden to the owner as well as in the level of owner's comfort with the administration of medications of a more expensive or experimental nature. Thus, specific decisions regarding the management of heart disease cannot always or equally fulfill the dual mission of the veterinarian's oath.*

The veterinarian must decide, in concert with the client's wishes, what is best. And what is best rarely means that everyone wins.

8.4 Quality Versus Quantity of Life

The delivery of healthcare often represents a precarious balance between quality of life and quantity of life. Quality more often trumps quantity. This requires the veterinary healthcare team, of which the client is a part of, to establish objective as well as subjective measures of what constitutes quality of life. The ability to make evidence-based, life-altering decisions for the patient depends heavily on it.

Although most of us have some understanding of what we mean when we use the term *quality of life*, the veterinary profession has yet to reach a consensus regarding what establishes and contributes to this state of existence.(26)

Many definitions for quality of life have been proposed. Most include other subjective determinations, including "pleasant affect, positive experiences, or overall well-being."(26)

The definition of quality of life by Taylor and Mills is perhaps the most descript:(27)

> ... *the state of an individual animal's life as perceptive by [it] at any one point in time. It is experienced as a sense of well-being which involves the balance between negative and positive affected states and any cognitive evaluation of these, where the animal has the capacity. To some extent, quality of life can be predicted by the fulfilment of basic and species specific health, social and environmental needs (and individual preferences for these) and is reflected in the animal's health and behaviour.*

As practitioners, we often struggle to identify and prioritize those factors that constitute quality of life. We each come to the table with different perspectives and experiences. These different perspectives and experiences enrich our profession and our ability to deliver care to a wide range of patients and clients. However, they may challenge us to come to consensus when we prioritize patient needs. Our colleague may feel that pain is the greatest determinant of quality of life while we may feel that mobility and its associated independence is key to quality living.

Neither of us is right nor wrong.

8.5 Assessing Quality of Life

It is our professional obligation to assess quality of life. According to Dr. Alice E. Villalobos, "the need is particularly acute when families are caring for aging, ailing, or terminally ill pets, especially pets with advanced or recurrent cancer ... ."(28)

Villalobos considers the growing complexity of quality of life (QoL) determinations when she shares the following:(28)

> *How do veterinarians know when a chronic, comorbid condition starts to ruin a pet's QoL? Most older pets have 1 or more comorbid conditions such as painful*

osteoarthritis (OA), obesity, or organ disease. When a life-limiting disease or cancer and its related treatment exert added burdens on a compromised pet, how will the effect on QoL be determined? Who is capable of monitoring that pet? How are they making their decisions? At what point should caregivers abandon further curative therapy? What obligation does the V-team have to provide palliative care or preserve their clients' hope for a beloved pet's well-being? Veterinarians are frequently asked, 'When is the right time to euthanize my beloved pet? How will I know?' These questions can be emotionally draining and difficult to answer without assessment guidance.

The development of quality-of-life scales in veterinary practice is an active area of research because they help the veterinarian and the client make determinations about a patient's trajectory.

Quality-of-life questionnaires for the veterinary team often ask about the following parameters:(29–52)

- attitude/temperament
- non-verbal cues
  - ear carriage
    - Are the ears facing forward?
    - Are the ears pulled apart?
    - Are the ears flattened and rotated outwards?
  - facial changes
    - muzzle tension
    - orbital tightening
  - squinted eyes
  - tautness of the whiskers
  - pupil size/shape
  - posture
    - Is the patient prostrate?
    - Is the patient tucked up with all four feet under the body?
    - Is the patient hunched at the shoulders?
    - Is the head held lower than the shoulders?
- changes to routine
  - Is the patient pacing?
- behavioral changes
  - growling, hissing, and other vocalizations
  - hiding
- reaction to palpation
  - biting
  - avoidance
- perception of anxiety

- perception of mental state
  - o Does the patient seem confused?
- appetite and ability to keep food down
- ability to maintain weight/degree of weight loss
- mobility
  - o Is the patient able to get around?
  - o Does the patient require assistance or support to get around?
- activity or energy level
  - o Is the patient sleeping more?
  - o Is the patient playing less?
- desire to interact with surroundings
- response to the client's presence
  - o Does the patient interact with the client in the same way as before?
  - o Is the patient apathetic to the client's presence?
- thirst
- respiratory rate, depth, quality, and ease
- perception of pain
- elimination habits
  - o urination
  - o defecation
- hygiene
  - o Is the patient developing pressure sores?
  - o Is the patient soiling itself?
  - o Is the patient grooming?
    - ▪ quality of fur coat
      - □ Is the patient unkempt?
      - □ Is the fur matted?
      - □ Is the fur soiled?
      - □ Is the coat piloerect?

To initiate conversation, we may provide clients with a visual analog scale. These tend to be specific to a given species. For instance, the following scales are used to assess quality of life with respect to acute pain in cats:

- Feline Grimace Scale (FGS)(53)
- UNESP-Botucatu cat pain scale (UCAPS)(54)
- Glasgow composite measure pain scale – Feline (CMPS – Feline)(49, 55)
- Colorado State University Feline Acute Pain Scale(48)

Alternatively, we may simply give clients a checklist and ask them to assign points based upon specific categories. For instance, points may be assigned to:(45)

- our overall perception of the patient's well-being
- their elimination habits and associated behaviors
- the patient's mental health
- the patient's social functions.

Depending upon how many points are assigned at that particular moment in time, the patient may be considered to have:(45)

- adequate quality of life
- questionable quality of life
- concerning quality of life.

Note that these types of scales can be challenging in that they reflect only a snapshot in time. For that reason, we may ask clients to rate their pet not only in the moment, but also when the pet is at their best (32), and to compare the two:

- Is one rating consistently better?
- Is one rating consistently worse?
- How does today stack up to yesterday?
- How does today compare to last week? Last month?

After all, we all can have a bad day … or two … or three. Day-to-day life for people is not consistently a ten out of ten on a 1–10 scale, so we need to provide some leeway in the event that a pet has an "off" week.

Sometimes, rather than assigning points to specific characteristics or traits, we ask clients to consider their pet's quality of life more broadly. We may ask them a more global question with respect to overall health: *do they perceive their pet to be having more good days than bad days?*

We may ask clients to count the number of good days and compare that count to the number of bad days. As time passes, we partner with our clients to identify any trends. When the number of bad days consistently exceeds the number of good days, then we need to engage in serious dialogue concerning quality of life.

Some scales combine techniques to broaden the scope of coverage. For instance, the HHHHHMM quality of life scale combines an assessment of good days versus bad with the following categories:(28, 56)

- hurt
- hunger
- hydration
- hygiene

- happiness
- mobility
- more good days than bad.

Each category of HHHHHMM, including "more good days than bad," is weighted equally; clients are tasked with providing a score for each on a scale of 1–10. A cumulative score of 35 or more suggests that palliative care, as provided through pet hospice ("Pawspice"), is acceptable to continue.(28)

If on the other hand the cumulative score for a patient on the HHHHHMM scale falls below 35, the number represents a starting point for conversation.

8.6 Initiating Conversations about Quality of Life

Beyond inviting conversations that transition from quality of life to end of life, the HHHHHMM scale also provides an opportunity for support and education. For example, the veterinary team may find that a patient is really struggling with one or more aspects of HHHHHMM.

Maybe the patient has sustained pressure sores from recumbency and the recumbency has also compromised the patient's hygiene. In these instances, the HHHHHMM scoring system becomes an easy approach to identifying problem areas and partnering with the family to both acknowledge and address these.

Villalobos shares how the HHHHHMM scale provides an opportunity to navigate such challenges in patient care as a team:(28) "When discussing hygiene, staff can demonstrate wound care techniques; teach clients to prevent decubital ulcers by using egg crate mattresses, soft bedding, and body rotation; and teach clients to prevent self-soiling with strategic elevation, absorbent towels, diapers, and so forth."

In this respect, the HHHHHMM scale opens the door for education and improvements in patient care:(28)

When family members use the [HHHHHMM] scale to assess the basic criteria, they may realize that they need to improve certain aspects of their home care to properly maintain their pet's comfort. A well-managed end-of-life care program allows more quality time … to be shared between family members and their beloved pet.

Note that this chapter is not intended to serve as a comprehensive review of the veterinary medical literature with respect to quality-of-life scoring or scales. It is intended to heighten awareness that the evolution of the human–animal bond has driven healthcare providers to develop and validate more quality-of-life measures for pets, particularly at end of life.(28)

8.7 The Struggle to Embrace Challenging Conversations about Quality of Life

Quality of life conversations challenge the veterinarian–client–patient relationship (VCPR). They require ample time to engage in conversation in which each party has an opportunity to express themselves fully. Dialogue is likely to stray from factual content concerning case management to touch upon the underlying emotions that case trajectories are provoking.

Past experiences, thoughts, considerations, concerns, and assumptions may play a role as veterinary team members (including the client) consider patient interventions and anticipated outcomes. It can be tempting to make assumptions about client needs/wants/expectations and gloss over the conversation altogether; however, these conversations are an essential part of clinical practice. Doctors must become comfortable with discomfort by broaching topics that they might otherwise shy away from, in a way that is both skillful and sensitive.(57)

Human medical doctors acknowledge that fear is the primary emotion that challenges bad news delivery(58): fear of the patient's response; fear of their own emotional triggers; fear of the unknown; and fear of having to admit defeat.(59–63)

Discomfort for the veterinarian is heightened by:(57)

Lack of training, being short of time, practice culture, feeling responsible for the patient's illness, perceptions of failure, unease with death and dying, lack of comfort with uncertainty, impact on the veterinarian-client-patient relationship, worry about the patient's quality of life, and concerns about the client's emotional response and [their] own emotional response to the circumstances.

According to Dr. Jane Shaw:(57) "Some of the same reasons account for client anxiety in receiving bad news. These include self-blame, unease with death and dying, anticipatory grief, effect on the human–animal bond, impact on the veterinarian-client-patient relationship, pet's quality of life, and concerns about their emotional response to the situation."

Because of barriers on all sides of the VCPR, quality-of-life conversations are often sub-optimal and may or may not effectively transition to talk about end-of-life.(57)

When end-of-life conversations go poorly, the impact is bidirectional. (57) How healthcare news is delivered and received impacts both the recipient and the messenger.(64–66) The human patient/veterinary client's prior life experiences, philosophical and/or spiritual beliefs, coping strategies, and the perceived presence or absence of support networks impact how the patient experiences and processes bad news delivery.(64)

The emotional toll on human medical patients and physicians is particularly steep when bad news delivery involves conversations about grief and grieving, death and dying.(63, 67, 68)

Veterinary clients may depart from the consultation room feeling dissatisfied or disappointed with care.(57) When clients do not feel heard, their grief is compounded.(57) They are at increased risk for complicated grief, and they may be more likely to pursue litigation.(57, 69–73)

Few human physicians express comfort and confidence with respect to quality of life and end of life discussions, and few feel adequately prepared to initiate this task.(62, 74, 75) Some clinicians have reported being weighed down emotionally in the aftermath by feelings of guilt, anger, anxiety, and exhaustion.(64, 76, 77) Many recall their first experiences with breaking bad news as being uncomfortable and unsettling.(74, 78) Over time, repeated experiences with difficult conversations contribute to the physician's dissatisfaction with clinical practice, burnout, and psychological distress.(79, 80)

The same can be said in veterinary practice. When conversations don't go as planned, again and again, veterinary team members risk dissatisfaction with their profession, burnout, and compassion fatigue.

8.8 Lessons from Human Healthcare

Because of their discomfort, doctors have historically been reluctant to deliver bad news.(64) Although informed consent has ethically tied physicians to the patients' right to know the details about their condition (81, 82), human physicians still struggle with bad news delivery and may choose censorship over full disclosure.(64) Even physicians working in hospices are not always frank with patients: only 37% honor patients' requests for an upfront survival estimate.(83) This paternalistic approach to protecting the patient persists despite patients' desire for the truth(64): as early as the 1980s, 85% of patients expected to receive facts from their physicians including realistic estimates of lifespan in the face of a cancer diagnosis.(84)

Because bad news delivery can adversely impact the patient and the patient's family, several studies have examined the patient's preferred approach.(58, 85–89) This evolving body of research has identified several common themes. Patients want physicians to be direct, patients want privacy, and patients want to be involved in decision-making regarding treatment plans.(58) Patients want the authority to control what they can. That means providing them with the information they need to plan for the future.(58)

8.9 What Do Veterinary Clients Want?

When it comes to conversations about grief and grieving, death and dying, companion animal owners seek transparency. Dog owners who participated in a focus group study expressed that they did not want facts withheld, even when such details conveyed bad news such as a cancer diagnosis.(90)

The following quotes from participants emphasize their desire that the veterinary team be direct in their approach to quality of life/end of life conversations:(90)

> *Don't beat around the bush. I already know it's cancer. I know what that means. So, get to the point of what needs to be done. We know what needs to be done. We just need to hear you say it.*
>
> *Don't soften things up. I want to know exactly what's happening with the dog and what the worst outcome could be.*
>
> *Tell me the news straight up. If it could be cancer, then don't be afraid to use the 'C' word – cancer.*
>
> *I need to hear the truth. I may not want to hear it, but I need to … in order to process and ultimately accept it.*

When information is withheld either about prognosis or terminal diagnosis, dog-owning participants felt offended. To these individuals, the doctor's failure of disclosure implied that the veterinary team did not feel they could handle the facts. Dog-owners also felt denied the opportunity to make informed decisions about their pet's care because they lacked the details that would have facilitated decision-making.(90)

8.10 Goals of Care (GOC) Conversations

In their 2019 article in the Veterinary Clinics of North America, Dr. Katherine J. Goldberg refers to this critical exchange of dialogue as Goals of Care (GOC) conversations. In Dr. Goldberg's words:(91)

GOC conversations focus on what is most important to patients and their families as they face serious illness. They do not presume that the only priority is living longer, but rather recognize that medical treatment plans may, and ought to be, altered depending on individual goals and preferences. They foster and prioritize "the ask," the simple yet revolutionary act of asking patients and families what is important to them as their lives are impacted by their illness and its treatment.

Goldberg adds:(91) "Although this may sound too simple to warrant scientific inquiry, those who have had a seriously or terminally ill (human) family member know that the impact of these conversations, or lack thereof, is significant."

Goldberg believes that these conversations are "low-risk, high-value."(91) They elicit perspective in terms of the client's wants, needs, and expectations early on in the course of life-limiting illness.(91) They offer the client the chance to be heard, and they offer the clinician the opportunity to clarify any questions or concerns that are unclear. This allows for clarity and enhances partnership. Patient care is more likely to align with the client's goals for the patient, and clients report improved quality of life measures.(91)

Veterinary team members who are interested in integrating GOC into clinical practice may draw upon the Serious Illness Conversation Guide (SICG), which was developed for human healthcare and has since been modified for veterinary use. The Serious Veterinary Illness Conversation Guide (SVICG) provides veterinary teams with guidance in navigating the complexities of quality of life/end of life dialogue.

8.11 Anticipatory Grief

As we engage veterinary clients in constructive dialogue about quality of life, what we often discover is that grief manifests itself long before a companion animal dies. The term, anticipatory grief, was first applied in 1994 by Lindemann to describe the onset of bereavement in advance of the actual loss.(92) Thereafter, anticipatory grief has on occasion been referred to as *premature* mourning. However, the word choice, *premature*, implies that grief is "too soon," when in fact it is right on schedule.

In veterinary practice, loss is an everyday occurrence. As veterinarians, we lose our patients to death more often than we can count. It is almost a given that most of our clients will outlive most of our patients, and that we will play a primary role in the passage from life to death for many pets.

Reflecting upon my time in practice, I have seen many patients age before my eyes. I can recall the names and faces of so many who came into my clinic as kittens or puppies only to grow up in what felt like the blink of an eye.

If time passed at lightning-fast speed for me, in the role of clinician, can you imagine how fast time flies for our clients?

I think back to my own personal experience shepherding my two Tonks, Nina and Bailey, through kittenhood to end of life. Nina was with me for 15 of those years and Bailey for 18.

It's hard to believe that Bailey spent the better part of roughly two decades by my side and now she's gone. Just like that.

It is a fact of life: kittens become cats who become seniors seemingly overnight.

When they live with you, day after day, you don't notice it all in the moment. Then, suddenly, one day, you turn around and bear witness to the greying muzzle and the silvery lenses of the eyes that stare back at you, peacefully, unafraid, and you realize that their chapter with you is almost over.

It is a natural recognition that many of us come to, whether others want to shield us from it or not.

Everyone asked me how old Bailey was, at each passing birthday, until she reached 14 and then they didn't.

It was almost as though if no one asked the question that was on everyone's minds, it wouldn't come to fruition.

What everyone wanted to ask, but didn't, for fear that it would put the idea in my head, was "How much longer does Bailey have by Ryane's side?" … which translated into "How much time do we have to prepare? Because if anything happens to her, I don't know what Ryane will do … ."

The funny thing about cats and aging and lifespans is that they didn't need to ask me anything. I already knew.

They didn't need to fear putting the idea in my head because it was already there. And with every passing birthday of hers, it got stronger.

I anticipated that I would one day turn around and Bailey wouldn't be there.

I anticipated that Bailey would one day die, leaving me to pick up the pieces and figure out that next chapter.

I didn't want to experience that chapter without her. At the same time, I knew I didn't have a choice.

I didn't know when that day would arrive. I just knew that it wasn't an "if." It was reality.

Anticipatory grief is much like that, for clients and for veterinarians alike.

There is never a question of *if* death will happen. It's a question of *when*. And most of us live to see the sunrise the day after our beloved companion leaves this world.

Because that is a given, for most of us, we think about it long before that day appears on the horizon.

It starts as a little wrinkle in the tapestry of our imagination and grows, over time, as the reality crystallizes in our mind.

At first, assuming that our senior companion is in good health, we may wonder, *What if?*

- *What if we were to come home and find that they had passed in their sleep?*
- *What if we were to wake up in the middle of the night and find that they had stopped breathing?*

What if?

We wrestle with the idea and toss it back into the ocean of our minds like "catch and release" fish, except the fish keep coming back, bigger, and stronger.

Then one day, we again wonder, *What if?*

- *What if they don't pass in their sleep?*
- *What if we must make the decision for them?*

Anticipatory grief is a wrestling match that we cannot win. And given that most of us come to know and love more than one pet over the course of our lifetime, it is something we will encounter again and again.

Barring critical emergencies in which time is of the essence in terms of decision-making, we experience anticipatory grief as if to prepare ourselves for the process.

Grief in veterinary practice is frequently tied to anticipation:

- anticipation of an undesirable diagnosis
- anticipation of an undesirable prognosis
- anticipation of decision-making surrounding euthanasia
- anticipation of loss before euthanasia has taken place.

8.12 A Case Study in Anticipatory Grief: Peabody, the Bichon Frise

To consider what anticipatory grief may look like in clinical practice, imagine that a new client presents Peabody, their 11-year-old castrated male Bichon Frise dog, to you for evaluation of halitosis. They may be anticipating that the dog needs a dental cleaning.

On physical examination, you auscultate a Grade III out of VI left-sided systolic heart murmur. This is the first time that the client has been told any concerns about Peabody's heart.

When you ask if the dog has a history of coughing spells or exercise intolerance, the client says that Peabody doesn't do all that much these days but can guarantee that he has not been coughing. At least not excessively so.

The client authorizes you to proceed with screening bloodwork (CBC, chemistry profile) and urinalysis to evaluate the dog's candidacy for anesthesia if you elect to proceed with dentistry.

The client also consents to orthogonal thoracic radiographs to evaluate Peabody's heart. The radiographic findings disclose left atrial enlargement based upon the clockface analogy of the heart as well as dorsal deviation of the trachea. You discuss these results and recommend referral to a board-certified veterinary cardiologist for echocardiography.

Echocardiography confirms the definitive diagnosis, mitral valve disease (MVD), with moderate left atrial enlargement. Enalapril therapy is initiated by the cardiologist for its cardioprotective effects.

The cardiologist tells the client that:

- MVD is common in adult, small-breed dogs
- although it can be medically managed, MVD cannot be cured
- MVD is likely to progress to congestive heart failure (CHF).

Knowing what the client has been told and knowing what they are currently processing about Peabody's condition:

- What concerns do you think the client has with respect to the diagnosis of MVD?
- What concerns do you think the client has with respect to the likely progression to CHF?

Although CHF could be years away, the client's conversation with the cardiologist has likely triggered questions about *when*, rather than *if*.

The client will likely leave the cardiologist wondering how long it will be before the disease progresses and the dog becomes symptomatic.

The client is likely to grieve the anticipation of disease progression whether CHF happens tomorrow, next week, next month, or next year, because they know that it is coming.

Now imagine that we fast-forward time. Consider that it is one year later.

Peabody represents to you for evaluation of a five-day history of progressive cough, intermittent tachypnea with increased respiratory effort, lethargy, and no interest in eating or drinking over the course of the past 12 hours.

On examination, he is anxious and shaking. Heart rate is 210 beats per minute. Respiratory rate is 65 breaths per minute. Peabody is normothermic and normotensive.

You detect a grade IV/VI systolic heart murmur with a point of maximal intensity over the left apical region; heart rhythm is regular, and pulses are strong and synchronous. Lung sounds are increased, with no crackles or wheezes.

Thoracic radiographs disclose progressive left atrial and ventricular enlargements, mildly enlarged pulmonary veins, a moderate patchy interstitial pattern in the right caudal lung lobe, and a mild interstitial pattern in the left caudal lung lobe. The lung patterns are consistent with pulmonary edema. Caudal mainstem bronchi are also compressed on lateral projections secondary to the cardiomegaly and left atrial enlargement. Radiographic findings are compatible with left-sided CHF secondary to MVD.

You place Peabody in an oxygen cage and administer the following drugs:

- injectable furosemide to manage this dog's cardiogenic pulmonary edema
- low-dose injectable butorphanol as a sedative and antitussive
- nitroglycerin to reduce preload.

These drugs make Peabody comfortable while you engage in dialogue with Peabody's owner.

You tell Peabody's owner that you are hopeful that you can stabilize Peabody to overcome this episode. However, you are concerned about the rapidity of this progression and want to prepare the client that Peabody may not have much time left.

- *How do you think the client will interpret the news that "Peabody may not have much time left"?*

You also share that it is likely that Peabody will decompensate again, in which case some "difficult decisions" will need to be made.

You skirt around the obvious, as we so often do, when in fact the client's mind has already gone there.

It is apparent to the owner that Peabody's lifespan is finite. Before this episode, MVD may have seemed abstract. Now, they recognize the severity of this disease.

Almost as soon as they do, they start planning. The following questions are likely running through their minds in the moment:

- What symptoms do they need to look for in Peabody at home that indicate he needs to seek medical attention right away?
- What is Peabody's quality of life (QoL) moving forward?
- Will they ultimately need to make the decision to end Peabody's life?
- What other challenging decisions might they need to make along the way?

Anticipatory grief is common among veterinary clients who often grapple with thoughts, feelings, and concerns that are associated with poor patient outcomes.

Anticipatory grief is equally common among veterinary clients who are faced with difficult decisions surrounding euthanasia. They may ask themselves:

- Does their pet have good quality of life?
- Is their pet suffering?
- How much time do they have with their pet?
- Why didn't they notice the symptoms sooner?
- Could they have done more to help their pet?
- Are they making the right decisions?
- When should they euthanize?
- Is there a "right time" to euthanize?
- What if they choose to euthanize too soon?
- What if they wait too long to euthanize?

Clients may ask you, the veterinarian, "*What would you do if my dog were yours?*"

Many veterinarians dread this question above all. What we hate to admit is that we're already thinking about the situation as if this were our dog. Our mind has already gone there, too.

And just like that, in the blink of an eye, we walk the walk alongside of our client as we companion them through the grief journey that is only just beginning.

It is a grief journey that is as normal as it is common. Some walks are shorter than others, but they all end the same way.

It's our role and our responsibility as veterinarians to guide our clients and our patients there with open minds and gentle hearts. The best we can offer them is compassionate transparency in those final minutes, hours, or days.

Accept them where they are at in their grief journey, even when that grief begins long before their loved one's final breath.

References

1. Veterinarian's oath. American Veterinary Medical Association. Available from: https://www.avma.org/resources-tools/avma-policies/veterinarians-oath.
2. Kurtz SM, Silverman J, Draper J, Silverman J. Teaching and learning communication skills in medicine. 2nd ed. Abingdon, Oxon: Radcliffe Medical Press; 2005.
3. Englar RE. A guide to oral communication in veterinary medicine. Sheffield: 5m Publishing; 2020.
4. Arborelius E, Bremberg S. What can doctors do to achieve a successful consultation? Videotaped interviews analysed by the "consultation map" method. Fam Pract. 1992;9(1):61–6. https://doi.org/10.1093/fampra/9.1.61, PMID 1634030.
5. Eisenthal S, Lazare A. Evaluation of the initial interview in a walk-in clinic. The patient's perspective on a "customer approach". J Nerv Ment Dis. 1976;162(3): 169–76. https://doi.org/10.1097/00005053-197603000-00003, PMID 1255147.
6. Eisenthal S, Koopman C, Stoeckle JD. The nature of patients' requests for physicians' help. Acad Med. 1990;65(6):401–5. https://doi.org/10.1097/00001888-199006000-00010, PMID 2372350.
7. Korsch BM, Gozzi EK, Francis V. Gaps in doctor-patient communication. 1. Doctor-patient interaction and patient satisfaction. Pediatrics. 1968;42(5):855–71. https://doi.org/10.1542/peds.42.5.855, PMID 5685370.
8. Shilling V, Jenkins V, Fallowfield L. Factors affecting patient and clinician satisfaction with the clinical consultation: can communication skills training for clinicians improve satisfaction? Psychooncol. 2003;12(6):599–611. https://doi.org/10.1002/pon.731, PMID 12923800.
9. Larsen KM, Smith CK. Assessment of nonverbal communication in the patient-physician interview. J Fam Pract. 1981;12(3):481–8. PMID 7462949.
10. DiMatteo MR, Hays RD, Prince LM. Relationship of physicians' nonverbal communication skill to patient satisfaction, appointment noncompliance, and physician workload. Health Psychol. 1986;5(6):581–94. https://doi.org/10.1037//0278-6133.5.6.581, PMID 3803351.
11. Weinberger M, Greene JY, Mamlin JJ. The impact of clinical encounter events on patient and physician satisfaction. Soc Sci Med E. 1981;15(3):239–44. https://doi.org/10.1016/0271-5384(81)90019-3, PMID 7323845.
12. Griffith CH, 3rd, Wilson JF, Langer S, Haist SA. House staff nonverbal communication skills and standardized patient satisfaction. J Gen Intern Med. 2003;18(3):170–4. https://doi.org/10.1046/j.1525-1497.2003.10506.x, PMID 12648247.
13. Inui TS, Yourtee EL, Williamson JW. Improved outcomes in hypertension after physician tutorials. A controlled trial. Ann Intern Med. 1976;84(6):646–51. https://doi.org/10.7326/0003-4819-84-6-646, PMID 937876.

14. Maiman LA, Becker MH, Liptak GS, Nazarian LF, Rounds KA. Improving pediatricians' compliance-enhancing practices. A randomized trial. Am J Dis Child. 1988;142(7):773–9. https://doi.org/10.1001/archpedi.1988.02150070087033, PMID 3381783.

15. Schulman BA. Active patient orientation and outcomes in hypertensive treatment: application of a socio-organizational perspective. Med Care. 1979;17(3):267–80. https://doi.org/10.1097/00005650-197903000-00004, PMID 763004.

16. Little P, Williamson I, Warner G, Gould C, Gantley M, Kinmonth AL. Open randomised trial of prescribing strategies in managing sore throat. BMJ. 1997;314(7082):722–7. https://doi.org/10.1136/bmj.314.7082.722, PMID 9116551.

17. Stewart M, Brown JB, Donner A, McWhinney IR, Oates J, Weston WW, et al. The impact of patient-centered care on outcomes. J Fam Pract. 2000;49(9):796–804. PMID 11032203.

18. Kaplan SH, Greenfield S, Ware JE, Jr. Assessing the effects of physician-patient interactions on the outcomes of chronic disease. Med Care. 1989;27(3);Suppl:S110–27. https://doi.org/10.1097/00005650-198903001-00010, PMID 2646486.

19. Rost KM, Flavin KS, Cole K, McGill JB. Change in metabolic control and functional status after hospitalization. Impact of patient activation intervention in diabetic patients. Diabetes Care. 1991;14(10):881–9. https://doi.org/10.2337/diacare.14.10.881, PMID 1773686.

20. Fallowfield LJ, Hall A, Maguire GP, Baum M. Psychological outcomes of different treatment policies in women with early breast cancer outside a clinical trial. BMJ. 1990;301(6752):575–80. https://doi.org/10.1136/bmj.301.6752.575, PMID 2242455.

21. Englar RE. Common clinical presentations in dogs and cats. Hoboken, NJ: Wiley/Blackwell; 2019.

22. Shaw JR, Adams CL, Bonnett BN, Larson S, Roter DL. Use of the roter interaction analysis system to analyze veterinarian-client-patient communication in companion animal practice. J Am Vet Med Assoc. 2004;225(2):222–9. https://doi.org/10.2460/javma.2004.225.222, PMID 15323378.

23. Murphy SA. Consumer health information for pet owners. J Med Libr Assoc. 2006;94(2):151–8. PMID 16636707.

24. Oyama MA, Rush JE, O'Sullivan ML, Williams RM, Rozanski EA, Petrie JP, et al. Perceptions and priorities of owners of dogs with heart disease regarding quality versus quantity of life for their pets. J Am Vet Med Assoc. 2008;233(1):104–8. https://doi.org/10.2460/javma.233.1.104, PMID 18593317.

25. Cassell EJ. Diagnosing suffering: a perspective. Ann Intern Med. 1999;131(7):531–4. https://doi.org/10.7326/0003-4819-131-7-199910050-00009, PMID 10507963.

26. Spofford N, Lefebvre SL, McCune S, Niel L. Should the veterinary profession invest in developing methods to assess quality of life in healthy dogs and cats? J Am Vet Med Assoc. 2013;243(7):952–6. https://doi.org/10.2460/javma.243.7.952, PMID 24050560.

27. Taylor KD, Mills DS. Is quality of life a useful concept for companion animals? Anim Welf. 2007;16(S1):55–65. https://doi.org/10.1017/S0962728600031730.

28. Villalobos AE. Quality-of-life assessment techniques for veterinarians. Vet Clin North Am Small Anim Pract. 2011;41(3):519–29. https://doi.org/10.1016/j.cvsm.2011.03.013, PMID 21601744.

29. How do I know when it's time? Ohio State University Press Veterinary Medical Center. Available from: https://vet.osu.edu/vmc/sites/default/files/import/assets/pdf/hospital/companionAnimals/HonoringtheBond/HowDoIKnowWhen.pdf.

30. Mullan S. Assessment of quality of life in veterinary practice: developing tools for companion animal carers and veterinarians. Vet Med (Auckl). 2015;6:203–10. https://doi.org/10.2147/VMRR.S62079, PMID 30101107.

31. Yeates J, Main D. Assessment of companion animal quality of life in veterinary practice and research. J Small Anim Pract. 2009;50(6):274–81. https://doi.org/10.1111/j.1748-5827.2009.00755.x, PMID 19527420.

32. Mullan S, Main D. Preliminary evaluation of a quality-of-life screening programme for pet dogs. J Small Anim Pract. 2007;48(6):314–22. https://doi.org/10.1111/j.1748-5827.2007.00322.x, PMID 17490443.

33. McMillan FD. Maximizing quality of life in ill animals. J Am Anim Hosp Assoc. 2003;39(3):227–35. https://doi.org/10.5326/0390227, PMID 12755194.

34. Wiseman-Orr ML, Nolan AM, Reid J, Scott EM. Development of a questionnaire to measure the effects of chronic pain on health-related quality of life in dogs. Am J Vet Res. 2004;65(8):1077–84. https://doi.org/10.2460/ajvr.2004.65.1077, PMID 15334841.

35. Wojciechowska JI, Hewson CJ, Stryhn H, Guy NC, Patronek GJ, Timmons V. Development of a discriminative questionnaire to assess nonphysical aspects of quality of life of dogs. Am J Vet Res. 2005;66(8):1453–60. https://doi.org/10.2460/ajvr.2005.66.1453, PMID 16173493.

36. Freeman LM, Rush JE, Farabaugh AE, Must A. Development and evaluation of a questionnaire for assessing health-related quality of life in dogs with cardiac disease. J Am Vet Med Assoc. 2005;226(11):1864–8. https://doi.org/10.2460/javma.2005.226.1864, PMID 15934254.

37. Wojciechowska JI, Hewson CJ, Stryhn H, Guy NC, Patronek GJ, Timmons V. Evaluation of a questionnaire regarding nonphysical aspects of quality of life in sick and healthy dogs. Am J Vet Res. 2005;66(8):1461–7. https://doi.org/10.2460/ajvr.2005.66.1461, PMID 16173494.

38. Yazbek KV, Fantoni DT. Validity of a health-related quality-of-life scale for dogs with signs of pain secondary to cancer. J Am Vet Med Assoc. 2005;226(8):1354–8. https://doi.org/10.2460/javma.2005.226.1354, PMID 15844428.

39. Budke CM, Levine JM, Kerwin SC, Levine GJ, Hettlich BF, Slater MR. Evaluation of a questionnaire for obtaining owner-perceived, weighted quality-of-life assessments for dogs with spinal cord injuries. J Am Vet Med Assoc. 2008;233(6):925–30. https://doi.org/10.2460/javma.233.6.925, PMID 18795853.

40. Favrot C, Linek M, Mueller R, Zini E. International Task Force on Canine Atopic Dermatitis. Development of a questionnaire to assess the impact of atopic dermatitis on health-related quality of life of affected dogs and their owners. Vet Dermatol. 2010;21(1):63–9. https://doi.org/10.1111/j.1365-3164.2009.00781.x, PMID 20187912.

41. German AJ, Holden SL, Wiseman-Orr ML, Reid J, Nolan AM, Biourge V, et al. Quality of life is reduced in obese dogs but improves after successful weight loss. Vet J. 2012;192(3):428–34. https://doi.org/10.1016/j.tvjl.2011.09.015, PMID 22075257.

42. Freeman LM, Rush JE, Oyama MA, MacDonald KA, Cunningham SM, Bulmer B, et al. Development and evaluation of a questionnaire for assessment of health-related quality of life in cats with cardiac disease. J Am Vet Med Assoc. 2012;240(10):1188–93. https://doi.org/10.2460/javma.240.10.1188, PMID 22559108.

43. Parker RA, Yeates JW. Assessment of quality of life in equine patients. Equine Vet J. 2012;44(2):244–9. https://doi.org/10.1111/j.2042-3306.2011.00411.x, PMID 21767299.

44. Yeates JW, Mullan S, Stone M, Main DC. Promoting discussions and decisions about dogs' quality-of-life. J Small Anim Pract. 2011;52(9):459–63. https://doi.org/10.1111/j.1748-5827.2011.01094.x, PMID 21896019.

45. Pet quality-of-life scale: lap of love. Available from: https://www.lapoflove.com/how-will-i-know-it-is-time/lap-of-love-quality-of-life-scale.pdf.

46. Epstein M, Rodan I, Griffenhagen G, Kadrlik J, Petty M, Robertson S, et al. 2015 AAHA/AAFP pain management guidelines for dogs and cats. J Am Anim Hosp Assoc. 2015;51(2):67–84. https://doi.org/10.5326/JAAHA-MS-7331, PMID 25764070.

47. Epstein ME, Rodanm I, Griffenhagen G, Kadrlik J, Petty MC, Robertson SA, et al. 2015 AAHA/AAFP pain management guidelines for dogs and cats. J Feline Med Surg. 2015;17(3):251–72. https://doi.org/10.1177/1098612X15572062, PMID 25701863.

48. Shipley H, Guedes A, Graham L, Goudie-DeAngelis E, Wendt-Hornickle E. Preliminary appraisal of the reliability and validity of the Colorado State University Feline Acute Pain Scale. J Feline Med Surg. 2019;21(4):335–9. https://doi.org/10.1177/1098612X18777506, PMID 29848148.

49. Nicholls D, Merchant-Walsh M, Dunne J, Cortellini NP, Adami C. Use of mechanical thresholds in a model of feline clinical acute pain and their correlation with the Glasgow Feline Composite Measure Pain Scale scores. J Feline Med Surg. 2022;24(6):517–23. https://doi.org/10.1177/1098612X211035051, PMID 34328358.

50. Boesch JM, Roinestad KE, Lopez DJ, Newman AK, Campoy L, Gleed RD, et al. The Canine Postamputation Pain (CAMPPAIN) initiative: a retrospective study and development of a diagnostic scale. Vet Anaesth Analg. 2021;48(6):861–70. https://doi.org/10.1016/j.vaa.2021.07.003, PMID 34483040.

51. Della Rocca G, Di Salvo A, Marenzoni ML, Bellezza E, Pastorino G, Monteiro B, et al. Development, preliminary validation, and refinement of the composite oral and maxillofacial pain Scale-Canine/feline (COPS-C/F). Front Vet Sci. 2019;6:274. https://doi.org/10.3389/fvets.2019.00274, PMID 31508431.

52. Piotti P, Albertini M, Lavesi E, Ferri A, Pirrone F. Physiotherapy improves dogs' quality of life measured with the Milan Pet quality of life scale: is pain involved? Vet Sci. 2022;9(7). https://doi.org/10.3390/vetsci9070335, PMID 35878353.

53. Feline Grimace Scale: Zoetis. Available from: https://www.felinegrimacescale.com/.

54. Belli M, de Oliveira AR, de Lima MT, Trindade PHE, Steagall PV, Luna SPL. Clinical validation of the short and long Unesp-Botucatu scales for feline pain assessment. PeerJ. 2021;9:e11225. https://doi.org/10.7717/peerj.11225, PMID 33954046.

55. Moody CM, Niel L, Pang DJ. Is training necessary for efficacious use of the Glasgow Feline Composite Measure Pain Scale? Can Vet J. 2022;63(6):609–16. PMID 35656525.

56. Gardner M, McVety D. Treatment and care of the geriatric veterinary patient. Vol. xi. Hoboken, NJ: Wiley-Blackwell; 2017.

57. Shaw JR, Lagoni L. End-of-life communication in veterinary medicine: delivering bad news and euthanasia decision making. Vet Clin North Am Small Anim Pract. 2007;37(1):95–108; abstract viii:abstract viii–ix. https://doi.org/10.1016/j.cvsm.2006.09.010, PMID 17162114.

58. Ambuel B, Mazzone MF. Breaking bad news and discussing death. Prim Care. 2001;28(2):249–67. https://doi.org/10.1016/s0095-4543(05)70021-x, PMID 11406434.

59. Curtis JR, Patrick DL, Caldwell ES, Collier AC. Why don't patients and physicians talk about end-of-life care? Barriers to communication for patients with acquired immunodeficiency syndrome and their primary care clinicians. Arch Intern Med. 2000;160(11):1690–6. https://doi.org/10.1001/archinte.160.11.1690, PMID 10847263.

60. Ellis PM, Tattersall MH. How should doctors communicate the diagnosis of cancer to patients? Ann Med. 1999;31(5):336–41. https://doi.org/10.3109/0785 3899908995900, PMID 10574506.

61. Lo B, Quill T, Tulsky J. Discussing palliative care with patients. ACP-ASIM end-of-life care consensus panel. American College of Physicians-American Society of Internal Medicine. Ann Intern Med. 1999;130(9):744–9. PMID 10357694.

62. Ptacek JT, Ellison NM. Health care providers' perspectives on breaking bad news to patients. Crit Care Nurs Q. 2000;23(2):51–9. https://doi.org/10.1097/00002727-200008000-00007, PMID 11853027.

63. Quill TE, Townsend P. Bad news: delivery, dialogue, and dilemmas. Arch Intern Med. 1991;151(3):463–8. https://doi.org/10.1001/archinte.1991.00400030033006, PMID 2001128.

64. Fallowfield L, Jenkins V. Communicating sad, bad, and difficult news in medicine. Lancet. 2004;363(9405):312–9. https://doi.org/10.1016/S0140-6736(03)15392-5, PMID 14751707.

65. Ptacek JT, Fries EA, Eberhardt TL, Ptacek JJ. Breaking bad news to patients: physicians' perceptions of the process. Support Care Cancer. 1999;7(3):113–20. https://doi.org/10.1007/s005200050240, PMID 10335928.

66. Davies R, Davis B, Sibert J. Parents' stories of sensitive and insensitive care by paediatricians in the time leading up to and including diagnostic disclosure of a life-limiting condition in their child. Child Care Health Dev. 2003;29(1):77–82. https://doi.org/10.1046/j.1365-2214.2003.00316.x, PMID 12534569.

67. Arnold RL, Egan K. Breaking the 'bad' news to patients and families: preparing to have the conversation about end-of-life and hospice care. Am J Geriatr Cardiol. 2004;13(6):307–12. https://doi.org/10.1111/j.1076-7460.2004.03913.x, PMID 15538066.

68. Buckman R, Kason Y. How to break bad news: a guide for health care professionals. Vol. x. Baltimore: Johns Hopkins University Press; 1992.

69. Adams CL, Bonnett BN, Meek AH. Predictors of owner response to companion animal death in 177 clients from 14 practices in Ontario. J Am Vet Med Assoc. 2000;217(9): 1303–9. https://doi.org/10.2460/javma.2000.217.1303, PMID 11061379.

70. Antelyes J. Difficult clients in the next decade. J Am Vet Med Assoc. 1991;198(4): 550–2. PMID 1953846.

71. Roberts CS, Cox CE, Reintgen DS, Baile WF, Gibertini M. Influence of physician communication on newly diagnosed breast patients' psychologic adjustment and decision-making. Cancer. 1994;74(1);Suppl:336–41. https://doi.org/10.1002/cncr.2820741319, PMID 8004605.

72. Cameron C. Patient compliance: recognition of factors involved and suggestions for promoting compliance with therapeutic regimens. J Adv Nurs. 1996;24(2):244–50. https://doi.org/10.1046/j.1365-2648.1996.01993.x, PMID 8858426.

73. Safran DG, Taira DA, Rogers WH, Kosinski M, Ware JE, Tarlov AR. Linking primary care performance to outcomes of care. J Fam Pract. 1998;47(3):213–20. PMID 9752374.

74. Orlander JD, Fincke BG, Hermanns D, Johnson GA. Medical residents' first clearly remembered experiences of giving bad news. J Gen Intern Med. 2002;17(11):825–31. https://doi.org/10.1046/j.1525-1497.2002.10915.x, PMID 12406353.

75. Firth-Cozens J. Emotional distress in junior house officers. Br Med J (Clin Res Ed). 1987;295(6597):533–6. https://doi.org/10.1136/bmj.295.6597.533, PMID 3117213.

76. Bousquet G, Orri M, Winterman S, Brugière C, Verneuil L, Revah-Levy A. Breaking bad news in oncology: A metasynthesis. J Clin Oncol. 2015;33(22):2437–43. https://doi.org/10.1200/JCO.2014.59.6759, PMID 26124489.

77. Dean A, Willis S. The use of protocol in breaking bad news: evidence and ethos. Int J Palliat Nurs. 2016;22(6):265–71. https://doi.org/10.12968/ijpn.2016.22.6.265, PMID 27349844.

78. Fallowfield L. Giving sad and bad news. Lancet. 1993;341(8843):476–8. https://doi.org/10.1016/0140-6736(93)90219-7, PMID 8094499.

79. Ramirez AJ, Graham J, Richards MA, Cull A, Gregory WM. Mental health of hospital consultants: the effects of stress and satisfaction at work. Lancet. 1996;347(9003):724–8. https://doi.org/10.1016/s0140-6736(96)90077-x, PMID 8602002.

80. Tesser A, Rosen S, Tesser M. Reluctance to communicate undesirable messages (mum effect) – field study. Psychol Rep. 1971;29(2):651–4. https://doi.org/10.2466/pr0.1971.29.2.651&.

81. Schildmann J, Cushing A, Doyal L, Vollmann J. Breaking bad news: experiences, views and difficulties of pre-registration house officers. Palliat Med. 2005;19(2):93–8. https://doi.org/10.1191/0269216305pm996oa, PMID 15810746.

82. Novack DH, Plumer R, Smith RL, Ochitill H, Morrow GR, Bennett JM. Changes in physicians' attitudes toward telling the cancer patient. JAMA. 1979;241(9):897–900. https://doi.org/10.1001/jama.1979.03290350017012, PMID 762865.

83. Lamont EB, Christakis NA. Prognostic disclosure to patients with cancer near the end of life. Ann Intern Med. 2001;134(12):1096–105. https://doi.org/10.7326/0003-4819-134-12-200106190-00009, PMID 11412049.

84. Abram MB. Making healthcare decisions. The ethical and legal implications of informed consent in the practitioner-patient relationship. President's commission for the study of ethical problems in medicine and biomedical and behavioral research. Superintendent of Documents U.S. Government Printing Office Washington, D.C. 20402. 1982.

85. Sharp MC, Strauss RP, Lorch SC. Communicating medical bad news: parents' experiences and preferences. J Pediatr. 1992;121(4):539–46. https://doi.org/10.1016/s0022-3476(05)81141-2, PMID 1403386.

86. Kutner JS, Steiner JF, Corbett KK, Jahnigen DW, Barton PL. Information needs in terminal illness. Soc Sci Med. 1999;48(10):1341–52. https://doi.org/10.1016/s0277-9536(98)00453-5, PMID 10369435.

87. Kim MK, Alvi A. Breaking the bad news of cancer: the patient's perspective. Laryngoscope. 1999;109(7 Pt 1):1064–7. https://doi.org/10.1097/00005537-199907000-00010, PMID 10401842.

88. Jurkovich GJ, Pierce B, Pananen L, Rivara FP. Giving bad news: the family perspective. J Trauma. 2000;48(5):865–70; discussion 70–3. https://doi.org/10.1097/00005373-200005000-00009, PMID 10823529.

89. Krahn GL, Hallum A, Kime C. Are there good ways to give "bad news"? Pediatrics. 1993;91(3):578–82. https://doi.org/10.1542/peds.91.3.578, PMID 8441562.

90. Englar RE, Williams M, Weingand K. Applicability of the Calgary-Cambridge guide to dog and cat owners for teaching veterinary clinical communications. J Vet Med Educ. 2016;43(2):143–69. https://doi.org/10.3138/jvme.0715-117R1, PMID 27075274.

91. Goldberg KJ. Goals of care: development and use of the serious veterinary illness conversation guide. Vet Clin North Am Small Anim Pract. 2019;49(3):399–415. https://doi.org/10.1016/j.cvsm.2019.01.006, PMID 30853241.

92. Thomas AE. Liquid. In: Ryan T, editor. Love publishing – Grief, loss, animal companions, and the social worker. Animals in social work: why and how they matter. Houndmills, Basingstoke, Hampshire; New York, NY: Palgrave Macmillan; 2014. p. 199–214.

Part Two

Communication Skills and Other Tools That Build Partnership with Clients During Times of Loss

CHAPTER 9

Shared Decision-Making Before, During, and After Euthanasia

In Chapter 7, I introduced the case of Nina, my then 15-year-old female spayed Tonkinese cat with respect to the grief I experienced surrounding her death.

The pertinent aspects of her case files are cold and clinical, a stark contrast to the warmth that Nina exuded, but nonetheless, they are significant when viewing her presentation through the lens of a veterinarian.

- Subjective:
  - ○ 12-hour history of inappetence progressing to four episodes of emesis overnight.
- Objective:
  - ○ skin tenting
  - ○ tacky mucous membranes with icteric undertones
  - ○ visual and palpable abdominal distension

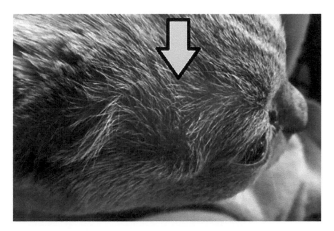

Figure 9.1 Practitioners must evaluate the peri-aural region for evidence of icterus. Icterus cannot be conveyed in a black and white photo such as this; however, in real life this cat's icterus was quite pronounced.

- o   pain elicited on cranial abdominal palpation
- o   bilaterally symmetrical peri-aural icterus.
- Complete Blood Count (CBC):
  - o   mild nonregenerative anemia
  - o   leukocytosis with neutrophilia.
- Serum biochemistry profile:
  - o   increased ALK PHOS, ALT, and bilirubin.
- Abdominal radiographs:
  - o   mass effect in the cranial abdomen.
- Sonography of the abdomen:
  - o   hepatic involvement.
- Presumptive diagnosis:
  - o   primary feline hepatobiliary neoplasia of liver, gall bladder, or bile duct origin
  - o   secondary hepatic lipidosis.

As a veterinarian, I could have offered myself, the client, the following options:

- hospitalization
- intravenous (IV) catheterization
- general anesthesia
- exploratory laparotomy with surgical biopsies
- esophageal feeding tube (E-tube) placement for nutritional support.

The attending veterinarian who was overseeing Nina's case did offer these options and she wasn't wrong to do so.

I would have offered them, too, as just that. Options.

But I didn't see the case as Nina's *veterinarian*.

I saw the case as Nina's *mother*.

As her *mother*, I had to ask myself, "*What would Nina want?*"

As her *mother*, I was her advocate, not my own.

As her *mother*, I had to elevate her needs above mine and make the choice that was *right* for her.

What was *right* and what was *easy* were two entirely different things.

The night before I made the choice to end Nina's suffering, I sat up all night to be with her. I laid flat on my back in my bedroom, where she had spent so many of her days, and she chose my stomach as her final resting place. There, she laid, stiller than she had ever been, hour after hour, until night had passed.

In those early morning hours, I hoped and prayed that Nina would make the choice for me, to pass in her sleep. Her breathing was shallow,

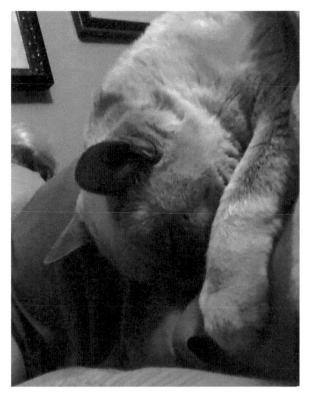

Figure 9.2 Nina's final resting place on the night before she was euthanized.

and she was barely responsive. She no longer acknowledged my presence with the slow blink of her eyes. She no longer acknowledged my voice with the perk of her ears. She appeared to recognize only the warmth of my body and the touch of my skin against her fur. I left her side only to use the facilities. When this required me to move her away from me, albeit temporarily, that is the only time she ever stirred. Beyond that, she had reached a state of obtundation from which very little roused her or seemed to matter.

When morning came, I knew what I had to do.

Making the choice to euthanize Nina was one of the most difficult decisions that I have ever had to make.

It wasn't that I questioned whether it was the right choice to make. *I didn't.*

I knew in my heart that it was right for her the moment we got to the clinic and experienced her brief burst of terminal lucidity – a final rallying of mental clarity and spirit – when she seemingly awoke from her coma to look at me, as if to say, "Thank you, Mom, for doing right by me."

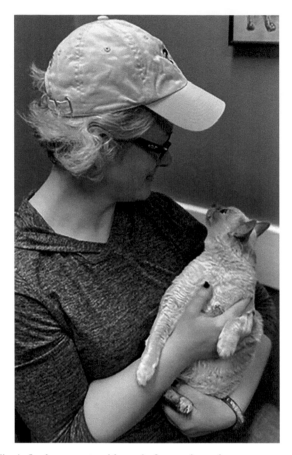

Figure 9.3 Nina's final moments with me before euthanasia.

Euthanizing Nina was not difficult because I questioned its rightness. It was right for her, always.

Euthanizing Nina was difficult because I knew what it meant for me.

It meant that I would be coming home from the clinic without her and that home, as I knew it, would never be the same again.

It meant that I would never again come home to Nina by the door waiting to greet me after a long day.

It meant that I would never again toss a Halls cough drop to Nina for her to fetch and retrieve.

And it meant that I would be moving cross-country without my empathetic Other Half.

In my role as veterinarian, I often share with my clients that euthanasia is the most selfless gift that we can give our loved one during their most critical time of need.

I believed that then, as I do now.

9.1 Euthanasia, Defined

The word, *euthanasia*, has its origins in the Greek language.(1) It is a combination of the terms, *eu*, meaning good and *thanatos*, meaning death. Combined into one word, *euthanasia* translates directly into *good death*.(1, 2)

What it means to have a *good death* is subject to interpretation. Recall from Chapter 2 that cultural and religious conceptions about death and dying influence what it means for people to both live and die well.(3–9)

When we consider the construct of *good death* in human healthcare, it often concentrates on the survivors' needs, wants, and expectations with respect to saying goodbye.(3) Death is often deemed to be *good* if it affords ample time for those left behind to prepare.(3)

Human hospice has in many ways elevated the consideration that society gives to death by refocusing healthcare onto the quality of the patient's dying experience.(10) Hospice improves quality of death(11, 12) through:(10, 13–22) "Good pain and symptom management; clear decision-making; respect for one's personhood; trust in health care providers; a sense of closure, completion or preparedness; minimizing family burden; being able to contribute to others; and maintaining control."(10)

When we think about *good death* in the context of veterinary practice, what we are hoping to achieve is an expedient end to life that minimizes, if not eliminates, pain and distress.(1) According to the American Veterinary Medical Association (AVMA), this requires two primary duties of veterinarians:(1)

1. humane disposition
2. humane technique.

Humane disposition means that the decision to euthanize was made in the best interest of the animal.(1) In other words, euthanasia was selected among other options because it was said to bring about the best outcome.(1)

According to the AVMA Guidelines for the Euthanasia of Animals:(1)

When animals are plagued by disease that produces insurmountable suffering, it can be argued that continuing to live is worse for the animal than death or that the animal no longer has an interest in living. The humane disposition is to act for the sake of the animal or its interests, because the animal will not be harmed by the loss of life. Instead, there is consensus that the animal will be relieved of an unbearable burden.

The Guidelines provide the following example:(1)

> *When treating a companion animal that is suffering severely at the end of life due to a debilitating terminal illness, a veterinarian may recommend euthanasia, because the loss of life (and attendant natural decline in physical and psychological faculties) to the animal is not relatively worse compared with a continued existence that is filled with prolonged illness, suffering, and duress. In this case, euthanasia does not deprive the animal of the opportunity to enjoy more goods of life (i.e., to have more satisfactions fulfilled or enjoy more pleasurable experiences). And, these opportunities or experiences are much fewer or lesser in intensity than the presence or intensity of negative states or affect. Death, in this case, may be a welcome event and euthanasia helps to bring this about, because the animal's life is not worth living but, rather, is worth avoiding.*

Sometimes clinical cases are not so clear-cut, and it can be challenging for the veterinarian to decide whether euthanasia is in fact the best treatment outcome.(1) In these situations, it is important to reference quality of life scales(23–46) and to consider animal welfare.(1) Animal welfare has been described as a function of health: the animal is able to feel well and demonstrate behaviors that are innate.(1)

Humane technique requires that death be expedient, ethical, and minimize suffering.(1) In the words of the AVMA:(1) "As veterinarians and human beings it is our responsibility to ensure that if an animal's life is to be taken, it is done with the highest degree of respect, and with an emphasis on making the death as painless and distress free as possible."

For this to occur:(1) "The technique employed should result in rapid loss of consciousness followed by cardiac or respiratory arrest and, ultimately, a loss of brain function. In addition, animal handling and the euthanasia technique should minimize distress experienced by the animal prior to loss of consciousness."

The concept of *prinum non nocere* – "First, do no harm" – may have been conceptualized in the writings of Hippocrates as a means to guide one's approach to the delivery of human healthcare.(47) However, it is applicable across health professions, particularly to the common veterinary practice of inducing humane death.

9.2 Euthanasia as a Medical Procedure

Euthanasia can be thought of as an act of service.

It is an act of service to the *animals*, so that they do not endure unnecessary suffering.

It is an act of service to the *human companions* of that animal, so that they do not have to watch the patient endure suffering.

It is an act of service to the *community*, by upholding the oath we took as veterinarians to set the standard for the "protection of health and welfare" as well as the "prevention and relief of animal suffering."(48)

As much as it is an act of service, it is a medical procedure, too. In the same way that we prepare for dentistry or surgery, so, too, must we prepare to perform euthanasia.

There are two stages to preparation:

1. We must prepare as a veterinary team for the procedural aspects of euthanasia.
2. We must prepare the veterinary client for the process in a way that conveys compassionate care, humility, medical competence, professionalism, and the highest regard for the human–animal bond.

Note that this chapter intends to provide an overview with respect to both the procedural and interpersonal aspects of euthanasia by taking into consideration that it is a legitimate treatment option and that guidelines are available to support the veterinary team's approach.

9.3 The Roles and Responsibilities of the Veterinary Team to the *Patient* at End of Life

Our primary responsibility, as the veterinary team, is to the patient. The patient's comfort and dignity should always come first.(1) That means that we should prepare for the procedure. The veterinary team should have a plan in place as well as options for how to flex if the need arises during euthanasia.

Many clinics have established a standard operating procedure (SOP) for companion animal euthanasia to be certain that all essential tasks are accounted for. In addition to preparing the drug of choice for the final injection, euthanasia-associated tasks typically include the following:

- Whether or not to utilize pre-euthanasia sedation.
  - o If yes, which drug(s) and route(s) of administration?
  - o If yes, when should you administer relative to the final injection of euthanasia solution to achieve the desired effect?
- Whether or not to utilize an intravenous (IV) catheter.
  - o If yes, will the catheter be placed in front of the client or out of view?

- o If the IV catheter will be placed out of view of the client:
  - Will you ask the client to step out of the consultation room?
  - Alternatively, will you ask the client for permission to bring the patient into the treatment area for IV catheter placement?
  - How will you explain this to the client?
  - How will you handle the hand-off of the patient from the client to the veterinary team to minimize impact?
  - How will you handle the patient to minimize fear, anxiety, and stress?
- o Will anxiolytics be administered to facilitate IV catheter placement?
  - If yes, the owner needs to be aware that medications may alter the patient's mental state and disposition.
  - Owners may wish to spend time with the patient *before* medications have been administered so that they have the opportunity to say goodbye while the patient is still lucid.

Both private practices and university teaching hospitals that I practiced at routinely made use of an anxiolytic (e.g., benzodiazepines), sedative/ anxiolytic combination, and/or injectable anesthetic agent (e.g., propofol) to facilitate the transition from life to death.

Oral medication may also be prescribed for at-home use, prior to coming into the clinic, to take the edge off.

For cats, these medications may include oral:(49, 50)

- alprazolam
- lorazepam
- buprenorphine
- gabapentin.

For dogs, these medications may include oral:(49)

- trazodone
- gabapentin.

For dosing information, please consult a veterinary pharmacology text.

Medications need to be given well in advance of the visit (e.g., 30 minutes to 2 hours, depending upon the drug of choice(50)) to maximize efficacy. Ideally, medications are administered at home, and the patient is provided with a quiet, dimly lit space to unwind. Medicated pets should be kept away from steps and staircases because they are likely to lose their balance.

The AVMA Guidelines for the Euthanasia of Animals reminds us that:(1) "A common characteristic of both sedatives and tranquilizers is that arousal to a conscious state can occur with sufficient stimulation, such that animals sedated or immobilized with these agents may still be consciously aware of, and connected to, their environment."

Thus, owners should be instructed that the response to medication may be variable, cat to cat, dog to dog, and that patients can override the medication once they encounter a stressful environment (e.g., the drive into the clinic, for many cats; or walking into the clinic waiting room).

In-clinic protocols are frequently used in combination with at-home protocols to smooth out any additional stress that the clinic experience may induce.

Feline-friendly pre-sedation in-clinic protocols include, but are not limited to, a combination of:(49, 50)

- ketamine, acepromazine, and tiletamine-zolazepam
- ketamine, butorphanol, acepromazine, and midazolam
- ketamine, butorphanol, and dexmedetomidine
- tiletamine-zolazepam, reconstituted with acepromazine +/- ketamine
- dexmedetomidine, ketamine, and butorphanol.

Canine pre-sedation in-clinic protocols may include, but are not limited to, combinations of:(49)

- dexmedetomidine or xylazine, nalbuphine or butorphanol, and acepromazine
- tiletamine-zolazepam, xylazine, and acepromazine
- acepromazine, ketamine, and midazolam.

Canine and feline-appropriate in-clinic protocols include, but are not limited to:(49)

- acepromazine, ketamine, and midazolam
- tiletamine-zolazepam and acepromazine
- butorphanol and acepromazine.

The advantage of injectable combinations, administered either subcutaneously (SC) or intramuscularly (IM), is that they take a few minutes to take effect. They act more quickly than oral medications to induce their effects, but the onset of effects is still gradual. In essence, this smooths out the transition between awake and decreased consciousness. The patient appears to be relaxing into sleepiness.

Many clients appreciate the apparent peacefulness of this time and are able to themselves settle in more comfortably during a time of acute discomfort. The client may feel comforted that the patient is more relaxed. When the patient's non-verbal cues reflect a calm state, the client may feel at peace with their decision. The client may appreciate that the patient appears to be drifting off to the sound of their voice.

As a veterinarian, I prefer to administer in-clinic pre-euthanasia sedation for all these reasons. When I consider that euthanasia means *good death*, the word, *peaceful*, comes to mind. Peaceful, to me, conjures up the image of falling asleep.

The illusion that our patient is *falling asleep* facilitates the perception among the veterinary team, including the client, that the transition from life to death will be smooth and peaceful.

The rationale for pre-euthanasia sedation is that it may:

- decrease fear, anxiety, and pain in the patient
- lessen the need for restraint during the Final Injection
  - this allows the patient to remain close to their caregiver
- reduce unwanted side effects from the administration of euthanasia solutions
  - e.g., jerky motions, reflex responses, and agonal breathing.

Just as I shared with respect to at-home sedation protocols, in-clinic sedation is imperfect. I think of its use as increasing the likelihood that euthanasia will proceed smoothly. However, every patient responds to every drug differently.

Depending upon which combination of drugs is administered, the patient may seem disoriented, rather than groggy, as if they're coming out of anesthesia. This may alter the client's perception of patient comfort. If clients have not adequately been prepared for this, it may be unsettling for them to observe. Seeing their disoriented cat attempt a drunken walk, for instance, may not be the lasting image that the client wants to preserve.

To minimize these unsettling effects, some clinicians opt to administer IV propofol alone, in lieu of a SC or IM drug cocktail.

The difference between IV propofol and a SC/IM injectable combination is that IV propofol takes the patient from awake to asleep near instantaneously. Pre-euthanasia sedation with propofol exhibits rapid onset that is profound. The patient skips over the disoriented phase and is instead rendered unconscious within seconds.

Which path towards euthanasia is preferred should depend upon individual patient considerations:

- How stressed does the patient get in the clinic?
- How has the patient responded to medications in the past?
  - Are there medications that the patient has responded well to, in the past, for instance, during pre-medication or induction for general anesthesia?
  - Are there medications that the patient has had adverse reactions to that we would like to avoid?
- Does the patient have any underlying conditions that may be improved by the administration of certain medications?
- Does the patient have any underlying conditions that may be exacerbated by the administration of certain medications?
- Which protocol is most likely to contribute to good death?

Although our primary responsibility is to the patient, we must also consider the client's presence – should they choose to witness the euthanasia – as well as what we want the client's lasting image to be of the patient as the patient passes.

We must consider the client's emotional state and how that may impact our patients as we transition them nearer to death. A client who is emotionally spent may not tolerate a drawn-out procedure and may themselves benefit – which in turn benefits the patient – from rapid induction of unconsciousness with propofol. On the other hand, a client who is not ready to say goodbye may benefit from the additional time that non-propofol protocols afford. Such a client may appreciate the added time to sit with, sit beside, talk to, and/or stroke their loved one.

In addition to the client, the following considerations influence which path towards euthanasia is preferred:

- clinic support
- clinician preference
- support staff preference
- stocked in-house pharmacy, in terms of drug availability
- cost to client.

Cost is a reality of veterinary practice. Because propofol has a short shelf-life, it is cost-prohibitive to open a single bottle of propofol for the sole purpose of augmenting euthanasia, particularly if the patient's body weight dictates a small dose. However, if the clinic knows in advance that propofol is a preferred choice among its doctors and propofol is used routinely on-site to induce general anesthesia for in-house surgical procedures, then expired propofol can be retained in the refrigerator to support in-house euthanasia.

These considerations should be discussed openly within the veterinary team. Individual clinicians are likely to have preferences and it is important that clinics honor these preferences whenever possible.

Euthanasia can be an incredibly stressful process for all members of the veterinary team, particularly when its role repeats multiple times within a given workday. For the team to sustain itself throughout the process, all team members must feel supported.

The best way to provide support is to allow for flexibility within SOPs. Individual team members are then able to provide optimal care in the best way that they see fit.

Individual team members may or may not elect to use pre-euthanasia sedation. It is important to acknowledge that the use of pre-euthanasia sedation, prior to the Final Injection, is a preference, not a requirement, as per the AVMA Guidelines for the Euthanasia of Animals:(1) "Barbiturates administered IV may be given alone as the sole agent of euthanasia or as the second step after sedation or general anesthesia."

As stated in the guidelines above, the preferred method for canine and feline euthanasia is to inject a barbituric acid derivative (e.g., pentobarbital or pentobarbital combination product) intravenously.(1) Pentobarbital is a fast-acting barbiturate that causes rapid loss of consciousness, followed by cardiac arrest.

Within the United States, federal drug regulations require strict accounting for barbiturates. Only those personnel who have specifically applied for and received a license by the Drug Enforcement Agency (DEA) can maintain a supply of these drugs and supervise their use.(1)

Within the United Kingdom, strict regulations with respect to controlled drugs also apply.(51) As Schedule 3 controlled drugs, barbiturates are required to be stocked under lock and key, and record-keeping is mandated to track drug usage.(51)

There are many different brands of commercially available euthanasia solution for veterinary practices. Some products contain exclusively pentobarbital. Others have been combined with a local anesthetic or phenytoin sodium. Phenytoin sodium hastens the loss of electrical activity in the heart during the deep anesthesia stage that is induced by the pentobarbital. This action speeds death.

One product is not superior to another; however, it is critical to familiarize yourself with the label of your practice's product of choice for details concerning product characteristics.(1) For instance, Sleepaway®, which is no longer manufactured, was a clear solution. Most solutions in veterinary medicine are clear. This reinforced the need to label all needles and syringes in clinical practice and not lay down anything unlabeled on the countertop. A clear solution could be mistaken for nearly any other drug.

Today, most euthanasia solutions are intentionally colored with a distinct pigment that is not seen in any other drug that is commercially available. The color has been added to the product to prevent accidental administration to the wrong patient:

- Euthasol®, Beuthanasia, and Somnasol are bright pink solutions
- Socumb® and FatalPlus® are distinctly blue
- Pentoject® has a distinctive yellow color.

Prior to participating in any euthanasia procedure, the veterinary team should familiarize themselves not only with the brand of choice, but also with the labelled dose. Products vary in terms of dosage. For instance, Socumb® is labelled for use at 1cc per 10lb of body weight. So, a 10lb cat should be administered a *minimum* of 1.0cc and a 20lb dog should be administered a *minimum* of 2.0cc. This initial dose is an estimate of the average volume of solution that is said to be effective.

You never want to put yourself in such a precarious situation as when you do not draw up enough solution. So, veterinarians typically round up. Some of my colleagues add an additional 0.5mL to the calculated dose, based upon patient body weight: they would administer 1.5cc of Socumb® to the 10lb cat and 2.5cc of Socumb® to the 20lb dog.

I was taught early on in my education that "You cannot overdo death." Therefore, I am always overly cautious and add at least 1.0mL–2.0mL more than what the label indicates. I would administer 3.0cc of Socumb® to the 10lb cat.

Once you have selected your drug of choice and drawn up the patient's dose in a syringe, you need a means by which to get the solution into the patient.

The goal of the barbituric acid derivative is to suppress the patient's nervous system. The ideal euthanasia solution is one that stops the brain before it stops the heart such that cerebral death is experienced by the patient before cardiovascular collapse. In laymen's terms, we want the patient to be unconscious so that the patient is unaware that death is coming.

The best way for any drug to reach the patient's brain quickly is through the circulatory system. Therefore, under ideal circumstances, we administer the Final Injection intravenously (IV).

The vessels of choice in companion animals are:

- cephalic vein (cats and dogs)
- lateral saphenous vein (typically reserved for dogs)

- medial saphenous vein (typically reserved for cats)
- lateral ear vein (typically reserved for rabbits and the occasional Bassett Hound).

Which vessel you access is typically based upon the clinician's preference.

If the veterinary technician is asked and consents to performing euthanasia under the supervision of a veterinarian, then they should have the choice of which vessel they prefer to access.

Personally, I prefer to access medial saphenous vessels in cats and lateral saphenous vessels in dogs when owners are present for euthanasia, assuming that the patient is laying on an examination room table. Doing so places me at the caudal half of the patient. This positioning affords the client space to be at the patient's head. If the client wants to stand at the head of the patient during the procedure and I were to use the cephalic vein instead, I tend to feel that I am in the client's way.

One way around that would be for me to place an extension set. The extension set allows me to stand at some distance away from the patient. This requires me to have an IV catheter in place.

When I have an IV catheter in place, I always carry at least one syringe of physiologic saline flush (0.9% NaCl) with me into the consultation room. I inject the flush into the vessel via the IV catheter immediately after injecting the euthanasia solution to help push the solution through the system. This speeds the delivery of the solution, via the circulatory system, to the brain, to induce cerebral death.

It is important to note that not every clinic includes IV catheterization as part of their SOP for owner-present euthanasia.

Not every clinician prefers IV catheterization as part of their SOP for owner-present euthanasia.

Not every owner is keen on having an IV catheter placed in the patient prior to euthanasia; most worry that it adds additional, unnecessary anxiety, fear, stress, or hurt.

Whether to place an IV catheter depends upon many factors including, but not limited to the following.

- Confidence and skill of the person who will be administering the Final Injection.
- Whether the patient's circulatory system is hemodynamically unstable (e.g., compromised), in which case I am much more concerned about my ability to find a vessel in the moment, in a consultation room, without an IV catheter having been placed.

Administering the Final Injection directly into the vessel of choice may seem preferable in that it (ideally) requires a single poke, and it is arguably a lot more comfortable than placing an IV catheter.

However, if the patient moves, then the needle is likely to slip out of the vein. This in essence ruptures the vein, causing blood (and the euthanasia solution) to leak into tissues that are immediately adjacent to the insertion site. We say that the vessel has "blown," which means that unless we can insert the needle proximal to the "blown" site to reinject, we will have to go fishing for another vessel. This delay in the euthanasia process intensifies the stress for the veterinary client, who may not understand why the procedure is taking so long. There is also significant impact on the veterinary team, who may feel that they fell short in their delivery of a good death.

I have experienced situations without IV catheters in which I've gotten "some" of the drug into circulation, but not enough before the vessel "blows." When any euthanasia solution seeps out into surrounding tissues, it burns. The patient may react to the unpleasant sensation. Whether their reactions are subtle or whether the patient actively tries to kick their leg to get away, the owner may question the patient's comfort. The owner is also likely to fixate on the patient's reaction as their final memory of how the patient passed.

For these reasons, many veterinarians and their support staff prefer that an IV catheter be placed prior to every euthanasia. The placement of an IV catheter makes the vessel instantly accessible. This reduces the likelihood that something will go wrong including, but not limited to the following:

- Not being able to find a blood vessel.
- Not having enough euthanasia solution drawn up and needing to administer more quickly, particularly to quiet agonal breathing episodes that may occur peri-mortem.
- Needing additional flush to push the euthanasia solution into circulation in a patient who is severely dehydrated, hypotensive, or both.
- Needing additional flush to push the euthanasia solution through an extension set.

What I appreciate most about placing IV catheters for euthanasia is that I don't have to go fishing for a vessel in the consultation room, in front of the client, and if I need to administer additional solution, I am able to do so because my access to the patient's circulatory system has been maintained through the IV catheter.

I personally have never felt confident enough in my skillset to hit a vessel each time, every time in front of a grieving client. Because of this, I defaulted to asking that an IV catheter be placed prior to every euthanasia. Granted, I had the advantage of working with all-star technicians who could place an IV catheter in any patient, at any time.

Placing an IV catheter allowed me to concentrate on the owner and their needs during the euthanasia process rather than focusing on trying to hit the vessel, which would have only compounded my stress.

In retrospect, my request for IV catheter placement was largely out of consideration for my own sake rather than my patient's. What I hope it allowed me to do was to provide my client with a smoother transition in the consultation room from life to death.

Not all my colleagues might feel the same way. Many of my colleagues would prefer a clean stick in the examination room rather than drawing out the procedure further, by placing an IV catheter, and many of my colleagues are far better phlebotomists than I will ever be.

An additional consideration is cost. For some clinic pricing structures, placing an IV catheter represents an additional charge to the client and this in and of itself may influence whether you proceed with one or not.

What is important to take away from this section is that IV catheter placement is a choice, not a mandate. Choices are just that. Choices. Options.

Options are meant to be considered. Each time you choose. Every time.

I respect the right of my colleagues to make choices that they feel are in the best interest of the patient. Every patient is unique. Every euthanasia is unique. We should tailor choices to the patient rather than adopt the same patient care plan in all instances. Such pet-specific care is a practice philosophy that is growing in popularity because it customizes the approach to healthcare delivery.(52) Rather than prescribing one approach to care, veterinarians can deliver a continuum of acceptable care options that can meet the needs of a diverse population of patients.(53)

Regardless of whether you use an IV catheter, you should dilute the euthanasia solution. No matter what brand you purchase, euthanasia solution is thick and sticky. These properties make it immensely challenging to inject the solution through our patients' small veins, particularly if our patients are hypotensive. Don't give the vessel any other reason to "blow." Dilute the solution so that it pushes like water rather than honey.

As a safety precaution, use syringes with Luer Lock tips to inject euthanasia solution whenever possible to prevent accidental exposure of the client and/or the veterinary care team due to needle/syringe separation. Pentobarbital will sting and/or numb any cuts, scrapes, or mucous membranes (e.g., conjunctival, nasal, oral) that it contacts. I have myself been splashed in the eye with pentobarbital and it is not a pleasant feeling. In the moment, it stung appreciably. After the fact, the affected eye felt unpleasantly numb for the better half of a day, even after using eyewash extensively.

Death via injectable IV barbiturates is rapidly achieved. It takes 1–3 minutes on average for the patient to be rendered unconscious and 3–5 minutes to reach cardiac arrest.

Following injection and prior to disposal of animal remains, death should be confirmed. It is essential that confirmation includes a combination of criteria such as:

- lack of pulse
- lack of breathing
- lack of corneal reflex
- lack of response to firm toe pinch
- inability to hear respiratory sounds and heartbeat via a stethoscope
- graying of the mucous membranes
- rigor mortis.

In considering route of administration for euthanasia solution, IV access is preferred, but not always possible. This route may be impractical, for instance, in neonatal puppies or kittens.(1) In these patients, barbiturates and barbituric acid derivatives can be administered via the intraperitoneal (IP) route.(1)

Note that the IP route is not advised for use in larger patients because higher volumes of euthanasia solution are necessary to induce death.(1) The time between IP injection and death in medium-sized or large-breed dogs is too extensively prolonged.(1) In such patients, intra-organ routes of administration may be advised.(1, 50) These include:(1, 50)

- intra-cardiac
- intra-hepatic
- intra-renal.

These routes of administration hasten death by speeding the rate of barbiturate uptake.(1) However, they are not particularly comfortable for the patient; therefore, the patient should be rendered unconscious prior to administration.(1)

Additional considerations for alternative routes of administration must include who will be present to witness the euthanasia. In owner-present euthanasia, the intra-cardiac route is not preferred by me because it is particularly unpleasant for most owners to witness.

The AVMA Guidelines for the Euthanasia of Animals also supports the use of nonbarbiturate anesthetic overdose (e.g., combination of ketamine and xylazine given IV, IP, or IM or propofol given IV) to induce death.(1)

On occasion, ovariohysterectomy (OVH) may be performed on a pregnant queen or bitch.(54)

Dr. Sara White explains two circumstances in which the need may arise:(54)

For feral cat control programs, ovariohysterectomy of pregnant females furthers the mission of population control and allows all animals brought to the clinic to be spayed the same day, eliminating the need for retrapping or extensive foster care. In the case of owned animals, owners may request pregnancy termination, and ovariohysterectomy is considered the best alternative for termination of unwanted pregnancies in cats and dogs not intended for breeding.

In either circumstance, the pregnant uterus is removed and thus the pregnancy is terminated.

In recent years, concern has been raised as to whether the fetuses contained within should be euthanized.(54, 55)

According to the Association of Shelter Veterinarians' 2016 Veterinary Medical Care Guidelines for Spay-Neuter Programs, euthanasia of fetuses is not necessary, provided that the uterus remains closed following OVH. (55)

The guidelines state their rationale as follows:(55) "Mammalian fetuses remain in a state of unconsciousness throughout gestation and, therefore, cannot consciously perceive pain. When a gravid uterus is removed en bloc, fetuses will not experience consciousness regardless of stage of gestation and death will occur without pain."

Even so, some veterinarians still elect to inject euthanasia solution through the wall of the closed uterus or into each closed fetal sac, as appreciated through palpation of the intact, whole uterus. Dr. White suggests that this final act may "speed the cessation of the spontaneous in utero fetal movements that some veterinarians and staff find troubling."(54)

9.4 The Roles and Responsibilities of the Veterinary Team to the *Client* at End-of-Life Consultations

The patient's comfort and dignity should be prioritized throughout the euthanasia process; however, end-of-life consultations impact far more than the patient. It is vital that the veterinary team acknowledge, validate, and affirm that the decision to euthanize is life-changing for those who will survive the pet's death.

The decision to euthanize often represents a precarious balance between the client's desire to extend their companion's life and the desire not to see their companion suffer.(56) Saying goodbye to their pet may be a deliberate choice to prioritize quality of life over quantity, and requires emotional support and regard from the entire veterinary team.(57)

The need for survivors to feel supported in their decision-making cannot be understated.(57) At least half of pet owners will experience and/or express guilt about making the choice to euthanize.(57, 58) Seven out of ten owners acknowledge that they are emotionally impacted by the death of their pet and one in three will experience severe grief.(58) How well owners feel supported influences their respective journeys through grief.(59)

At any given time throughout the euthanasia process, the veterinary team fulfills several roles that collectively meet each client's needs:(56, 60–62)

- educator
- supporter
- patient advocate
- advisor
- listener
- facilitator
- partner
- caretaker.

The professional obligation to provide emotional support to every grieving client can be overwhelming for the veterinary team, who experiences patient death at a rate of five times what other healthcare professionals experience.(59, 63, 64) Self-care and work-life balance is essential to guard against burnout and compassion fatigue.(59, 65, 66) At the same time, death, which has become so commonplace for veterinarians, is entirely unique when viewed through the client's lens. That patient is not just another cat or just another dog. That patient is someone's loved one. Someone's "sibling." Someone's "child." Someone's "family."

Every experience with that family member, including death, is unique for survivors, whose grief will either be supported or aggravated by the perceived manner in which the veterinary team offers support.(59)

Veterinary teams who demonstrate willingness to accompany the survivors in their respective journeys through grief demonstrate immense commitment to relationship-centered care.

Companioning clients through grief is not easy.

Companioning clients through end-of-life consultations can be one of the most challenging tasks of a veterinarian's day.

Companioning clients through end-of-life consultations requires the team to put aside their perceptions of what needs to be done and instead sit with the client as they work through the process at their own pace. This requires patience and compassion, as well as the desire to partner with and connect to clients on an inherently human level.

The need for patients to establish a connection with their doctors is not a new concept.(47) As early as the 1940s, internist and psychiatrist George Engel emphasized client communication as a means of relating to the patient.(67) Engel's biopsychosocial vision of healthcare delivery highlighted a humanistic approach to medicine.(68) His work at the University of Rochester, New York linked physician–patient bonds to successful patient outcomes and physician resilience.(68) By the late 20th century, it was believed by many more than Engel that "before anything else, a good doctor must be a good communicator."(69)

This perspective persisted and was influential in establishing the relationship-centered approach to present day healthcare delivery in which:

> *The patient is not just a group of symptoms, damaged organs and altered emotions. The patient is a human being, at the same time worried and hopeful, who is searching for relief, help and trust. The importance of an intimate relationship between patient and physician can never be overstated because in most cases an accurate diagnosis, as well as an effective treatment, relies directly on the quality of this relationship.(70)*

Strong relationships between provider and patient foster trust and security. Human medical patients value and recall, with gratitude, those instances when their physicians demonstrated concern, empathy, regard, sensitivity, sincerity, and/or warmth.(71–73)

This constellation of valued traits is what we have historically referred to as "bedside manner." A doctor with good "bedside manner" was said to apply compassion to patient care. The doctor with good "bedside manner" was said to meet patient care needs more effectively because they took the time to elicit the patient's perspective. When the patient shared what they valued most, the doctor actively listened. Moreover, the doctor demonstrated that the patient was heard by taking measures to incorporate what mattered most to the patient into the patient care plan. Patients interpreted this as a sign of respect. They appreciated being treated as a significant part of the healthcare team.

Indeed, the ways in which providers relate to their clients and communicate drive patient outcomes. Research consistently demonstrates in human healthcare that effective communication improves:(74–80)

- accuracy of diagnosis
- interpersonal relationships and professional relationship-building(81, 82)
  - o patients feel connected
  - o patients feel understood
  - o patients feel validated
- patient adherence to treatment plans
- patient compliance
- patient coping skills
- patient outcomes(79, 80)
  - o emotional health
  - o function
  - o mental health
    - ▪ acceptance of disease process
    - ▪ reduction of anxiety
    - ▪ understanding treatment options and risks associated with treatment
  - o physiologic health
    - ▪ blood pressure
    - ▪ blood sugar regulation
  - o symptom management, including pain
  - o symptom resolution.

The link between effective communication and positive patient outcomes is not unique to human healthcare.(83, 84) Effective communication drives client satisfaction in veterinary practice as well, and clients seek rapport-building when establishing veterinarian–client–patient relationships (VCPRs).(83, 84)

Nowhere in veterinary practice is relationship-building more critical than end-of-life consultations. End-of-life consultations are make-it-or-break-it visits for many VCPRs. After all, how they and their loved ones were treated at end of life is what clients remember. The memory of that final moment is so powerful that it is capable of enduring for days, weeks, months, even years after euthanasia.

Matte et al. explain that:(56) "When euthanasia-related care is managed well, a client's grief may be [more easily managed], their concerns acknowledged, emotions supported and difficult decisions, such as the transition to end-of-life, can be more easily negotiated."

On the other hand, when end-of-life consultations are handled poorly:(56) "Clients may experience dissatisfaction with their veterinarian, have a decreased willingness to continue a relationship with that veterinarian or veterinary hospital and be at a greater risk for complicated forms of grief."

Because our actions and words impact their journey through grief, we owe it to our clients to be skillful in our approach. We benefit clients during end-of-life consultation when they:(59)

- have an opportunity to voice questions and/or concerns
- feel heard
- hear us acknowledge the difficulty of decision-making
- hear us affirm and/or validate their emotions
- are given an opportunity to engage in shared decision-making
- feel that their decisions are respected.

9.5 Making the Choice to Euthanize

For the purposes of this chapter, we will exclude emergency situations in which time is of the essence and euthanasia must be performed with urgency as a medical necessity, rather than a choice.

In all other cases, the choice to euthanize is part of the shared decision-making process in which the client–veterinarian partnership makes a joint determination that the patient's life is served best by facilitating that patient's death.

Making that choice is inherently unique to the individual patient, client, and the human–animal bond that they share.

Some choices are inherently more challenging than others to make, from the perspective of the veterinarian.

Some choices are inherently more challenging than others to make, from the perspective of the client.

Some choices are riddled with shades of grey and clouded with "*What ifs?*":

- *What if* the cat with urinary tract obstruction (UTO) is medically managed and never were to block again?
- *What if* we knew for sure that the dog with gastric dilatation and volvulus (GDV) with severe increases in plasma lactate concentration (>10mmol/L) would survive surgical correction without developing gastric necrosis?

Young pets with serious medical conditions are particularly troubling for clients and veterinarians alike.(85) On the one hand, we see a patient who has yet to experience much of life and potentially has much more life to live. On the other hand, we must consider both diagnosis and prognosis:(85)

- Can the patient recover? If so:
  - Is treatment curative or palliative?
  - What is the best-case scenario?
  - What is the worst-case scenario?
  - What is the anticipated timetable for recovery?
  - What are potential complications that the patient could experience?
  - Are potential complications treatable?
  - Is there a possibility that the patient could relapse?
  - What would a relapse in condition look like?
  - How would a relapse in condition be managed?
    - Would a relapse necessitate medical intervention?
    - Would a relapse necessitate surgical intervention?
    - Would a relapse necessitate both?
- What is the short-term prognosis?
- What is the long-term prognosis?
- Is the client prepared to handle the worst-case scenario?
- Is the patient likely to experience any mobility and/or elimination issues that might adversely affect the human–animal bond?
- Will the patient have any lasting adverse effects of this clinical condition and/or the treatment that is medically indicated?
- Will the patient require any long-term treatments, including medications?
- What are client-specific constraints in terms of immediate, short-term, and long-term aftercare?
- Clients may need to also factor in financial considerations:(85)
  - How much can they commit financially now?
  - How much can they commit financially later in the event that complications arise or in the event that the patient relapses?
  - Does investing in healthcare now preclude treatment later? If so, to what extent?

Whether the patient is young, with a serious medical condition; geriatric with a terminal disease; or geriatric without a terminal condition, it is essential that parameters for quality of life be defined based upon the pet's current clinical presentation.

Recall quality-of-life parameters that were first introduced in Chapter 8:(23–46)

- attitude/temperament
- non-verbal cues
  - ear carriage
  - facial changes
  - squinted eyes
  - tautness of the whiskers
  - pupil size/shape
  - posture
- changes to routine
- behavioral changes
- reaction to palpation
- perception of anxiety
- perception of mental state
- appetite and/or ability to keep food down
- ability to maintain weight/degree of weight loss
- mobility
- activity or energy level
- desire to interact with surroundings
- response to the client's presence
- thirst
- respiratory rate, depth, quality, and ease
- perception of pain
- elimination habits
- hygiene.

It may be helpful to provide the client with a quality-of-life scale that you prefer, or you can partner with the client to create your own. Assessing the patient based upon the parameters that you and the client agree to, on a routine basis, can assist with decision-making and provide a more objective means by which to evaluate the patient's quality.

Quality-of-life scales are imperfect. However, what they achieve is opening the door to dialogue so that clients' expectations can be explored, acknowledged, and addressed. Sometimes clients' expectations are unrealistic. These require the veterinarian to navigate challenging conversations in which they and the client may not see eye to eye.

Goals of care (GOC) conversations can be a meaningful place to begin because they set the tone in terms of transparency:

- "This is what I want …"
- "This is what I don't want …"
- "This is what I'm hearing that you want …"
- "This is what I'm hearing that you don't want …"
- "This is what I'm hearing that we both want …"

Sometimes it is helpful to hear from the client what their past experiences have been with loss:(86)

- Have they lost pets before and, if so, how?
- Have they had to make a choice to euthanize in the past? If so, how did they feel about having to make that decision? Did they feel at peace with the decision, or did they harbor regret? If there is a history of regret, what specifically did the client wish had gone differently and why?
- What, if anything, helped them to make the decision to euthanize, in the past, and could they draw inspiration from that to help them make the choice today?
  - o How did they know it was time *then*?
  - o How might that help them *now*?
- When their last pet passed, what stood out to them about the pet's passing?
  - o What would they like to replicate about that experience for this pet?
  - o What might they like to avoid and/or forget?

Sometimes we need to ask the client what or who would be most helpful to point them in the direction of what is "right" for them. It may be that a vital person needs to weigh in on the conversation but has not yet been invited to participate. One owner may have brought the patient in to be seen; a second owner may need to be present for end-of-life decision-making to proceed.

Ask your client who else is involved in decision-making. Ask who else needs to be present for life-altering decisions and who else might the client need for additional support.(86)

Everyone who needs to be a part of the conversation should be encouraged to participate. This may require rearranging schedules and/or accommodating more than one consultation.

Create a safe, supportive space in which the client may answer the following questions freely:(86)

- What makes the pet happy?
- What makes the pet's days enjoyable?

- What does quality of life mean to the client?
- Does the pet have quality now?
- Is the pet enjoying life in the moment?
- Is the pet happy?
    - o If not, what needs to be done to create the ideal circumstances under which the pet can be happy?
    - o Can something be done to create the ideal circumstances under which the pet can be happy?
    - o If nothing can be done to create the ideal circumstances under which the pet can be happy, how can we make the pet more comfortable?
- Is the pet suffering?

Allow the client to share their story. Elicit the client's perspective. Help them share with you what they perceive their pet to be experiencing and what, if anything, concerns them.

Be open to seeing the pet through their perspective.

Ask for permission to share your own perspective with them about the patient.

Acknowledge emotions as they arise. Normalize and validate emotions. Demonstrate empathy. Ask the client for permission to broach sensitive subjects, including how the client is feeling. Permission statements might take the form of:

- "Would it be alright if I … ?"
- "Would you like me to talk you through … ?"

Visible sadness can be acknowledged directly, but the likely presence of other emotions, such as anger, are better suggested than identified.

- "I can see you are distressed."
- "I can see you're upset."
- "Many pet owners in this situation would feel angry, understandably. I wonder if you might be feeling this way?"

Empathic displays of support might include statements of acknowledgment and/or affirmation. For instance, you might share that:

- "It's very upsetting when you receive bad news like this."
- "It's heart-breaking to have to think about saying goodbye."
- "I'm so sorry we are having this conversation."
- "I cannot imagine what you are going through."

Find out as best you can what the owner is feeling and how those feelings are translating into actions.

Do what is essential to ensure that there is clarity about any decisions that are made and that everyone understands the path moving forward. This means that we, the veterinary team, must take care to be exceptionally clear in our explanations and with our language. Avoid metaphors when possible and euphemisms, too. "Put to sleep" or "Put out of their misery" may have very clear meanings to the healthcare team, but these phrases run the risk of being misunderstood, particularly in times of distress when the client may not be thinking clearly.

Don't be afraid to use the word, *euthanasia*, or the verb, *euthanize*, and check for understanding. It is vital that you and your client be on the same page before moving forward with protocol.

Moving forward does not mean that the client is at peace with the decision, that the client will not grieve the loss of their pet, and/or that the client will not question the decision after-the-fact. Second-guessing after euthanasia is common and is a part of many grief journeys.

What moving forward does mean is that the client and veterinarian are both in agreement to proceed with euthanasia as the treatment option, and that this patient will be euthanized with legal permission from the owner after appropriate paperwork has been signed.

9.6 Deciding Where to Euthanize

After deciding to euthanize the patient, clients face a second critical choice:

- where to euthanize
  - euthanasia on-site at the clinic
  - at-home euthanasia.

Owners who elect to euthanize *at home* often share the following:

- They perceive that travelling to the veterinary clinic will create unnecessary fear, anxiety, and stress that they do not want their loved one to experience in their final moments.
- They perceive that entering the veterinary clinic will create unnecessary fear, anxiety, and stress that they do not want their loved one to experience in their final moments.
- They want their pet to die in the comfort of their home surrounded by family.

- They want their pet to die in a space that is warm and inviting rather than cold and clinical.
- They want their pet to die in their own bed.
- They want their pet not to know that their life is ending, by falling asleep in their owner's arms on the couch rather than on a stainless-steel exam table.
- They want to experience their pet's death in a safe and comfortable space where it feels okay to let emotions out.
- They do not want to have to face the public and/or drive home after euthanasia.

Owners with larger families have also shared that being at home is advantageous in that the entire family doesn't have to cram into one small exam room or risk having to ask people to step outside.

Owners who elect to euthanize *at the clinic* often share the following:

- They perceive that having the veterinarian come to the home will create unnecessary fear, anxiety, and stress that they do not want their loved one to experience in their final moments. This may be especially true for a dog who hides at the sound of a doorbell or becomes anxious in the presence of visitors within the home environment.
- They perceive that having the veterinarian come to the home may be unsafe in cases where the patient exhibits territorial aggression and/or resource guarding within the confines of their own home.
- They perceive that having daily reminders within the home of where the pet was euthanized would be too difficult to bear.

When owners ask me which site for euthanasia is preferrable, I tell them that the best place is wherever they and the pet feel comfortable.

Owners who have time to consider what is "right" for their pet are able to process what each site would require of their pet and which setting is least likely to induce stress.

Note that some owners may not have a choice. Their pet may already be critically ill and hospitalized, in which case, transferring the patient home could create additional unnecessary stress. In this circumstance, bringing a piece of home into the clinic could be valuable to facilitate the transition from life to death. You might suggest that a client bring in the pet's favorite blanket, bed, or treats. This small taste of home can go a long way in terms of making the pet and the client feel more comfortable.

9.7 Deciding Whether to Be Present for Euthanasia

After deciding to euthanize the patient, clients face a third critical choice: whether to be present for the procedure.

Being present for the procedure means that they will bear witness to the event and observe their pet transition from life to death.

Owners who elect to be present often share the following:

- They want their pet to know that they were there.
- They want their pet to know that their "preferred people" were at their side.
- They want to alleviate the pet's anxiety, stress, or fear that may be exacerbated if the pet is without their presence.
- They want their pet to feel reassurance from them that they're going to be okay.
- They want to gain a sense of closure in knowing that the pet has passed and that they are free from pain and discomfort.
- They want to be a part of their pet's transition from life through a peaceful passing.
- They want their face to be the last face that the pet sees.

Owners who elect *not* to be present often share the following:

- They are afraid that they may react explosively with emotion that they cannot control.
  - They may not want to break down in tears.
  - They may feel embarrassed about the intensity of their emotions.
- They are afraid that their pet will pick up on their own anxiety, fear, or stress and that this might adversely affect their peaceful passing; they don't want them to die afraid.
- They are afraid of watching death happen; some have previously witnessed a bad death (human or non-human animal) and do not wish to replicate the experience.
- They don't want their last memory of their pet to be watching them die.

Clients often feel very strongly one way or the other about whether they ought to be there or not.

Clients within the same family may not always agree; some family members may choose to be present while other family members may choose not to be.

Whether owning a pet obligates the client to be present for death has sparked intense debate both within the veterinary community and within the public eye. A pet owner captured the intensity of this debate in the following tweet that took place over the summer of 2018:(87)

> *Asked my vet what the hardest part was about his job & he said when he has to put an animal down 90% of owners don't actually want to be in the room when he injects them so the animal's last moments are usually them frantically looking around for their owners & [to be honest] that broke me.*

This one tweet led to a series of posts and articles by veterinarians across the globe who decided to weigh in on whether clients should be allowed to choose. One anonymous veterinarian posted their plea to owners:(87)

> *Do not make them transition from life to death in a room of strangers in a place they don't like. The thing you people need to know that most of you don't is that THEY SEARCH FOR YOU WHEN YOU LEAVE THEM BEHIND!!!!*

Whether we agree with this statement or not, it is ultimately the client's decision. It is important that we, the veterinary team, provide the opportunity for clients to consider all choices and to make the "right" decision for them.

It is also important to note that being present does not have to be all or none. Some of my clients have decided to be partially present, meaning that they have stayed up through the administration of injectable propofol. Once the patient has reached a state of unconsciousness, the client departs from the consultation room, prior to the Final Injection. These clients have felt comforted in knowing that their pet drifted off with a loved one nearby but could not bear to be present when the patient was pronounced dead.

This is an easy-to-achieve viable option that you might consider offering to clients who want to find middle ground in their decision to be there for their pet without breaking themselves in the process.

9.8 Preparing the Client for Euthanasia

Clients who elect to be present for euthanasia need to be prepped so that they know what to expect. In order to prepare our clients effectively, we need to hear from them how they have experienced loss in the past.

Have they been through the euthanasia process before?

- If so, was it at the same clinic?
  - o Which patient and when?
    - ▪ Have the protocols remained the same?
    - ▪ If not, how are they different?
- If the euthanasia took place at a different clinic, what do they recall about the process?
  - o What did they experience?
  - o What would they like to replicate about that experience for this pet?

Eliciting their perspective about euthanasia invites the client to share their past experiences. You may elicit their perspective by asking the closed-ended question, "Have you ever gone through this process before?"

If the answer is "yes," then you can follow-up with the open-ended statement: "Share with me what that experience was like for you."

Alternatively, you might ask, "What are you comfortable sharing with me about that experience that might help to guide our approach with [insert pet's name here]?"

By hearing from the client directly, we gain a foundational understanding as to what their experience with euthanasia has been. Our client's past experiences offer a starting point so that we know where we need to begin in terms of our explanation and what we may be able to leave out. For example, if the client mentions that they are familiar with and agreeable to IV catheter placement, then you do not have to spend time trying to convince them why you would like to use one. You simply build upon their past knowledge by sharing that, "We also make use of IV catheters to support the process of euthanasia and, with your permission, would like to place one in [insert pet's name here]."

When explaining the euthanasia process, my goal is to give the owner peace of mind. I explain that we are going to work together to make the transition from life to death as peaceful as possible for [insert pet's name here].

I intentionally name the patient when describing the procedure. In this moment, I do not want to sound clinical. I want to sound reassuring and conversational. I explain that the medication is an overdose of anesthesia and that [insert pet's name here] will fall into a deep sleep from which they can't awake.

Note that I use this description for teenagers and adults.

Recall from Chapter 4 that when navigating pet loss among young children, adults should avoid saying that the dog or cat will be "put to sleep." Children between the ages of three and five may subsequently fear bedtime thinking that they can be "put to sleep," too. You should also avoid sharing with the same age group that a loved one is "sleeping" or "resting."(88, 89) That may precipitate fear that if they sleep or rest, then they, too, will die.

As a novice veterinarian, I used to go into much more detail with clients than I do now.

As I gained experience, I thinned out my description.

I don't want to list every side effect or adverse reaction that can occur as the pet dies.

Instead, I limit preparation to this:

> *The two things I will prepare you for are that Nina's eyes won't close all the way and she may lose control over her bladder and her bowels as her body relaxes and let's go. If anything else happens, I'll be right here beside you and I will explain it at that time.*

For example, in the moment, should an agonal breath arise, I may explain it as "a spasm of the diaphragm, the muscle that helps us to breathe. It's kind of like a hiccup; it's uncommon but normal and does not cause Nina any pain."

As a second example, if the patient begins to twitch, I may explain that "Death is a phase, not a moment, and this is normal as different areas of the body shut down."

Every veterinarian develops their own euthanasia "script" that they walk through. Your "script" may be different from mine. Your phraseology should be your own. Make it authentic to you. Describe the process as you see fit, provided that you check in throughout your explanation to see if your clients have any questions or concerns.

Answer any questions or concerns as transparently and as simply as possible so that your clients feel heard, supported, and understood.

When questions or concerns have been answered, you may ask the client if they would like any additional time with the patient before they are ready to begin.

Once the client signifies to you that they are ready, the process can commence.

Paperwork authorizing euthanasia can be signed while the IV catheter is being placed, in clinics that provide IV catheters.

A sample form is published by the AVMA to provide guidance to clinics who may be in the process of developing their own.(90)

Euthanasia paperwork typically includes:(90)

- practice name
- case/client number
- patient description
  - signalment (age, sex, sexual status, breed, species)
  - color or other identifying features
  - weight
- owner name and contact information

- a certification statement
  - "I certify that I am the legal owner / duly authorized agent for the owner of the animal described above and do hereby give Dr. _____, the [insert Veterinary Business Name] and any authorized agents, staff, or representatives full and complete authority to euthanatize and dispose or arrange for cremation of said animal in a humane manner."(90)
- a legal statement with respect to rabies
  - "State law requires post euthanasia rabies testing of any animal who has bitten people/other animals or been exposed to rabies virus in the last _____ days.
    - I do also certify to the best of my knowledge the said animal has not bitten any person or animal during the last _____ days and has not been exposed to rabies virus.
    - Said animal has bitten a person or animal or been exposed to rabies virus in the last days. I understand that said animal must be tested for rabies virus after euthanasia. Remains cannot be returned after rabies testing. Ashes may be returned if specified below."(90)
- aftercare options(90)
  - "I request that this animal's remains be cared for in the following manner.
    - Private cremation with return of ashes.
    - Cremation with no return of ashes. My pet's remains will not be returned to me.
    - Home burial. I wish to take my pet's body home. I further authorize the attending veterinarian to dispose of remains in accordance with hospital policy."
- necropsy preference(90)
  - "I decline the option of necropsy (autopsy)."
  - "I authorize a necropsy. I understand it may not be possible to have the remains returned to me."
- owner signature and date
- clinician signature and date
- witness signature and date.

After the euthanasia paperwork has been completed and the IV catheter has been placed, the patient is returned to the client.

It is routine to again ask if the client would like some additional time alone with the patient.

Not every client will say "yes." Those who do appreciate and remember those final moments.

9.9 Walking the Client Through Euthanasia

Prior to starting the process of euthanasia, communicate with the rest of your team that you are re-entering the room to perform euthanasia and are not to be disturbed.

Turn off your cell phone, turn your cell phone to "do not disturb," or leave your cell phone outside of the room so that the phone does not ring in the middle of euthanasia.

Re-enter the exam room and ask the client if they are ready to begin.

If you are going to be injecting pre-euthanasia medication (e.g., propofol), explain what it is that you are doing and why in easy-to-understand terms. For example, "I am going to administer the sedative now. This is going to make [insert pet's name] sleepy."

It is okay to name the drug as long as you share what the goal of drug administration is in terms that the client can understand. For instance, "I am going to administer the first medication, propofol. Propofol is a sedative. I am giving this medication to [insert pet's name] so that they are comfortable before we administer the Final Injection."

When it comes time for the Final Injection, it is important to let the owner know that you are proceeding.

I prepare the clients that "This is a very peaceful process" and I reiterate that [insert pet's name] will drift off to sleep.

I emphasize the peacefulness rather than accentuating negative word associations (e.g., "It doesn't hurt," or "He won't be in pain.")

I allow the client to position themselves wherever they want to be relative to the patient. This is where the extension set on the IV catheter can be of significant help: it gives the client a chance to be near the patient's head and/or the patient can rest comfortably on their lap.

I affirm throughout the process that "[insert pet's name] knows you're here; they can hear you," particularly if the client is talking to the pet.

Be sure to use the pet's correct pronouns. In this day and age where non-binary names are commonplace, I tend to use the patient's name much more frequently, in lieu of pronouns, when I am concerned about getting them wrong. For example, my 18-year-old cat was named Bailey. My Bailey was a she, but I have known many Baileys in my lifetime that were assigned he/him pronouns. If I were the veterinarian overseeing this case, then I would likely refer to Bailey by name more so than by pronouns for fear that I might call Bailey by he/him pronouns instead of she/her or vice versa. We tend to default to what we are used to. Because my Bailey went by she/her pronouns, I have a tendency to call all Baileys by she/her pronouns. In the moment of Bailey's passing, the clinician doesn't want to get it wrong. The client may be significantly impacted if we use incorrect pronouns. Therefore, I tend to use proper names more so than pronouns, and I double-check the paperwork always.

I tell clients when I am ready to administer the Final Injection. I share simply that "I am injecting the euthanasia solution now."

After administration of the Final Injection, I listen to the patient's heart with my stethoscope.

Listen with effort and deliberation. I tend to listen for longer than I need to, to be certain that the patient has passed before I express the finality of the procedure aloud.

I tend to share aloud that the patient is no longer with us, taking care to use the pet's name, or that "[insert name here] has passed."

I tend *not* to say, "[insert name here] has earned their wings," or "[insert name here] has reached the rainbow bridge."

I do not want to make assumptions about the client's afterlife beliefs.

I stay present in the room for a few minutes as I gather the syringe and supplies. While I am gathering supplies, I watch for agonal breath(s), twitching, or any other movements, which generally happen within 1–5 minutes postmortem.

Since I do not recommend warning about every potential side effect of euthanasia solution before it is administered, this is the time to explain any adverse effects if they occur.

Before I leave the client alone in the consultation room, I ask the client if they want to spend any additional time in private with their pet.

It is important to note that not every client wants alone time with the deceased.

If the client does want time alone with the body, consider implementing a system that helps them to communicate with team members when they are "ready" to depart from the hospital.

One clinic that I worked at had a wireless doorbell assigned to each of the euthanasia/grief rooms. We could hand the "ringer" portion of the wireless doorbell to our clients. We then handed over the bell portion to the technician assigned to the case. The client could "ring" us when they were ready for us to return to the consultation room.

This system prevents the client from having to leave their pet's body alone to find someone when they need additional support or are ready to depart.

When the client leaves the clinic, they may say, "thank you." I avoid the default responses such as "my pleasure" or "you're welcome."

Instead, I simply say, "I'm very sorry for your loss. Take care and let us know if we can help in any way."

9.10 Aftercare

Aftercare options are discussed with the client prior to euthanasia to allow the client to fully consider their approach to managing their pet's remains.

Many clients attend the end-of-life consultation already knowing which aftercare option they would like to explore. Many clients default to what they have always done – for instance, some clients always bury their pets; others always opt for cremation with ashes returned.

It is important not to make assumptions. A client may never have opted for ashes to be returned in the past, yet this patient may hold special meaning to them, necessitating a change in aftercare plans.

Other clients may be new to the process and uncertain what your clinic offers.

Approach each clinical case as its own entity and be transparent about cost. Cost does play a role in the decision-making process for some, so it is important that you and your team be transparent and approximate what final expenses for the pet will be based upon which aftercare option the client has selected.

In Section 9.8, I allude to the fact that most practices offer three options for aftercare:

1. individual cremation with return of ashes
2. group ("communal") cremation, without return of ashes
3. home burial.

When describing aftercare options, familiarize yourself with the local crematoriums that service your practice. Many will allow the veterinary team to tour the facilities if doing so will help you and your team to feel confident partnering with them.

Know what your partnered crematoriums do with communal ashes. If ashes are truly scattered at a butterfly garden, then let the client know, but avoid making things up if you are uncertain.

Acknowledge the difficulty of this line of questioning. I often share with my clients, "This is a very personal decision, and there's no right answer, only what's right for you."

When I discuss aftercare in advance of euthanasia, I avoid saying the word, "body."

For example, I may ask, "Do you know how you would like to care for Nina after euthanasia?" rather than "Do you know what you would like to do with Nina's body?"

To the family, it's not Nina's body. It's still Nina.

If a family asks if it's legal to bury at home, you might say, "I buried my little one in my backyard. You can check your county ordinances and do what you feel is best for you."

Pets are property. Even when ordinances dictate very clearly that you are not legally allowed to bury an animal, the fact of the matter is that you cannot demand that a pet's body remain at your clinic. Horses and other livestock are euthanized with barbiturates and buried all the time. It is the clients' choice to bury, cremate, or otherwise honor their pets in whatever way they see fit and at their own risk. It is your responsibility to educate the owner on proper burial techniques. Pets should be buried at least three feet below ground to prevent other animals from digging up remains. This would not only be traumatic to the bereaved, it would also be potentially hazardous to wildlife who might then consume barbiturates and/or barbiturate acid derivatives.

Some clients may invest in pet-specific coffins. Some of these have been advertised as eco-friendly pods that becomes compost within five years of burial. Other clients may repurpose infant caskets for small dogs and cats.

As an alternative to at-home burials, clients may elect to purchase a plot at a pet cemetery.(91)

For example, in my home state of Maryland, Dulaney Valley Memorial Gardens offers pet burial.(91) Pet Haven, the cemetery's first pet memorial garden, opened in 1967.(91) It became so popular that it expanded to Pet Sanctuary in 2010.(91) Also, in 2010, Dulaney Valley Memorial Gardens opened Faithful Friends, which allows people to be interred with their companion animals resting at their feet.(91)

Amy Shimp, the cemetery's general manager, explains that: "Over the years, and particularly since the pandemic, we have seen growth exponentially in this area as pets have become more a part of families, and now, their owners want to celebrate their lives."(91)

For those clients who are unable to bury, but fear cremation, there is a newer option. Aquamation has been described as an "eco-friendly alternative."(91) Aquamation is a new age process that is synonymous with alkaline hydrolysis.(91) It accelerates decomposition through water and alkaline agents rather than traditional flame cremation.(91)

9.11 Memorialization

Memorialization is the way in which we honor the memory of someone or something. When we talk about memorialization with respect to pet loss, we are considering the many ways in which owners choose to preserve the memory of their beloved pet.

Memorialization is a critical part of the grieving process because it creates ritual. It is how we begin to wrap our heads around the permanence of our loss while at the same time cherishing the memories of the one we loved.

Memorialization is how we center our emotions during a time of inner turmoil to focus on those moments, times, places, and spaces that we shared with our loved one.

Memorialization is one way that we come together in grief. It is how we celebrate our loved one while still being respectful of the ways in which each of us individually grieve.

Memorialization comes in many shapes and forms and may include one or more of the following.

- Host a memorial service.
- Select an urn that represents your pet.
- Scatter your pet's ashes at a favorite spot.
- Light a candle.
- Write a letter to your pet.
- Write a poem about your pet.
- Find a quote that makes you think about your pet or one that acknowledges the depth of the grief that you are feeling in the moment.
- Find a song that makes you think about the relationship that you shared with your pet.
- Get a memorial bird feeder (e.g., if your cat loved to watch the birds).
- Create a photo album or photo collage.
- Create a memorial slideshow.
- Create a memory chest.
- Create a post on an online pet memorial website.
- Create an outdoor memorial.
  - It could be something as simple as a stone that you add to your garden or a tree that you plant in honor of the pet.
  - It could be a plaque that you designed in honor of them that you put in the yard.
  - It could be that you bury the urn in your yard and mark the resting place.
  - It could be a bench that you engrave with the pet's name.
  - Outfit a resin stone with your pet's image and name.
  - Hang wind chimes.
- Create an indoor memorial.
  - It could be something as simple as a candle (lit or unlit).

    o   It could be a pet memorial shelf that you place significant objects on (e.g., the pet's cremation urn and/or photographs).

- Preserve their paw print or nose print in ink or with a simple salt dough. You can also purchase a commercially available product (e.g., Clay Paws) that can help you capture the print.
- Preserve a clipping of fur.
- Grow a tree from the pet's ashes.
- Turn your favorite photo into a pet portrait or caricature.
- Turn your favorite photo into a memorial pillow that you can hug when you are missing your pet.
- Turn your favorite photo into a laser-engraved crystal (e.g., Crystal Clear Memories, https://www.crystalclearmemories.com/).
- Customize jewelry that is created using your pet's ashes.
- Create a custom paperweight or other treasured memento using your pet's ashes.
  - o   Blown-glass stones.
  - o   Blown-glass ornaments.
- Create an abstract image from your pet's ashes (e.g., EverAfter, https://everafterart.com/).
- Create a customized stuffed animal replica of your pet.
- Get a tattoo to honor your pet.
- Celebrate their birthday.
- Do something special for you on the anniversary date of their passing.

Memorialization is common among dog and cat owners. The American Pet Products Association (APPA) reported that: "52% of dog owners in 2018 said they would purchase something upon the death of their pet, while 2020 saw 61% and, for cat owners, 42% to 57% for the same years."(91)

According to the 2020 APPA survey: "Most people would buy an urn for ashes or a memorial stone for the home or yard and caskets. Just under 10% of pet owners say they would purchase memorial jewelry upon the death of their pet."(91)

9.12 Ways that the Veterinary Team Can Honor the Patient After Death

As we saw in the preceding section, memorialization plays an important part of the grief journey for the bereaved.

Memorialization is also one of the ways that the veterinary team can contribute. In this way, the team companions the bereaved through their grief journey through actions or words that honor the pet's memory.

Many veterinary clinics will offer to provide pawprints and/or clippings of the fur to the bereaved. It is vital to ask the bereaved if either is something that would be helpful to them because not everyone feels comforted by these mementos.

Many veterinary clinics will mail out a condolence card to the bereaved after euthanasia.

Cards may be printed with stock messages. For example:

- "We extend heartfelt condolences."
- "Our hearts are saddened by your loss."
- "With thoughts of peace and courage during this most difficult time."
- "Words cannot express our feelings of sorrow over the loss of your companion."

Cards tend to be most meaningful when team members individually sign and when the patient is referred to by name. For instance:

- "Bailey touched so many lives."
- "Nina will be remembered always and forever loved."

Author Dr. Englar's line of Empathy Cards can be found here: www.intheirpaws.com

References

1. AVMA guidelines for the euthanasia of animals: 2020 Edition. American Veterinary Medical Association (AVMA); 2020. Available from: https://www.avma.org/sites/default/files/2020-02/Guidelines-on-Euthanasia-2020.pdf.
2. Sife W. The loss of a pet: a guide to coping with the grieving process when a pet dies. 4th ed. New York. Vol. xii. New York: Howell Book House; 2014.
3. Gire J. How death imitates life: cultural influences on conceptions of death and dying. Online readings in psychology and culture; 2014.
4. Cain CL, McCleskey S. Expanded definitions of the "good death"? Race, ethnicity and medical aid in dying. Sociol Health Illn. 2019;41(6):1175–91. https://doi.org/10.1111/1467-9566.12903, PMID 30950077.
5. Broom A, Cavenagh J. Masculinity, moralities and being cared for: an exploration of experiences of living and dying in a hospice. Soc Sci Med. 2010;71(5):869–76. https://doi.org/10.1016/j.socscimed.2010.05.026, PMID 20573434.
6. Carr DA. "Good death" for whom? Quality of spouse's death and psychological distress among older widowed persons. J Health Soc Behav. 2003;44(2):215–32. https://doi.org/10.2307/1519809, PMID 12866391.
7. Zimmermann C. Denial of impending death: a discourse analysis of the palliative care literature. Soc Sci Med. 2004;59(8):1769–80. https://doi.org/10.1016/j.socscimed.2004.02.012, PMID 15279932.

8. Zimmermann C. Acceptance of dying: a discourse analysis of palliative care literature. Soc Sci Med. 2012;75(1):217–24. https://doi.org/10.1016/j.socscimed.2012.02.047, PMID 22513246.

9. Kellahear A. Dying of cancer: the final year of life. London: Harwood Academic Publishers; 1990.

10. Cagle JG, Pek J, Clifford M, Guralnik J, Zimmerman S. Correlates of a good death and the impact of hospice involvement: findings from the national survey of house-holds affected by cancer. Support Care Cancer. 2015;23(3):809–18. https://doi.org/10.1007/s00520-014-2404-z, PMID 25194877.

11. Teno JM, Clarridge BR, Casey V, Welch LC, Wetle T, Shield R, et al. Family perspectives on end-of-life care at the last place of care. JAMA. 2004;291(1):88–93. https://doi.org/10.1001/jama.291.1.88, PMID 14709580.

12. Wallston KA, Burger C, Smith RA, Baugher RJ. Comparing the quality of death for hospice and non-hospice cancer patients. Med Care. 1988;26(2):177–82. https://doi.org/10.1097/00005650-198802000-00008, PMID 3339915.

13. Kehl KA. Moving toward peace: an analysis of the concept of a good death. Am J Hosp Palliat Care. 2006;23(4):277–86. https://doi.org/10.1177/1049909106290380, PMID 17060291.

14. Downey L, Curtis JR, Lafferty WE, Herting JR, Engelberg RA. The Quality of Dying and Death Questionnaire (QODD): empirical domains and theoretical perspectives. J Pain Symptom Manage. 2010;39(1):9–22. https://doi.org/10.1016/j.jpainsymman.2009.05.012, PMID 19782530.

15. Heckel M, Bussmann S, Stiel S, Weber M, Ostgathe C. Validation of the German ver-sion of the quality of dying and death questionnaire for informal caregivers (QODD-D-Ang). J Pain Symptom Manage. 2015;50(3):402–13. https://doi.org/10.1016/j.jpainsymman.2015.03.020, PMID 26079825.

16. Pérez-Cruz PE, Padilla Pérez O, Bonati P, Thomsen Parisi O, Tupper Satt L, Gonzalez Otaiza M, et al. Validation of the Spanish version of the quality of dying and death questionnaire (QODD-ESP) in a home-based cancer palliative care program and development of the QODD-ESP-12. J Pain Symptom Manage. 2017;53(6):1042–9.e3. https://doi.org/10.1016/j.jpainsymman.2017.02.005, PMID 28323080.

17. Steinhauser KE, Bosworth HB, Clipp EC, McNeilly M, Christakis NA, Parker J, et al. Initial assessment of a new instrument to measure quality of life at the end of life. J Palliat Med. 2002;5(6):829–41. https://doi.org/10.1089/10966210260499014, PMID 12685529.

18. Steinhauser KE, Christakis NA, Clipp EC, McNeilly M, Grambow S, Parker J, et al. Preparing for the end of life: preferences of patients, families, physicians, and other care providers. J Pain Symptom Manage. 2001;22(3):727–37. https://doi.org/10.1016/s0885-3924(01)00334-7, PMID 11532586.

19. Steinhauser KE, Christakis NA, Clipp EC, McNeilly M, McIntyre L, Tulsky JA. Factors considered important at the end of life by patients, family, physicians, and other care providers. JAMA. 2000;284(19):2476–82. https://doi.org/10.1001/jama.284.19.2476, PMID 11074777.

20. Steinhauser KE, Voils CI, Clipp EC, Bosworth HB, Christakis NA, Tulsky JA. "Are you at peace?": one item to probe spiritual concerns at the end of life. Arch Intern Med. 2006;166(1):101–5. https://doi.org/10.1001/archinte.166.1.101, PMID 16401817.

21. Steinhauser KE, Clipp EC, McNeilly M, Christakis NA, McIntyre LM, Tulsky JA. In search of a good death: observations of patients, families, and providers. Ann

Intern Med. 2000;132(10):825–32. https://doi.org/10.7326/0003-4819-132-10-200005160-00011, PMID 10819707.

22. Cagle JG, Munn JC, Hong S, Clifford M, Zimmerman S. Validation of the quality of dying-hospice scale. J Pain Symptom Manage. 2015;49(2):265–76. https://doi.org/10.1016/j.jpainsymman.2014.06.009, PMID 25057986.

23. How Do I Know When it's Time? Ohio State University Press Veterinary Medical Center. Available from: https://vet.osu.edu/vmc/sites/default/files/import/assets/pdf/hospital/companionAnimals/HonoringtheBond/HowDoIKnowWhen.pdf.

24. Mullan S. Assessment of quality of life in veterinary practice: developing tools for companion animal carers and veterinarians. Vet Med (Auckl). 2015;6:203–10. https://doi.org/10.2147/VMRR.S62079, PMID 30101107.

25. Yeates J, Main D. Assessment of companion animal quality of life in veterinary practice and research. J Small Anim Pract. 2009;50(6):274–81. https://doi.org/10.1111/j.1748-5827.2009.00755.x, PMID 19527420.

26. Mullan S, Main D. Preliminary evaluation of a quality-of-life screening programme for pet dogs. J Small Anim Pract. 2007;48(6):314–22. https://doi.org/10.1111/j.1748-5827.2007.00322.x, PMID 17490443.

27. McMillan FD. Maximizing quality of life in ill animals. J Am Anim Hosp Assoc. 2003;39(3):227–35. https://doi.org/10.5326/0390227, PMID 12755194.

28. Wiseman-Orr ML, Nolan AM, Reid J, Scott EM. Development of a questionnaire to measure the effects of chronic pain on health-related quality of life in dogs. Am J Vet Res. 2004;65(8):1077–84. https://doi.org/10.2460/ajvr.2004.65.1077, PMID 15334841.

29. Wojciechowska JI, Hewson CJ, Stryhn H, Guy NC, Patronek GJ, Timmons V. Development of a discriminative questionnaire to assess nonphysical aspects of quality of life of dogs. Am J Vet Res. 2005;66(8):1453–60. https://doi.org/10.2460/ajvr.2005.66.1453, PMID 16173493.

30. Freeman LM, Rush JE, Farabaugh AE, Must A. Development and evaluation of a questionnaire for assessing health-related quality of life in dogs with cardiac disease. J Am Vet Med Assoc. 2005;226(11):1864–8. https://doi.org/10.2460/javma.2005.226.1864, PMID 15934254.

31. Wojciechowska JI, Hewson CJ, Stryhn H, Guy NC, Patronek GJ, Timmons V. Evaluation of a questionnaire regarding nonphysical aspects of quality of life in sick and healthy dogs. Am J Vet Res. 2005;66(8):1461–7. https://doi.org/10.2460/ajvr.2005.66.1461, PMID 16173494.

32. Yazbek KV, Fantoni DT. Validity of a health-related quality-of-life scale for dogs with signs of pain secondary to cancer. J Am Vet Med Assoc. 2005;226(8):1354–8. https://doi.org/10.2460/javma.2005.226.1354, PMID 15844428.

33. Budke CM, Levine JM, Kerwin SC, Levine GJ, Hettlich BF, Slater MR. Evaluation of a questionnaire for obtaining owner-perceived, weighted quality-of-life assessments for dogs with spinal cord injuries. J Am Vet Med Assoc. 2008;233(6):925–30. https://doi.org/10.2460/javma.233.6.925, PMID 18795853.

34. Favrot C, Linek M, Mueller R, Zini E, International Task Force on Canine Atopic Dermatitis. Development of a questionnaire to assess the impact of atopic dermatitis on health-related quality of life of affected dogs and their owners. Vet Dermatol. 2010;21(1):63–9. https://doi.org/10.1111/j.1365-3164.2009.00781.x, PMID 20187912.

35. German AJ, Holden SL, Wiseman-Orr ML, Reid J, Nolan AM, Biourge V, et al. Quality of life is reduced in obese dogs but improves after successful weight loss. Vet J. 2012;192(3):428–34. https://doi.org/10.1016/j.tvjl.2011.09.015, PMID 22075257.

36. Freeman LM, Rush JE, Oyama MA, MacDonald KA, Cunningham SM, Bulmer B, et al. Development and evaluation of a questionnaire for assessment of health-related quality of life in cats with cardiac disease. J Am Vet Med Assoc. 2012;240(10): 1188–93. https://doi.org/10.2460/javma.240.10.1188, PMID 22559108.

37. Parker RA, Yeates JW. Assessment of quality of life in equine patients. Equine Vet J. 2012;44(2):244–9. https://doi.org/10.1111/j.2042-3306.2011.00411.x, PMID 217 67299.

38. Yeates JW, Mullan S, Stone M, Main DC. Promoting discussions and decisions about dogs' quality-of-life. J Small Anim Pract. 2011;52(9):459–63. https://doi. org/10.1111/j.1748-5827.2011.01094.x, PMID 21896019.

39. Pet quality-of-life scale: lap of love. Available from: https://www.lapoflove.com/ how-will-i-know-it-is-time/lap-of-love-quality-of-life-scale.pdf.

40. Epstein M, Rodan I, Griffenhagen G, Kadrlik J, Petty M, Robertson S, et al. 2015 AAHA/AAFP pain management guidelines for dogs and cats. J Am Anim Hosp Assoc. 2015;51(2):67–84. https://doi.org/10.5326/JAAHA-MS-7331, PMID 257 64070.

41. Epstein ME, Rodanm I, Griffenhagen G, Kadrlik J, Petty MC, Robertson SA, et al. 2015 AAHA/AAFP pain management guidelines for dogs and cats. J Feline Med Surg. 2015;17(3):251–72. https://doi.org/10.1177/1098612X15572062, PMID 25701863.

42. Shipley H, Guedes A, Graham L, Goudie-DeAngelis E, Wendt-Hornickle E. Preliminary appraisal of the reliability and validity of the Colorado State University Feline Acute Pain Scale. J Feline Med Surg. 2019;21(4):335–9. https://doi. org/10.1177/1098612X18777506, PMID 29848148.

43. Nicholls D, Merchant-Walsh M, Dunne J, Cortellini NP, Adami C. Use of mechanical thresholds in a model of feline clinical acute pain and their correla-tion with the Glasgow Feline Composite Measure Pain Scale scores. J Feline Med Surg. 2022;24(6):517–23. https://doi.org/10.1177/1098612X211035051, PMID 34328358.

44. Boesch JM, Roinestad KE, Lopez DJ, Newman AK, Campoy L, Gleed RD, et al. The Canine Postamputation Pain (CAMPPAIN) initiative: a retrospective study and development of a diagnostic scale. Vet Anaesth Analg. 2021;48(6):861–70. https:// doi.org/10.1016/j.vaa.2021.07.003, PMID 34483040.

45. Della Rocca G, Di Salvo A, Marenzoni ML, Bellezza E, Pastorino G, Monteiro B, et al. Development, preliminary validation, and refinement of the composite Oral and maxillofacial pain Scale-Canine/feline (COPS-C/F). Front Vet Sci. 2019;6: 1–10. https://doi.org/10.3389/fvets.2019.00274, PMID 31508431.

46. Piotti P, Albertini M, Lavesi E, Ferri A, Pirrone F. Physiotherapy improves dogs' quality of life measured with the Milan Pet quality of life scale: is pain involved? Vet Sci. 2022;9(7):1–9. https://doi.org/10.3390/vetsci9070335, PMID 35878353.

47. Englar RE. A guide to oral communication in veterinary medicine. Sheffield: 5m Publishing; 2020.

48. Veterinarian's oath. American Veterinary Medical Association. Available from: https://www.avma.org/resources-tools/avma-policies/veterinarians-oath.

49. Cooney K. Oral and injectable pre-euthanasia sedatives/anesthetics for dogs and cats: companion animal euthanasia training academy; 2017. Available from: http:// caetainternational.com/wp-content/uploads/2017/10/CAETA-Program-Oral-Sedative-Handout.pdf.

50. End of life educational toolkit. American Association of feline practitioners. 2021. Available from: https://catvets.com/end-of-life-toolkit/.

51. Code of professional conduct for veterinary surgeons: veterinary medicines. Royal College of Veterinary Surgeons; 2022. Available from: https://www.rcvs.org.uk/setting-standards/advice-and-guidance/code-of-professional-conduct-for-veterinary-surgeons/supporting-guidance/veterinary-medicines/.

52. Ackerman LJ. Pet-specific care for the veterinary teams. Hoboken, NJ: John Wiley & Sons, Inc; 2021.

53. Fingland RB, Stone LR, Read EK, Moore RM. Preparing veterinary students for excellence in general practice: building confidence and competence by focusing on spectrum of care. J Am Vet Med Assoc. 2021;259(5):463–70. https://doi.org/10.2460/javma.259.5.463, PMID 34388008.

54. White SC. Prevention of fetal suffering during ovariohysterectomy of pregnant animals. J Am Vet Med Assoc. 2012;240(10):1160–3. https://doi.org/10.2460/javma.240.10.1160, PMID 22559103.

55. Association of Shelter. Veterinarians' veterinary task force to advance S-N, griffin B, Bushby PA, McCobb E, White SC, Rigdon-Brestle YK, et al. J Am Vet Med Assoc. 2016 Veterinary Medical Care Guidelines for Spay-Neuter Programs;249(2):165–88.

56. Matte AR, Khosa DK, Coe JB, Meehan MP. Impacts of the process and decision-making around companion animal euthanasia on veterinary wellbeing. Vet Rec. 2019;185(15):480–488. https://doi.org/10.1136/vr.105540, PMID 31409747.

57. Fernandez-Mehler P, Gloor P, Sager E, Lewis FI, Glaus TM. Veterinarians' role for pet owners facing pet loss. Vet Rec. 2013;172(21):555–564. https://doi.org/10.1136/vr.101154, PMID 23492929.

58. Adams CL, Bonnett BN, Meek AH. Predictors of owner response to companion animal death in 177 clients from 14 practices in Ontario. J Am Vet Med Assoc. 2000;217(9):1303–9. https://doi.org/10.2460/javma.2000.217.1303, PMID 11061379.

59. Shaw JR, Lagoni L. End-of-life communication in veterinary medicine: delivering bad news and euthanasia decision making. Vet Clin North Am Small Anim Pract. 2007;37(1):95–108; abstract viii:abstract viii–ix. https://doi.org/10.1016/j.cvsm.2006.09.010, PMID 17162114.

60. Bishop G, Cooney K, Cox S, Downing R, Mitchener K, Shanan A, et al. 2016 AAHA/IAAHPC end-of-life care guidelines. J Am Anim Hosp Assoc. 2016;52(6):341–56. https://doi.org/10.5326/JAAHA-MS-6637, PMID 27685363.

61. Lagoni L, Hetts S, Butler C. The human-animal bond and grief. Philadelphia: Saunders; 1994.

62. Shanan A, Pierce J, Shearer TS. Hospice and palliative care for companion animals: principles and practice. Vol. xxi. Hoboken, NJ: Wiley/Blackwell; 2017. 325 p.

63. Hart L. Hart B. Grief and stress from so many animal deaths. Companion Anim Pract. 1987;1:20–1.

64. Williams S, Mills JN. Understanding and responding to grief in companion animal practice. Aust Vet Pract. 2000;30:55–62.

65. Ratanawongsa N, Teherani A, Hauer KE. Third-year medical students' experiences with dying patients during the internal medicine clerkship: a qualitative study of the informal curriculum. Acad Med. 2005;80(7):641–7. https://doi.org/10.1097/00001888-200507000-00006, PMID 15980080.

66. Manette CS. A reflection on the ways veterinarians cope with the death, euthanasia,

and slaughter of animals. JAMA. 2004;225(1):34–8. https://doi.org/10.2460/javma.2004.225.34.

67. Engel GL. How much longer must medicine's science be bound by a seventeenth century world view? In: White KL, editor. The task of medicine: dialogue at Wickenburg. Menlo Park, CA: Henry J Kaiser Family Foundation; 1988. p. 133–77.

68. Epstein RM. Realizing Engel's biopsychosocial vision: resilience, compassion, and quality of care. Int J Psychiatry Med. 2014;47(4):275–87. https://doi.org/10.2190/PM.47.4.b, PMID 25084850.

69. Cohen-Cole SA. The medical interview: the three function approach. St. Louis: Mosby Year book; 1991.

70. Hellín T. The physician-patient relationship: recent developments and changes. Haemophilia. 2002;8(3):450–4. https://doi.org/10.1046/j.1365-2516.2002.00636.x, PMID 12010450.

71. O'Donnell M. The night Bernard Shaw taught us a lesson. BMJ. 2006;333(7582):1338–40. https://doi.org/10.1136/bmj.39062.728900.55, PMID 17185735.

72. Silverman JD, Kurtz SM, Draper J. Skills for communicating with patients. Oxford: Taylor & Francis Group; 2013.

73. Simpson M, Buckman R, Stewart M, Maguire P, Lipkin M, Novack D, et al. Doctor-patient communication: the Toronto consensus statement. BMJ. 1991;303(6814):1385–7. https://doi.org/10.1136/bmj.303.6814.1385, PMID 1760608.

74. Stein TS, Nagy VT, Jacobs L. Caring for patients one conversation at a time: musings from the interregional clinician patient communication leadership group. Permanente J. 1998;2(4):62–8. https://doi.org/10.7812/TPP/98.916.

75. Beckman HB, Frankel RM. The effect of physician behavior on the collection of data. Ann Intern Med. 1984;101(5):692–6. https://doi.org/10.7326/0003-4819-101-5-692, PMID 6486600.

76. Becker MH. Patient adherence to prescribed therapies. Med Care. 1985;23(5):539–55. https://doi.org/10.1097/00005650-198505000-00014, PMID 4010350.

77. Coleman VR. Physician behaviour and compliance. J Hypertens Suppl. 1985;3(1):S69–71. PMID 3870472.

78. Garrity TF. Medical compliance and the clinician-patient relationship: a review. Soc Sci Med E. 1981;15(3):215–22. https://doi.org/10.1016/0271-5384(81)90016-8, PMID 7323842.

79. Stewart MA. Effective physician-patient communication and health outcomes: a review. CMAJ. 1995;152(9):1423–33. PMID 7728691.

80. Travaline JM, Ruchinskas R, D'Alonzo GE, Jr. Patient-physician communication: why and how. J Am Osteopath Assoc. 2005;105(1):13–8. PMID 15710660.

81. Matthews DA, Suchman AL, Branch WT, Jr. Making "connexions": enhancing the therapeutic potential of patient-clinician relationships. Ann Intern Med. 1993;118(12):973–7. https://doi.org/10.7326/0003-4819-118-12-199306150-00010, PMID 8489112.

82. Suchman AL, Matthews DA. What makes the patient-doctor relationship therapeutic? Exploring the connexional dimension of medical care. Ann Intern Med. 1988;108(1):125–30. https://doi.org/10.7326/0003-4819-108-1-125, PMID 3276262.

83. Englar RE, Williams M, Weingand K. Applicability of the Calgary-Cambridge guide to dog and cat owners for teaching veterinary clinical communications. J Vet Med Educ. 2016;43(2):143–69. https://doi.org/10.3138/jvme.0715-117R1, PMID 27075274.

84. Show A, Englar RE. Evaluating dog- and cat-owner preferences for Calgary-Cambridge

communication skills: results of a questionnaire. J Vet Med Educ. 2018;45(4):534–43. https://doi.org/10.3138/jvme.0117-002r1, PMID 30285592.

85. Reck J. Facing farewell: making the decision to euthanize your pet. Wenatchee, Wash.: Dogwise Pub.; 2012.

86. Kogan L. Pet loss, grief, and therapeutic interventions: practitioners navigating the human-animal bond. New York: Routledge; 2020.

87. Sacks E. Is it OK for owners to leave while vet puts the pet down?; 2018. Available from: https://www.today.com/pets/vet-s-comment-about-pet-owners-leaving-room-euthanasia-sparks-t137331.

88. Jones AM, Deane C, Keegan O. The development of a framework to support bereaved children and young people: the Irish Childhood Bereavement Care Pyramid. Bereavement Care. 2015;34(2):43–51. https://doi.org/10.1080/0268262 1.2015.1063857.

89. Mahon MM. Death of a sibling: primary care interventions. Pediatr Nurs. 1994;20(3):293–5, 328. PMID 8008481.

90. Model euthanasia authorization. American Veterinary Medical Association. Available from: https://www.avma.org/sites/default/files/resources/model-euth-auth-form.pdf.

91. Ho N. As the pet industry grows, so does the business of pet death care. The Baltimore Sun; November 15 2022.

CHAPTER 10

When Loss is Sudden, Traumatic, or Unanticipated

Disenfranchised grief was first introduced in Chapter 6 as bereavement that occurs in the absence of social acknowledgement or validation.(1) Pet loss was explored as one of many types of disenfranchised grief, and both Chapters 7 and 8 covered the extent to which the loss that clients feel in anticipation of euthanasia plays a role in companion animal practice.

When we consider that veterinarians attend their patients' deaths at a rate of five times more than other healthcare professionals experience, we begin to recognize just how immersed veterinarians are in that life to death transition.(2–4) It is the regularity with which we companion clients through anticipatory grief that gives bereavement meaning.

We recognize the value of the human–animal bond and the years with which a companion animal has intertwined their life with our client's. We see over time the strength of attachment and the uniqueness of that bond. We witness patient transformations from kittenhood and puppyhood to adult and ultimately senior status and we feel privileged to have observed, from the outside in, the tremendous capacity for love that can radiate from such attachment. It is life-changing and inspiring.

When that earthly tie comes to an end, we feel the weight of that finale alongside of our clients.

We will never ever know what it is like to be them, but we understand and appreciate and accept the loss because it is valid and we ourselves bear witness to it each time, every time we euthanize one of our regulars.

When we watch our clients with whom we have built lifetime relationships prepare themselves for that final goodbye, we honor that departure as real loss. We know that although they will navigate loss constructively, learning to live with loss, the bereaved will never be the same again.

10.1 Empathizing with the Bereaved when Loss Involves a Lengthy or Otherwise Unique Relationship

When clients telephone me weeks after their pet was euthanized and complain that "no one gets it," we do.

The veterinary profession gets it, to the best of our ability, because we see it every day.

We see the bonds built from scratch and strengthened by blood, sweat, and tears.

A lifetime spent together is something we treasure. Those are the clients and the patients and the veterinary–client–patient relationships (VCPRs) that we remember, always.

We remember them because they are, in many ways, why we were drawn into the practice of veterinary medicine: to participate in a bond that not even death can sever.

The love that we bear witness to is truly forever.

10.2 The Struggle to Relate to Other Types of Loss that Clients Experience

Anticipatory grief is not the only form of grief that many of our clients experience during their lifetime, and death is not the only loss they grieve.

Sometimes, despite our compassion towards those who mourn the loss of their lifetime companion – their so-called "heart dog" or their "forever cat" – we forget, along with the rest of the world, to acknowledge and appreciate that other losses also come into play.

Sometimes, unless we ourselves have lived through the experience, we just can't "get it." Or worse, maybe we think we do, when we really don't.

Other pet losses that clients may experience in their lifetime include, but are not limited to:(5–9)

- death secondary to anaphylaxis
  - wasp and bee stings
  - vaccine hypersensitivity reactions
- unexpected anesthetic death during routine procedures (e.g., elective sterilization surgery)
- death secondary to exposure to the elements
  - accidental drowning
  - heatstroke
  - frostbite

- death by natural disaster
- sudden, traumatic death by predator (e.g., small-breed dog killed by coyote; outdoor cat carried away by bird of prey)
- sudden, traumatic death by other companion animal (same species)
  - dog fight involving pets that live under the same roof
  - dog fight involving neighbor's/friend's pet
  - dog fight involving stranger's pet
- sudden, traumatic death by other companion animal (other species; e.g., cat killed by dog)
  - mauling involving pets that live under the same roof
  - mauling involving neighbor's/friend's pet
  - mauling involving stranger's pet
- sudden, traumatic death by accident (e.g., dog got hit by a car)
- sudden, traumatic death by intent/cruelty (e.g., dog got shot; kittens killed by drowning)
- death owing to complications from trauma
  - diaphragmatic hernia
  - flail chest
- unexpected death by toxin
  - pet ate rodenticide
    - anti-coagulant varieties
    - bromethalin
    - cholecalciferol
    - corn cellulose
  - dog ate grapes or raisins
  - cat drank antifreeze
  - cat ate lilies
  - cat drank water from a vase that contained lilies
- sudden, unexpected death during parturition
- sudden, unexpected death from surgical condition
  - gastric dilatation-volvulus (GDV)
  - splenic torsion
  - splenic hemangiosarcoma
  - gastrointestinal foreign bodies with perforation leading to sepsis
- sudden, unexpected death from medical condition
  - status epilepticus
  - asphyxiation due to choking, as from an object inadvertently lodged within the throat
  - urinary tract obstruction (UTO)
  - dilated cardiomyopathy (DCM)
  - cardiac hemangiosarcoma
  - aortic stenosis

- o pulmonic stenosis
- o valvular endocarditis
- o hypertrophic cardiomyopathy (HCM)
- o aortic thromboembolism (ATE), including saddle thrombus
- o dyspneic cat with open mouth breathing
- o cerebral cuterebriasis
- o lyme nephritis
- o hemorrhage unrelated to trauma, such as that which occurs secondary to hemolytic anemia
  - *Babesia canis*
  - *Cytauxzoon felis*
- death due to sequelae associated with viral infection
  - o feline immunodeficiency virus (FIV)
  - o feline leukemia virus (FeLV)
    - lymphoma
    - erythemic myelosis
    - nonregenerative anemia
- stillbirth
- unexpected death in a young patient
  - o failure to thrive
  - o flea bite anemia
  - o canine parvovirus
  - o feline panleukopenia
  - o anasarca ("water puppies," "swimmer puppies," "walrus puppies")
    - these pups are born with severe edema
- separation because the pet ran away or otherwise went missing
- separation because the pet was stolen
- housing restrictions
- placing a pet for adoption
- losing custody (e.g., divorce settlements)
- relinquishment to a shelter
- forced relinquishment to Animal Control or comparable humane organization
- voluntarily signing over the rights to a patient (e.g., to the veterinary team) on account of cost of care.

10.3 The Impact of Finances on Patient Lifespan

Clients may be forced to make challenging choices about patient care under less-than-ideal circumstances. Financial constraints may preclude the ability to manage a treatable condition medically or surgically. A cat with a UTO is treatable, however it is costly, and there is potential for recurrence. A dog with exocrine pancreatic insufficiency (EPI) is treatable, however, it requires lifelong supplementation with pancreatic enzymes, the cost of which adds up over time, particularly for a large or giant-breed. When cost of care exceeds the client's capacity to afford what the patient needs in the short- or long-term to survive, the client's only available option may be euthanasia even though the patient's condition was "fixable."

10.4 Beyond Cost of Care

Cost of care is not the only obstacle in terms of healthcare delivery. Sometimes clients lack the means by which to appropriately manage care. A cat with diabetes mellitus is treatable; however, a client may be unable to physically administer injections. They may themselves have a medical condition that complicates the process of drug administration (e.g., rheumatoid arthritis) or they may be constantly on the road travelling on account of business, without the schedule flexibility and consistency that would effectively promote disease management. In either situation, they may be forced to consider rehoming – which is its own loss – or consider euthanasia of a patient that could have otherwise been medically managed.

10.5 Considering Client Choices and Redefining Ours

As veterinarians, we are more likely to understand and accept cost of care limitations because we experience these cases walking into our clinics each day, every day. However, we may not always consider other rationales for relinquishment and/or requests to proceed with euthanasia in an otherwise healthy patient. When we receive such a request, we may experience one or more gut reactions. We may experience significant emotional distress. We may question the client's judgment and/or cast our own judgments about the choices that the client has made, and the choices that they are asking us to make alongside of them. We may assume that euthanasia is for convenience when in fact underlying issues that are unbeknownst to us may well be at play.

This text is *not* intended to decide for you, the veterinarian, what is the best course of action medically or ethically. You and only you can decide how best to proceed clinically in partnership with any client, and you reserve the right to decline to euthanize.

The goal of this chapter is to acknowledge those instances when grief and/or loss is complicated by extenuating circumstances and to recognize that those circumstances are especially distressing to the client who has sought your counsel.

Clients often feel exceptional guilt when having to choose between a rock and a hard place. It can be especially devastating to contemplate or experience the loss of a pet that is young. Whether we choose to support clients' decisions in all situations and follow through with euthanasia requests, it is important that we come at each case with regard.(10)

10.6 Demonstrating Regard for Clients in Their Time of Need

Unconditional positive regard is a concept that was coined by Carl Rogers, a mental health expert in human healthcare.(10, 11) Although it is referenced most often by experts in the disciplines of psychiatry, social work, counseling, and psychology, the practice of unconditional positive regard applies to all healthcare professionals.(10) Those who practice regard for others approach each clinical case as an opportunity to suspend judgment and demonstrate respect. It is about seeing people as they are, rather than comparing them to others and holding them to impossibly high standards.(10, 12)

Not all human or veterinary patients are alike. Every patient is unique. Some patients may be "easier" than others. Some may require less of us; others may require more. More effort. More time. More patience.

It is important to recognize that those who require "more" are not inherently "difficult," though we have a tendency to label them as such. (10) Difficulties are not uncommon in healthcare; however, we need to shift our perspective to appreciate that it is more often the cases than the people, who challenge us.(10)

In those times when human patients, veterinary clients, and doctors do not see eye to eye, it is vital for practitioners to display positive regard. Refocus on the common ground. Ask yourself what both you and the patient/client wish to achieve and consider how you two can work together to achieve it.(10, 13)

Unconditional positive regard requires us to move from reaction to response.(10) It requires us to step away from judgment, which is part of human nature.(10) It is normal for us to label others, including our clients, or to judge them for the choices they make, especially when we disagree with them.(10)

In such circumstances, it is important to remember that: "Individual practitioners do not have to morally agree with an individual's behavior, nor should we avoid counseling for fear of intruding on individual values, but we must never view the individual as unworthy of conscientious care."(14)

Regard does *not* mean that we always agree with our client or their choices.

Regard *does* mean that we make every effort to pause and breathe and take all appropriate measures to understand the situation rather than judge.

10.7 Navigating Clients' Reactions to Sudden, Unexpected Loss, Part I: It's All *My* Fault

Veterinary clients fear being judged by other members of the veterinary team.(10) This fear may prevent them from being candid about their thoughts, feelings, and concerns about patient care.(10) They may worry about what will be said to them or about them behind closed doors.(10) Companion animal owners, particularly those with cats, appreciate when the veterinary team acknowledges their good intentions, even if in some cases their actions lead to missteps.(12)

One focus group participant of a 2015 research study shared the importance of being understood: "Have you ever done something stupid with your cat and you've got to go tell the vet you did something stupid? [Vets] don't look at you like you're crazy. They understand that we make mistakes."(12)

Another offered a specific example from their own case file: "[When] the cat [eats] a cardboard box and [swallows] it, [vets] don't say, 'why on earth did you let him eat the cardboard box?' Simply put, they understand."(12)

A third participant explained the significance of regard:

We need that understanding to apply at all stages of life, no matter how small and no matter how big. We need to know that the vet stands with us in solidarity no matter what, even when we were wrong. And sometimes we do goof. Sometimes we mess up, big time!(12)

Consider three additional examples.(10)

- The client who mistakenly gives the cat Tylenol® (acetaminophen or paracetamol) because the cat was in pain and there were no overnight emergency care options.
- The client whose dog ingested grapes, and who didn't seek medical care right away because they didn't realize that grapes could induce acute kidney injury (AKI).

- The client who accidentally hit their dog with their automobile, backing out of the driveway, or the client who didn't realize that their cat ingested antifreeze until their kidneys shut down.

All these clients may present to you in different emotional states.(10) Despite the variations in emotional displays, guilt is a common denominator.(10)

Guilt within the context of grief has been defined as a:(15) "[r]emorseful emotional reaction … with recognition of having failed to live up to one's own inner standards and expectations in relationship to the deceased and/ or the death."

Guilt is common following the death of a loved one, particularly for pet owners who feel that their actions may have prevented it.(16–18) Clients who make mistakes that jeopardize their pet's health often feel guilty about their actions, although there was no intent to cause harm. These clients may be angry with themselves, whether their anger is rational or not.(10) They often blame themselves for what happened, whether the blame is accurate or not, misplaced or not.(10)

Blame is a powerful reaction to grief. It is related to, yet distinct from regret. Both may play a significant part in the survivors' adaptation to life after loss.(16)

Stroebe et al. define regret as:(16) "involving painful thoughts and feelings about past actions and how one could have achieved a better outcome(19), and in the bereavement specific literature, as feelings associated with unfinished business with the deceased in general(20), or the perception that one could have done things differently."(21).

Stroebe et al. differentiate regret from self-blame:(16) "While self-blame stresses responsibility for the death, and implies accusation of oneself, regret in bereavement focuses more on possible better outcomes, without impaired sense of self."

Both regret and self-blame may contribute to bereavement; however, the latter has the potential to damage psychological well-being and complicate grief.(16)

Blame temporarily grants the illusion that the bereaved are in control at a time when they otherwise feel helpless. By blaming something or someone, the bereaved put themselves in the driver's seat. They get to determine who to find fault with and there is comfort in that. There's someone to go to, to blame, and that someone is usually themselves irrespective of whether blame is deserved.

Blame ignites magical thinking. The bereaved may articulate that, "If I had just done 'x', then [insert pet name] would be okay. They would still be here with me. They would still be alive."

Blame tells the client they had the power to effect change, but they blew it. Because of this, blame can give rise to self-loathing. Survivors may say that they "hate" themselves for what they've done even when harmful actions (e.g., delayed visit to the visits, administering the wrong drug, administering the right drug at the wrong dose) were unintentional.

Veterinary clients may verbalize self-hate, self-resentment, or self-blame. They may tell you that "It's all my fault."

There is immense sorrow and pain in that statement, and emptiness, too.

Now, it may be true, what they say. Maybe it is their fault. I have had clients who inadvertently ran over their dogs in the driveway. In that case, there is some truth to their statement. They were driving the car. If they hadn't gone out driving that day or night, then maybe, just maybe their dog would still be alive.

But playing "What if?" is a dangerous game.

Who truly knows what would have happened. It may be that the dog would have still run out into the road and been hit by someone else.

It may not have happened that same day. It could have happened tomorrow or the next day, next week, next month, or even next year.

That's why it is such a tragedy and why life is so unpredictable. There are too many variables to name. We can ask ourselves a hundred "What if's?"

None of us can say for sure what would have been, and none of us can ever reverse time to bring the deceased back to life.

When clients express that they take ownership of fault, what it means is, "I really need someone to blame right now and that someone is me. Blame gives me control and it's the only sense of control that I am clinging onto in the moment. If I let that part of me go, I don't know what will happen. I don't know what I'll do."

It is a cry of desperation. It is a cry for help. It is someone seeking to be accepted and loved unconditionally, even if they bear responsibility for any fraction of what went down.

When clients present this side of themselves to you, it is vital that you hear them out. Provide a safe, supportive space in which they can open up to you and your team.

Our knee-jerk reaction may be to say, "Don't be crazy."

Avoid that reaction. Suppress it. Do what you can to not say it aloud.

It may be true. It may be how we feel. But it negates what our clients are feeling in that moment. It invalidates what they have just shared with us about how they feel. It reinforces that their perception of reality is at odds with yours rather than assuages them of guilt.

Instead of defaulting to this phraseology, try the following approaches:

- "I can't even begin to imagine what you're going through. My heart breaks for you and all that you've experienced."
- "It is normal to feel that way. I might feel that way, too, if I were in your shoes."
- "I get where you are coming from; if I were in your shoes, I might also feel that I were responsible."
- "I can see how you might feel that way. May I share with you what I see differently?"
- "I can see why you might feel the way that you do. May I share with you how I see the situation, from my perspective? What I see is that …"

Be certain that they feel supported by you. You might share that:

- "You were only trying to help."
- "You did the best you could."
- "You did what you thought was best."
- "You did what anyone would have done in your shoes."
- "Of course, you didn't mean to …"
- "How would you have known …"
- "I could have done the same thing …"
- "I have done the same thing …"
- "I might have done the same thing …"
- "It happens – let me help you."

Verbalizing regard in such a way is demonstrative of respect, understanding, and empathy. We can further reinforce our support for the client through respectful pausing.

What do we mean by pausing?

[pause]

We mean just that.

A pause is a break in conversation. A pause is a spacer between words. A pause is a breath.

It allows the speaker to consider word choice and to consider intent upon delivery.

It allows the speaker time to contemplate how best to say what needs to be said in a way that will hopefully be received constructively, with the intention with which the message was delivered.

Pausing is not something that comes naturally to all of us, but it is an essential aspect of life. It's how we recharge. It's how we reboot. It's how we process all of life, not just life in veterinary practice.

Why is it so hard for us to pause? Why is it so hard to take that moment?

Veterinary medicine is a constant onslaught of activity. It's always *go, go, go*. Get patients in. Get them diagnosed. Get them treated. Get them out the door. Get them back in for follow-up. And that's on a good day. That's not even considering the work-in and work-around appointments, the walk-ins, the emergencies.

We rarely breathe because we rarely have the time. Yet pausing is vital to our health, to the well-being of our clients, and to the survival of the VCPR.

Pausing helps us to:

- consider all sides
- process what you've heard
- think before you speak
- choose words wisely, with care
- consider your intent
- consider the potential impact.

Pausing also allows the other person to speak. It cuts off our monologues. It reminds us to reengage the client.

Pausing is how we help the client when they are frozen with shock and not much is sinking in. Pausing is how we help the client when there is so much static and noise in the client's mind that they don't have the ability to process new words until their heart catches up with reality and they come out of the fog of shock or grief.

Pausing gives the client a moment to catch their breath. A moment to just be.

In this respect, pausing facilitates challenging conversations.

Maybe a mistake was made by the client, like giving Tylenol® to a cat. Now the cat is in liver failure, and you must explain that the cat's liver has failed because of the client's action.

That is a difficult conversation to have. Pausing helps before you deliver a "warning shot."

You can say, "I'm afraid what I have to share is not good news" or "I'm afraid that what I have to say may come as a shock."

Then you pause. Pausing helps to break the news more gently. Calmly.

In that way, Pausing can also help us during times of grief. As we've discussed in earlier chapters, there is no one right way to grieve. Everyone navigates that path differently, in their own way, on their own timetable.

Pausing gives that extra moment to absorb, to consider what one needs in their moment of grief.

Sometimes a pause is enough of a bridge to connect two people during a devastating time.

Often in grief there are no right answers, no right words to say, and nothing can make it better.

Sometimes all one needs is a partner in life, someone to sit beside – to know they're there, even when no words are shared.

A pause is that bridge, that lifeline.

Sometimes the most powerful thing in the world is just sitting beside our client and pausing to take in that moment of silence, together.

Pausing also provides an opportunity for the other person to collect their thoughts and share. Sharing inspires mutual understanding. Sharing allows you to consider someone else's perspective. Sharing allows you to understand the "why" behind one's actions.

Most importantly, sharing allows the other person to be understood. Sharing allows you to "get" another person fully.

Sharing is how we give the client an opportunity to let us know what is weighing on them.

If clients blame themselves, you cannot make them stop. Only they hold the power to put an end to the blame game that they started and directed at themselves.

Instead of trying to change them, hear their grief. It's about meeting them where they are at, in their grief. Rather than try to "fix" it, acknowledge it. Validate it.

That doesn't mean you agree with them and that they are to blame. It means you validate why they feel that way. You understand and accept that it is human to feel as they do. And that maybe, just maybe, you would, too.

That degree of understanding is what they are looking for, it is what they are after, it is what they need to take a step back and breathe, pause and reflect, and begin to heal.

10.8 Navigating Clients' Reactions to Sudden, Unexpected Loss, Part II: It's All *Your* Fault

Any death that occurs at the veterinary clinic other than planned, owner-consented euthanasia is unexpected.

Patients may present to the veterinary team on emergency status or at a "sick visit" in rough shape. Patients often present in compromised or in critical condition. Many are extremely dehydrated, hypotensive, and in varying degrees of shock, with altered mentation. Many arrive at the clinic moribund whether the client perceives them to be or not.

These patients do not always make it out of the clinic alive. Some do. A fraction of their owners decline care and take the patient home against medical advice (AMA). However, many patients are euthanized in the consultation room, after deliberate consideration, before they decompensate. Others may be euthanized on the surgical table pending a critical conversation with the client.

Patients often decompensate during triage and/or delivery of life-stabilizing care. They may arrest. Cardiopulmonary resuscitation (CPR) may be unsuccessful at reviving them. When such death occurs, there is significant underlying pathology that may or may not be outwardly apparent.

The veterinary team often senses that death is impending. It is akin to a sixth sense. But clients may not be aware of the severity of a given situation.

For the client, death often comes as a shock. It is not expected. It was not predicted. And it can be extraordinarily challenging for the client to move past that.

When clients receive news that is unexpected, particularly if it involves the death of their pet, they may react any number of ways. They may blame us for their loss, whether we were responsible for having caused it or not.

Blame may be immediate or blame may be delayed. It may not take shape until several days after the death, when the client resurfaces to share that they hold us accountable.

Sometimes they circle back to us after having talked with a family member, close friend, or neighbor about the case. Sometimes the other person asks questions that our client doesn't know the answers to.

That plants a seed of doubt. Doubt grows into something with roots. And those roots are hard to shake.

Being blamed for the death of a patient that wasn't our fault is impactful.

When you hear the words, "This is your fault," for the first time, they will haunt you. Even if you had absolutely nothing to do with the pet's death – even if they arrested before they walked in the front door to the clinic and even if they arrived DOA – you can't help but doubt yourself and your team.

Is there something you could have done?

Would you have done something, anything differently?

Could you have done more?

Those are the questions that we will take to our graves. They plague us because they are inconsistent with the driving force behind our reason for being. They are the opposite of why we come to work each day, every day.

We work to save lives; not to kill.

I have been called a "killer" and a "murderer" on two separate occasions, by two unrelated clients, and I have never forgotten.

Those terms have stuck with me for more than a decade because they hurt. They cut me to the quick.

The suckerpunch was intentional. Those words were meant to hurt.

In both cases, both clients were hurting. Neither client knew what to do with their hurt; they just knew that they wanted someone else to feel what they were feeling, too. That someone else just so happened to be me.

In the moment, I felt their hurt all too clearly, and I wanted more than anything else to take their pain away.

I wanted to tell them that it wasn't me, that it wasn't my fault.

I wanted to tell that them I had nothing to do with taking their pet away from them, that I had been there to help, that I did all in my power to make a difference, but that it was too late for help, that their pet was long gone by the time I set eyes on them.

I wanted to tell them anything and everything that I had done to reverse death.

I wanted to tell them that there was nothing anyone could have done.

I wanted to plead my case. I wanted to defend myself. I wanted them to wash my hands clean of the guilt they made me feel inside, for something I had nothing to do with, for something that I had no reason to feel guilty about.

The truth is, none of that would have helped the client in the moment.

It didn't matter to them that I had tried three rounds of CPR, unsuccessfully.

It didn't matter to them what drugs I had administered or for how long my team performed chest compressions.

It didn't matter to them that we had been able to successfully intubate or place a central line.

What mattered to them, the only thing that mattered to them, was that who they loved was gone.

No amount of detail as to what was done to try to cheat death would ever come close to bringing back who they loved. Their pet had died. Period. End of story. And they weren't coming back.

Death is scarring. What people say when they are grieving can be scarring, too.

Impact works both ways. The veterinary team can wrongfully impact the client through actions or statements. The client can do the same.

We are a partnership above all. We either soar together or sink each other.

When we are on the receiving end of blame, it is natural to react defensively. Adrenaline kicks in and we are ready to fight.

We would do better to first take a breath and check in with ourselves. We need to ask ourselves the following questions:

- Are you in the right frame of mind to entertain this conversation?
- Can you focus on what the client needs right now?
- Can you put the client's needs before your own?
- Have you reached out to available resources for support?

If we are not ready to take on the conversation in a way that will be productive, then we may need to hit the pause button on the conversation until we are "ready." We may need to schedule a meeting with the client so that we can check in at a time when we are fully present and in control rather than engage in "fight" mode, fists raised.

Note that if we postpone conversation, time is still of the essence:(22) "While allowing a client to cool off is sometimes warranted in an effort to ensure a productive conversation, committing to a timely response is important. Letting a client's emotions fester while you procrastinate over making an uneasy phone call is counterproductive."

We may never feel ready to check in with the client but doing so is essential. We can help ourselves by drawing from models in human healthcare to prepare for the conversation that we may be dreading.

The **SPIKES** and **ABCDE** models(23, 24) are the most often cited in the medical literature for bad news delivery although others have been more recently described.(25–27)

The **SPIKES** model stands for:

S – Setting

- create a supportive setting

P – Perspective

- elicit your client's perspective

I – Invitation to Share

- absorb what the client has chosen to share with you
- use what the client has shared with you as a foundation upon which to build
- ask for permission to share

K – Knowledge

- share what you know
- share what you don't know

E – Empathize
S – Summarize and Strategize

The SPIKES approach requires the clinician to establish a supportive setting in which to elicit the client's perspective, invite discussion about the case, and provide the client with details about the patient's condition(2). The physician must balance the need to be clinical against the need to be compassionate. Empathy is the primary communication skill that the SPIKES model employs to foster relationship-centered care. A final summary statement ties the conversation together and prevents key concepts from being lost in translation.(2, 23)

In addition to drawing upon the SPIKES model, which has been adapted for veterinary practice from human healthcare, you may need to invite a colleague, employer, practice manager, or better yet, a neutral third party – a mediator – to the table. This individual helps to navigate delicate situations and to refocus both you and the client when conversations take unfortunate turns.

From the beginning of engagement with the client, be very clear about boundaries to protect you and your team from verbal abuse. Demonstrate respect for the client; however, respect works both ways. If conversations get heated, then you may need to call a time-out.

Come prepared to discuss the case. If you are the employer or practice manager, find out the whole story first. Gather information. Review the chart. Connect with your employees. Discern the facts and come up with options for moving forward.(22)

Select a setting that is conducive to dialogue. "Hold the conversation in a quiet, private area where both parties can concentrate and where no audience can incite theatrical behavior."(22)

Keep your emotions in check and be open-minded: "Conjure up the ability to approach the client with your emotions in neutral and with an open mind. Strike a balance of compassion and confidence. Defensiveness has no place in productive conflict resolution."(22)

Begin with eliciting the client's perspective: let the client know that you are up to speed with respect to the situation, but want to hear from them what their experience has been.(22)

Listen carefully to what the client has to say and "make no attempt to justify or problem-solve. This is the time to let the client vent and for you to gather facts and truly understand the client's perspective."(22)

Make certain that the client feels heard and understood. Use active listening to check for accuracy in what you believe you heard the client say.(22)

Acknowledge the client's emotional state, using the client's words to complete this statement: "I can understand why you are _____."

If the client says that they are angry, use that word choice to reflect that that have been heard.

If the client does not select the word *angry*, then use what word they referenced instead to fill in the blanks.

Don't put words in their mouths. Listen to what they share and make use of their sentiments to connect yourself to them.

"Be respectful, but do not patronize."(22)

As the conversation is drawing to a conclusion: "Apologize for what needs an apology. Take responsibility when appropriate and be careful to not throw teammates under the bus. If an apology is unnecessary, you can always say, 'I am sorry that this has been so impactful' or 'I am sorry we made you feel this way.'"(22)

Ask what you and the team can do to support the client during their time of need.

Consult your insurance carrier if you suspect that you or your team may be accused of malpractice. This is especially vital when unexpected death at the veterinary clinic results from adverse effects of treatment following hospitalization, treatment complications, or medical error.(28)

When such death occurs, the client may or may not be present. In either case, the veterinarian is responsible for death notification.(28) Effective death notification is particularly critical in the disciplines of emergency medicine and surgery.(29–35)

Patient prognoses may be guarded in both the intensive care units (ICUs) and the peri-operative period, and patients are not guaranteed to survive procedural interventions.

Anesthesia is not without risk.(36) The primary anesthetic complications in veterinary medicine are intra-operative hypotension(37–39), opioid-induced dysphoria(40–42), cardiac dysrhythmias(39), post-operative regurgitation and vomiting(43), aspiration pneumonia(44), cerebellar dysfunction(45), blindness or deafness in cats(46–48), and death(49). With regards to anesthetic death, a recent study in the UK evaluated records from 98,036 cats and 79,178 cats between June 2002 and 2004 and found the risk in dogs and cats to be 0.17% and 0.24%, respectively.(50)

When patients were categorized by health status, the risk of anesthetic death in *healthy* dogs and cats dropped to 0.05% and 0.11% compared with 1.33% and 1.40% in ill dogs and cats.(50) These percentages are much higher than those that have been reported for anesthetized people, 0.02–0.05%,(51–53) yet veterinary clients are often not prepared for anesthetic death as a potential and devastating complication.

A 2016 survey questionnaire by my research team asked dog and cat owners to rank their level of concern with regards to their pet undergoing general anesthesia.(54) Pet-owners that scored their level of concern as an eight or higher on a scale of 1–10 gave the following reasons:(54)

- They considered their pet to be their child.
- They were aware that their pet had one or more risk factors.
- They were afraid of the unknown.

Yet, according to companion animal owners, one-in-three veterinarians and one-in-two veterinary technicians do not mention anesthetic risk during pre-surgical consults.(54) Although the majority of dog- and cat-owners are required to sign paperwork that acknowledges the potential for anesthetic risk, many clients either do not understand what they are signing or do not take the time to read the information that has been provided.(54)

When complications arise, clients often do not feel prepared to handle them.

We need to do a better job as a profession of anticipating risks and engaging clients in open conversations about patient prognosis in easy-to-understand language that is clear, concise, and direct. These conversations are not always possible in emergency situations during immediate patient stabilization; however, they must take place at some point so that the client has heard at least once, from at least one team member, what the expected outcome is.

In cases where the patient's prognosis is poor, clients often need to hear this news multiple times, from multiple people, in order for it to be processed through their shock and grief. Shock and grief prevent critical words that our clients need to hear from getting through and being absorbed. It is why we might discuss risks once, only to have a client react when they hear it for the second time, as if they're hearing it for the first time.

10.9 Loss of Pet Ownership

Pet ownership is not always forever, even if it intends to be.

Pets may be acquired throughout life as relationships and lives join hands. Partners may take on the responsibility of one or more pets as surrogate children, or they may combine households and in so doing, add pets to the family unit.

Relationships may break up; partners may divorce. When that happens, property is divided and partners must make arrangements to establish sole versus shared custody of pets and kids alike.(5)

In a divorce:(5)

A pet may become the focus of anger and resentment or it can remind a client of happier times shared with a spouse. Some clients genuinely love and want the pet, while others use the issue of custody to get back at their spouses. Some clients, in an ultimate act of cruelty, even euthanize or abandon the pets as a way to get back at a partner seeking a divorce.

Sometimes there are no custody battles between partners; however, divorced or separated couples often relocate. Many are forced to downsize owing to financial constraints. When relocation occurs, individuals may be limited in terms of what they can afford or where they geographically must reside. This may require them to sign a lease or rent a room/studio/apartment/home that does not allow pets. Or, some residences will allow pets, but only so many. Other residences may place other restrictions upon pet ownership. For instance, they may require a pet deposit (which may or may not be financially feasible), or they may preclude a certain species (e.g., no dogs), certain breeds (e.g., no Pit Bulls), or certain sizes (e.g., no dogs over 50 pounds).

These restrictions, individually or collectively, may preclude one or more pets from moving with the custodial "parent." If the noncustodial "parent" cannot accommodate the pets, then the partners may be forced to relinquish one or more pets to the shelter. Alternatively, they may seek to place their pet(s) up for adoption. In either case, they are hoping to find a good home.

Divorce and separation are not the only reasons why one might seek to relinquish their pet ownership rights. Other reasons for placing a pet up for an adoption include:(5)

- allergies to the pet
- behavioral issues(55, 56)
  - aggression
  - separation anxiety
  - inappropriate elimination(57–64)
- transitional periods in life
  - relocation of primary pet owner to extended care facility that does not allow pets
  - terminal illness and/or hospice care for the primary pet owner
  - relocation of primary pet owner to college and parents not being willing to take on the responsibility of one or more pets
  - unemployment and associated financial constraints
  - employment opportunities that are tied to frequent travel
  - death of the primary pet owner
  - birth within the family
    - pre-existing concerns about integrating the pet into households with children (e.g., pets with histories of aggression)

- pressure from neighbors
  - e.g., noise ordinances and excessive barking in outdoor dogs.

Finding a good home does not negate the grief that is associated with giving up a loved one.

10.10 Unresolved Grief When Patients Go Missing

Sometimes not knowing what happens to a beloved pet can be more devastating than learning of that pet's death. When a pet goes missing, it could be literally anywhere.

As hours pass into days, and as days pass into weeks, clients are left to wonder, "What if …"

- "What if the pet is lost?"
- "What if the pet is scared?"
- "What if the pet is hungry?"
- "What if the pet is cold?"
- "What if the pet is lonely?"
- "What if the pet is hurt?"
- "What if the pet got hit by a car?"
- "What if the pet cannot find its way back to me?"
- "What if the pet needs me; how will it find me?"
- "What if the pet is suffering and needs to be put down?"

These questions haunt our clients. Their minds may conjure up all kinds of images and nightmares that plague their thoughts. They may imagine the suffering that their pet is enduring, without them. This creates additional stress and, over time, repetitive trauma.

It is as if they are reliving the loss again and again because at any point, they could find out devastating news. They might stumble across their pet's body. They might find out by cold-calling shelters that their pet was found, without identification, and put to sleep. They might hear someone talking about how a cat or dog was hit on the road up the street. If any part of the description fits their pet (e.g., coloration, marking, size, breed), then they re-experience grief until they find out otherwise. Every close call is another time they are suspended in mid-air, holding their breath, hoping, praying that their pet was spared.

Sometimes the incident was no one's fault. A natural disaster may have come along and decimated the home, surrounding property, and neighboring communities. Consider, for instance, the destruction that Hurricane Katrina unleashed. Many pets went missing.

Consider other disasters such as house fires. Indoor pets may or may not have made it out alive. The client may hold out hope that the fire paved the way for escape and that they fled the scene and scattered. The client may never know. Their bodies may never be found. It then becomes unclear whether they died in the fire or got lost and so never came home.

Sometimes, pets go missing not because of a disaster but because of an accident. In these instances, guilt and blame may perpetuate and intensify grief. Perhaps the client left a gate open. Maybe they turned their back for a split second when the door was ajar. Maybe they left their dog unattended. Maybe their cat escaped through a window. Maybe they ran their dog off-leash, the dog spooked, and got away.

When their own actions caused the pet to go missing, they may struggle to forgive themselves.

When the actions of someone else they love caused the pet to go missing, then grief is compounded by the fact that other pivotal relationships are also impacted. The client may have preferred to lean on that other person to companion them through grief. Now, the client may see them as unreliable and distance themselves because that other person is a constant reminder of what went wrong. They blame them for the accident, even though it was just that, an accident. They may always blame them for the accident. That blame may weaken the bond they share and may adversely impact their capacity to relate to one another.

The lack of knowing and the persistent uncertainty may make it difficult to move forward. There is no end to the game of "What ifs" unless the pet is found.

When time stretches on and no pet is to be found, healing is hard to come by.

Others in our clients' lives will move on. They will forget the loss and the pain and the grief of the unknown.

But our clients cannot move on without knowing. They may hold out forever, waiting, wondering, always vigilant. Answers may never come.

We help these individuals by being patient. We help them by acknowledging the unknown and that uncertainty weighs them down.

Some clients may need to invent an ending to the story that they can live with, to move with grief.(5)

The client may or may not recover. It is not our job as veterinarians to fix them. All we can do is make time to listen and hear them out.

10.11 Unsolved Mysteries and the Role of Necropsies

Sometimes clients come home to find that their pet has passed away, unexpectedly. With respect to this situation, Dr. Margaret Stalker, a veterinary pathologist at the University of Guelph, explained that: "There are few things more traumatic for a pet owner than witnessing the completely unexpected death of a family pet, or finding a pet lying dead in the home, yard or neighborhood."(7)

Even though any of us can pass at any time, clients typically only reserve that expectation for elderly pets. When they own a dog or cat that is young to middle-aged and who exhibited no signs of being unwell prior to death, clients cannot wrap their heads around the loss. By their estimations, an otherwise healthy animal does not show up dead. Because the death is premature in their eyes and because premature death doesn't make sense, clients search for answers.

In their search to resolve the mystery, clients may grapple with the possibility that their pet encountered foul play. Clients may reach out to their veterinarians, teaching hospitals, and/or local diagnostic laboratories with questions about whether their pet's sudden death could have been maliciously induced.(7) It is not uncommon for clients to suspect their neighbors of poisoning their pet, particularly if there are ongoing rifts related to the pet having outdoor free rein. For instance, I have had clients question their neighbors upon finding their deceased cat in the backyard; the neighbors had threatened the week prior to the cat's death to "put an end to it" because the cat was stalking their birdfeeder. The clients consented to a necropsy, which provided the closure that they needed. The cat, as it turned out, did not die because of poisoning by neighbor. The cat died of HCM. Cardiomyopathy is second only to trauma among the most common cause of sudden, unexpected death in cats.(9) It is the primary cause of sudden, unexpected death in dogs.(8) The client was relieved to discover that the neighbor was innocent. It was an added relief to the client to know that cardiomyopathies rarely induce overt clinical signs. Symptoms can be subtle or even clinically silent.(7)

Postmortem examinations are the best way to provide clients with the answers that they are searching for. Clients may be referred to a pathologist through their primary care veterinarian or they may reach out to an affiliated animal diagnostic center on their own.(7)

Talking with clients about necropsies requires skillful conversations. Veterinarians need to elicit the client's perspective in terms of their expectations, wants, and needs. If the client's goal is to discover the cause of death and doing so will bring the client peace, then the best chance they have is to consent to postmortem examination.

Clients do not always understand what a postmortem examination entails. Anecdotally, in my experience, clients are more likely to relate to the word, *autopsy*, than *necropsy*, perhaps because the former word choice is recognizable from past experiences with human healthcare. In this respect, *autopsy* can be thought of as humanizing a very somber event. *Necropsy*, on the other hand, separates animal death from human death, when most clients who view pets as family perceive the impact of animal and human death to be the same.

Necropsies are an imperfect science. Clients need to know that there is a cost tied to the procedure and that there is no guarantee that a diagnosis will be made. An isolated study in 2000 disclosed that 19/151 (12.6%) of postmortem examinations did not establish the cause of death in dogs.(8) A follow-up study in 2001 disclosed that 10/79 (12.7%) of postmortem examinations did not establish the cause of death in cats.(9) However, in spite of diagnostic uncertainties that are beyond our control, in most cases an answer is found.(7)

Not every client will feel that answers are helpful. Some may feel that it is "too late" because knowing what precipitated death cannot reverse it. That being said, clients should be given the choice to determine for themselves what will be most helpful.

Sometimes in our discomfort with grief and in our haste to rush people through the sadness, we do not make every option available. Many of us do not offer necropsies. This is a disservice to clients when we make assumptions about what they would want and make the choice for them.

Pathologist Dr. Spangler shares that "veterinarians may underestimate the desire of pet owners to understand why their pet has died."

In Dr. Spangler's experience:

Our clients are generally very appreciative of knowing the specifics of what happened and being able to talk about it with a professional pathologist. These pets have been beloved members of the family, and the necropsy—and the answers that come with it—seems to really help the grieving process. It helps give them closure.(7)

References

1. Doka K. Disenfranchised grief: recognizing hidden sorrow. Lexington, MA: Lexingon Books; 1989.
2. Shaw JR, Lagoni L. End-of-life communication in veterinary medicine: delivering bad news and euthanasia decision making. Vet Clin North Am Small Anim

Pract. 2007;37(1):95–108; abstract viii:abstract viii–ix. https://doi.org/10.1016/j. cvsm.2006.09.010, PMID 17162114.

3. Hart L. Hart B. Grief and stress from so many animal deaths. Companion Anim Pract. 1987;1:20–1.

4. Williams S, Mills JN. Understanding and responding to grief in companion animal practice. Aust Vet Pract. 2000;30:55–62.

5. Barton Ross C, Baron-Sorensen J. Pet loss and human emotion: a guide to recovery. 2nd ed. Vol. xvii. New York: Routledge; 2007.

6. Stalker M. Causes of sudden unexpected death in dogs and cats – it's not the neighbour! Guelph, Ontario: Animal Health Laboratory, University of Guelph, ON. 2019.

7. Burns K. When death comes suddenly to a pet. American Veterinary Medical Association (AVMA); 2022. Available from: https://www.avma.org/news/whe n-death-comes-suddenly-pet#:~:text=In%20many%20cases%20of%20sud den,fatal%20progression%20of%20that%20condition

8. Olsen TF, Allen AL. Causes of sudden and unexpected death in dogs: a 10-year retrospective study. Can Vet J. 2000;41(11):873–5. PMID 11126495.

9. Olsen TF, Allen AL. Causes of sudden and unexpected death in cats: a 10-year retrospective study. Can Vet J. 2001;42(1):61–2. PMID 11195527.

10. Englar RE. A guide to oral communication in veterinary medicine. Sheffield, United Kingdom: 5m Publishing; 2020.

11. Amadi C. Clinician, society and suicide mountain: reading Rogerian doctrine of unconditional positive regard (UPR). Psychol Thought. 2013;6(1):75–89. https://doi. org/10.5964/psyct.v6i1.54.

12. Englar RE, Williams M, Weingand K. Applicability of the Calgary-Cambridge guide to dog and cat owners for teaching veterinary clinical communications. J Vet Med Educ. 2016;43(2):143–69. https://doi.org/10.3138/jvme.0715-117R1, PMID 27075274.

13. Gibson S. On judgment and judgmentalism: how counselling can make people better. J Med Ethics. 2005;31(10):575–7. https://doi.org/10.1136/jme.2004.011387, PMID 16199597.

14. Larkin GL, Iserson K, Kassutto Z, Freas G, Delaney K, Krimm J, et al. Virtue in emergency medicine. Acad Emerg Med. 2009;16(1):51–5. https://doi.org/10.1111/ j.1553-2712.2008.00315.x, PMID 19076103.

15. Li J, Stroebe M, Chan CL, Chow AY. Guilt in bereavement: a review and conceptual framework. Death Stud. 2014;38(1–5):165–71. https://doi.org/10.1080/07481187. 2012.738770, PMID 24524544.

16. Stroebe M, Stroebe W, van de Schoot R, Schut H, Abakoumkin G, Li J. Guilt in bereavement: the role of self-blame and regret in coping with loss. PLOS ONE. 2014;9(5):e96606. https://doi.org/10.1371/journal.pone.0096606, PMID 24819238.

17. Fleming S, Robinson. P. Grief and cognitive-behavioral therapy: the reconstruction of meaning. In: Stroebe MS, Hansson RO, Stroebe W, Schut H, editors. Handbook of bereavement research: consequences, coping, and care. Washington, DC: American Psychological Association; 2001. p. 647–70.

18. Parkes CM. Bereavement; studies of grief in adult life. Vol. xiii. New York: International Universities Press; 1972.

19. Rose NJ, Epstude KAI, Fessel F, Morrison M, Smallman R. Repetitive regret, depression, and anxiety: findings from a national representative survey. J Soc Clin Psychol. 2009;28:671–88.

20. Holland JM, Thompson KL, Rozalski V, Lichtenthal WG. Bereavement-related regret trajectories among widowed older adults. J Gerontol B Psychol Sci Soc Sci. 2014;69(1):40–7. https://doi.org/10.1093/geronb/gbt050, PMID 23766434.

21. Torges CM, Stewart AJ, Nolen-Hoeksema S. Regret resolution, aging, and adapting to loss. Psychol Aging. 2008;23(1):169–80. https://doi.org/10.1037/0882-7974.23.1.169, PMID 18361664.

22. Suiter A. Resolve to solve. Today's veterinary business [internet]; 2018. Available from: https://todaysveterinarybusiness.com/resolve-to-solve/.

23. Baile WF, Buckman R, Lenzi R, Glober G, Beale EA, Kudelka AP. SPIKES-A six-step protocol for delivering bad news: application to the patient with cancer. Oncologist. 2000;5(4):302–11. https://doi.org/10.1634/theoncologist.5-4-302, PMID 10964998.

24. Abdul Hafidz MI, Zainudin LD. Breaking Bad News: an essential skill for doctors. Med J Malaysia. 2016;71(1):26–7. PMID 27130740.

25. Ford S, Fallowfield L, Lewis S. Can oncologists detect distress in their out-patients and how satisfied are they with their performance during bad news consultations? Br J Cancer. 1994;70(4):767–70. https://doi.org/10.1038/bjc.1994.393, PMID 7917937.

26. Lind SE, DelVecchio Good MJ, Seidel S, Csordas T, Good BJ. Telling the diagnosis of cancer. J Clin Oncol. 1989;7(5):583–9. https://doi.org/10.1200/JCO.1989.7.5.583, PMID 2709087.

27. Seale C. Communication and awareness about death: a study of a random sample of dying people. Soc Sci Med. 1991;32(8):943–52. https://doi.org/10.1016/0277-9536(91)90249-c, PMID 2031210.

28. Englar RE. Using a standardized client encounter to practice death notification after the unexpected death of a feline patient following routine ovariohysterectomy. J Vet Med Educ. 2019;46(4):489–505. https://doi.org/10.3138/jvme.0817-111r1, PMID 30806560.

29. Lamba S, Tyrie LS, Bryczkowski S, Nagurka R. Teaching surgery residents the skills to communicate difficult news to patient and family members: A literature review. J Palliat Med. 2016;19(1):101–7. https://doi.org/10.1089/jpm.2015.0292, PMID 26575251.

30. Lamba S, Pound A, Rella JG, Compton S. Emergency medicine resident education in palliative care: a needs assessment. J Palliat Med. 2012;15(5):516–20. https://doi.org/10.1089/jpm.2011.0457, PMID 22577784.

31. Taylor D, Luterman A, Richards WO, Gonzalez RP, Rodning CB. Application of the core competencies after unexpected patient death: consolation of the grieved. J Surg Educ. 2013;70(1):37–47. https://doi.org/10.1016/j.jsurg.2012.06.023, PMID 23337669.

32. Benenson RS, Pollack ML. Evaluation of emergency medicine resident death notification skills by direct observation. Acad Emerg Med. 2003;10(3):219–23. https://doi.org/10.1111/j.1553-2712.2003.tb01994.x, PMID 12615586.

33. Iserson KV. The gravest words: sudden-death notifications and emergency care. Ann Emerg Med. 2000;36(1):75–7. https://doi.org/10.1067/mem.2000.107664, PMID 10874244.

34. Fallowfield L, Jenkins V. Communicating sad, bad, and difficult news in medicine. Lancet. 2004;363(9405):312–9. https://doi.org/10.1016/S0140-6736(03)15392-5, PMID 14751707.

35. Jurkovich GJ, Pierce B, Pananen L, Rivara FP. Giving bad news: the family perspective. J Trauma. 2000;48(5):865–70; discussion 70–3. https://doi.org/10.1097/00005373-200005000-00009, PMID 10823529.

36. Ackerman LJ. Blackwell's five-minute veterinary practice management consult. 3rd ed Hoboken NJ, editor. John Wiley & Sons, Inc; 2020.

37. Iizuka T, Kamata M, Yanagawa M, Nishimura R. Incidence of intraoperative hypotension during isoflurane-fentanyl and propofol-fentanyl anaesthesia in dogs. Vet J. 2013;198(1):289–91. https://doi.org/10.1016/j.tvjl.2013.06.021, PMID 23938002.

38. EM, AE W. Hypotension during anesthesia in dogs and cats: recognition, causes, and treatment. Compend Contin Educ Pract Vet. 2001;23:728–37.

39. Gaynor JS, Dunlop CI, Wagner AE, Wertz EM, Golden AE, Demme WC. Complications and mortality associated with anesthesia in dogs and cats. J Am Anim Hosp Assoc. 1999;35(1):13–7. https://doi.org/10.5326/15473317-35-1-13, PMID 9934922.

40. Becker WM, Mama KR, Rao S, Palmer RH, Egger EL. Prevalence of dysphoria after fentanyl in dogs undergoing stifle surgery. Vet Surg. 2013;42(3):302–7. https://doi.org/10.1111/j.1532-950X.2012.01080.x, PMID 23231071.

41. Väisänen M, Oksanen H, Vainio O. Postoperative signs in 96 dogs undergoing soft tissue surgery. Vet Rec. 2004;155(23):729–33. PMID 15623085.

42. Light GS, Hardie EM, Young MS, Hellyer PW, Brownie C, HAnsen BD. Pain and anxiety behaviors of dogs during intravenous catherization after premidication with placebo, acepromazine or oxymorphone. Appl Behav Anim Sci. 1993;37:331–43. https://doi.org/10.1016/0168-1591(93)90122-6.

43. Davies JA, Fransson BA, Davis AM, Gilbertsen AM, Gay JM. Incidence of and risk factors for postoperative regurgitation and vomiting in dogs: 244 cases (2000–2012). J Am Vet Med Assoc. 2015;246(3):327–35. https://doi.org/10.2460/javma.246.3.327, PMID 25587733.

44. Ovbey DH, Wilson DV, Bednarski RM, Hauptman JG, Stanley BJ, Radlinsky MG, et al. Prevalence and risk factors for canine post-anesthetic aspiration pneumonia (1999–2009): a multicenter study. Vet Anaesth Analg. 2014;41(2):127–36. https://doi.org/10.1111/vaa.12110, PMID 24588929.

45. Shamir M, Goelman G, Chai O. Postanesthetic cerebellar dysfunction in cats. J Vet Intern Med. 2004;18(3):368–9. https://doi.org/10.1892/0891-6640(2004)18<368:pcdic>2.0.co;2, PMID 15188828.

46. Barton-Lamb AL, Martin-Flores M, Scrivani PV, Bezuidenhout AJ, Loew E, Erb HN, et al. Evaluation of maxillary arterial blood flow in anesthetized cats with the mouth closed and open. Vet J. 2013;196(3):325–31. https://doi.org/10.1016/j.tvjl.2012.12.018, PMID 23394845.

47. Jurk IR, Thibodeau MS, Whitney K, Gilger BC, Davidson MG. Acute vision loss after general anesthesia in a cat. Vet Ophthalmol. 2001;4(2):155–8. https://doi.org/10.1046/j.1463-5224.2001.00170.x, PMID 11422998.

48. Jurk IR, Thibodeau MS, Whitney K, Gilger BC, Davidson MG. Acute temporary visual loss after general anesthesia in a cat. J Vet Clin. 2009;26:480–2.

49. Clarke KW, Hall LW. A survey of anaesthesia in small animal practice: AVA/BSAVA report.

50. Brodbelt DC, Blissitt KJ, Hammond RA, Neath PJ, Young LE, Pfeiffer DU, et al. The risk of death: the confidential enquiry into perioperative small animal fatalities. Vet Anaesth Analg. 2008;35(5):365–73. https://doi.org/10.1111/j.1467-2995.2008.00397.x, PMID 18466167.

51. Kawashima Y, Seo N, Morita K, Iwao Y, Irita K, Tsuzaki K, et al. [Annual study of perioperative mortality and morbidity for the year of 1999 in Japan: the outlines–report of the Japan Society of Anesthesiologists Committee on Operating Room Safety]. Masui Jpn J Anesthesiol. 2001;50(11):1260–74. PMID 11758340.

52. Biboulet P, Aubas P, Dubourdieu J, Rubenovitch J, Capdevila X, d'Athis F. Fatal and non fatal cardiac arrests related to anesthesia. Can J Anaesth. 2001;48(4):326–32. https://doi.org/10.1007/BF03014958, PMID 11339772.

53. Eagle CC, Davis NJ. Report of the Anaesthetic Mortality Committee of Western Australia 1990–1995. Anaesth Intensive Care. 1997;25(1):51–9. https://doi.org/10.1177/0310057X9702500110, PMID 9075515.

54. Englar RE, Show-Ridgway A, Jones J, editors. Communicating with clients about anesthetic risk. NAVC live. Portland, OR; 2017 8-22-17.

55. Duarte Cardoso S, da Graca Pereira G, de Sousa L, Faraco CB, Piotti P, Pirrone F. Factors behind the relinquishment of dogs and cats by their guardians in Portugal. J Appl Anim Welf Sci. 2022:1–12.

56. Salman MD, New JG, Jr., Scarlett JM, Kass PH, Ruch-Gallie R, Hetts S. Human and animal factors related to relinquishment of dogs and cats in 12 selected animal shelters in the United States. J Appl Anim Welf Sci. 1998;1(3):207–26. https://doi.org/10.1207/s15327604jaws0103_2, PMID 16363966.

57. Cooper LL. Feline inappropriate elimination. Vet Clin North Am Small Anim Pract. 1997;27(3):569–600. https://doi.org/10.1016/s0195-5616(97)50055-6, PMID 9170636.

58. Herron ME. Advances in understanding and treatment of feline inappropriate elimination. Top Companion Anim Med. 2010;25(4):195–202. https://doi.org/10.1053/j.tcam.2010.09.005, PMID 21147472.

59. Marder AR, Engel JM. Long-term outcome after treatment of feline inappropriate elimination. J Appl Anim Welf Sci. 2002;5(4):299–308. https://doi.org/10.1207/S15327604JAWS0504_04, PMID 16221080.

60. Vollmer PJ. Feline inappropriate elimination: Part 5–conclusion. Vet Med Small Anim Clin. 1979;74(10):1419–21. PMID 260997.

61. Vollmer PJ. Feline inappropriate elimination. Part 4–Marking. Vet Med Small Anim Clin. 1979;74(9):796–798. PMID 260558.

62. Vollmer PJ. Feline inappropriate elimination. Part 3. Vet Med Small Anim Clin. 1979;74(8):1101–2. PMID 260537.

63. Vollmer PJ. Feline inappropriate elimination. Part 2. Vet Med Small Anim Clin. 1979;74(7):928–30. PMID 257980.

64. Vollmer PJ. Feline inappropriate elimination. Part 1. Vet Med Small Anim Clin. 1979;74(6):796–8. PMID 256687.

Part Three

Accepting and Affirming That Healthcare Is Challenging: What it Takes to Rebuild the Veterinary Team

CHAPTER 11

When Caring Hurts

Acknowledging Burnout, Addressing Compassion Fatigue, and Building Resilience

Healthcare professionals are globally in demand, yet these professions are inherently demanding and potentially detrimental to the health of those who pursue healthcare as a career trajectory. From the moment that they choose this path, they place significant demands upon themselves to prioritize the well-being of others. Physicians take oaths to do no harm,(1) and veterinarians commit to "lifelong" obligations to continually apply professional knowledge and competence to the protection of "health and welfare" and the "prevention and relief of animal suffering."(2)

11.1 Expectations that Healthcare Workers Have for Themselves

Some healthcare workers consider their work to be a calling.(3, 4) At times, this can be a source of inner strength and resilience.(4) A calling can provide a sense of purpose. It gives life intrinsic value and meaning.

Many believe that they have a "duty of care" to their patients.(5, 6) As such, healthcare workers often expect themselves to be:

- patient advocates
- active listeners
- life-saving leaders
- passionate planners
- dedicated doctors and nurses
- omniscient critical thinkers
- quick-on-their-feet problem-solvers
- benevolent, compassionate caregivers
- warm, transparent communicators
- technically savvy doers
- highly functional professionals.

Patient care often comes before sleep, nourishment, and time with family and friends.(4) Despite best efforts to leave it at the door, many healthcare professionals take work home that keeps them up at night.

The selflessness of healthcare workers advances the needs of others and rises to meet the growing expectations of the public; however, it often means that healthcare workers care for themselves last.

While the desire to care for others is laudable, it often leads to self-sacrifice in the areas of mental, physical, emotional, and psychological health. In the short-term, that sacrifice seems like a worthy cause, and it drives those in healthcare forward to achieve selfless acts of care. However, it is not always sustainable in the long run. The trade-off is the physical, emotional, and psychological well-being of those who have invested their lives and their careers in healthcare.(4)

11.2 Daily Challenges Faced by Healthcare Workers

Healthcare workers are continually challenged by:(7–71)

- long hours
- irregular shifts
- staff sickness
- staff shortages and absenteeism
- high turnover rates
- sleep-deprivation and chronic fatigue
- skill underutilization
- inefficient work processes
- clerical burden
- patient-care interruptions
- real and perceived restrictions on autonomy
- role conflict and associated ambiguities
- pay inequity
- lack of career advancement opportunities
- co-worker conflicts and workplace ostracism
- as-needed scheduling
- unexpected double-shifts
- holiday shifts
- overnight or weekend duty
- unpaid overtime
- unpredictable on-call duties
- physical and emotional labor
- risks of occupational injury

- o risk of physical injury is 2.9 times higher for veterinarians than for human medical doctors in general practice(72)
- o physical hazards in veterinary practice include lifting patients and heavy objects and working with large animals(73, 74)
- diagnostic errors
- treatment errors
- near misses
- litigation
- exposure to patient pain, distress, and suffering
- increased risk of exposure to disease
  - o needle-stick injuries and bloodborne pathogens
  - o respiration and airborne pathogens
- increased risk of exposure to hazardous drugs
- increased exposure to controlled drugs and associated risk of substance abuse
- cardiopulmonary resuscitation (CPR) failures
- witnessing patient death
- work-home interference
- moral distress(75–79)
  - o knowing what the correct decision/action/statement/choice is for a given situation, yet having one's hands tied such that it is impossible to act on it
  - o in a 2018 study by Moses et al., 70% of veterinary participants reported that they had felt moderate to severe distress because obstacles precluded them from providing appropriate care(75)
- moral injury(80–96)
  - o unlike moral distress, which refers to a situational problem, moral injury refers to how one experiences the problem
  - o if moral injury is sustained, it can cause the following changes:
    - ▪ it may impair one's capacity to withstand stress
    - ▪ it may elicit disillusionment with healthcare
    - ▪ it may induce feelings of guilt and/or shame
    - ▪ it may make one feel that they have been betrayed by the profession.

11.3 Veterinary-Specific Challenges

Veterinary team members face additional challenges:(68, 97–109)

- animal cruelty
  - o treatment of animals is influenced by societal and cultural norms(110)
  - o there is no universal definition of animal cruelty(110)

- o the North American and European perspectives consider animal cruelty to be "socially unacceptable behavior that intentionally causes unnecessary pain, suffering or distress to and/or death of a non-human animal"(111)
- o subsets of animal cruelty include neglect, intentional abuse, animal hoarding, and organized abuse(110)
- o in the United States, all subtypes are ultimately defined by the legal system; however, statutory language varies between states and even by jurisdiction(110)
- o a link has been established between violent acts against animals and subsequent violence against people(110, 112–116)
- financial limitations/cost of care
- owner relinquishment
- broken human–animal bonds and ethical dilemmas regarding treatment options:
  - o economic euthanasia
  - o convenience euthanasia
    - ▪ according to the Voice of the Veterinary Profession survey by the British Veterinary Association (BVA), 98% of veterinarians have been asked to perform euthanasia of a healthy pet(117)
    - ▪ examples of requests often cite:
      - □ poor behavior
      - □ poor socialization.

Although both the BVA and the American Veterinary Medical Association (AVMA) provide guidelines and policies with respect to euthanasia, including that for convenience purposes, "determining whether or not an animal can be rehabilitated or re-homed is completely subjective and up to the individual veterinarian."(117)

Veterinarians are often conflicted by which choice is the "right" one to make in such situations. Many veterinarians express frustration that pets are seen as disposable and that companion animal owners may see euthanasia as a way to absolve their responsibilities towards owned pets.

One veterinarian who participated in a 2017 study explained that: "Euthanasia shows a degree of cowardice because the owner asks someone else to take responsibility for the healthy animal. It is the only method that he has found."(99)

Another participant shared that:

I remember one case; it was a couple with a young child. They decided to adopt a great Dane puppy. Before adopting the dog, they should have gotten information about great Danes. It is a big dog and he will grow faster than the child. They came for convenience euthanasia when the dog was 6 months old, because he was playing too roughly with the child ... A great Dane is not just great, he is going to eat a lot and he will need to play a lot also. It is not a delicate breed; he will wag his tail and whip everything around. We did find a new home for this puppy, because I refused to euthanize him. But once again, who was stuck with the problem? We were! This is what pisses me off and in the long-term it is burdensome. People do not take their responsibilities. They unload their responsibilities onto someone else.(99)

Many veterinarians express frustration that refusal to perform convenience euthanasia may not in fact change the outcome for the patient. One participant shared that:

I am thinking about what would happen if we refused to euthanize the animal. What will the owner do? The owner will go to the SPCA and the animal will stay there. He will not be adopted by another family and we as veterinarians think that we saved the animal's life.(99)

Others feel conflicted about whether convenience euthanasia negates the veterinary oath to protect and respect the animals' best interests.(99) Rathwell-Deault et al. explain the source of the conflict as follows: "The origin of the psychological stress surrounding the convenience euthanasia dilemma seems to arise from the conflict between the prioritization of the animal's interests and the willingness to satisfy the owner."(99)

Rathwell-Deault et al. acknowledge that: "Stress surrounding the decision [to euthanize may] also [be] amplified by the pressure of profitability coming from the owner of the veterinary facility."(99)

11.4 The Impact of Global Pandemic on Healthcare Workers

Prior to the COVID-19 pandemic, healthcare was experiencing an epidemic of its own: one-third to one-half of healthcare workers were reporting signs of:(118)

- emotional depletion
- physical exhaustion
- depersonalization
  - loss of connection to patients
  - loss of connection to themselves
  - loss of connection to relationships outside of the clinic

- loss of job satisfaction
- loss of passion for their respective professions.

The onset of the COVID-19 pandemic intensified the aforementioned challenges (see Sections 11.2 and 11.3). Ongoing shortages in staffing and fatigue, loss and grief have created new burdens for healthcare delivery.

Healthcare workers were expected to staff the frontlines and go head-to-head with an unknown illness, in an increasingly precarious landscape of uncertainty, often without support, often in isolation, and at great risk to their own lives and those they love.(119)

In return for their service, they have been on the receiving end of praise by some for their reportedly heroic actions:

> *In a disorienting experience like a pandemic, it's reassuring to talk of heroes. We can picture the mythic hero charging the battlefield despite the danger, getting the job done no matter the obstacles, and paying no heed to possible or actual injury. The hero image burns so bright that it eclipses any light shining on the failures of the system that could turn heroes into involuntary martyrs.(119)*

Yet, as Lewis et al. shared: "a paramedic friend privately shared with us that he'd gladly trade the hero label for the proper personal health equipment."(119)

Many healthcare workers compare themselves to others. When they aren't logging the hours that others do, they feel guilty: "A neurologist colleague shared that when she hears those nightly celebrations lauding essential workers as heroes, the pots and pans clanging outside her home bring her a daily dose of shame because her practice has temporarily closed and she isn't in the fight."(119)

Many healthcare workers express the internal conflict that they feel when their duty is labelled heroism, at a time when they feel anything but heroic:

> *We think of the physician who said that if she really was a hero, her patients wouldn't have died. Or the many colleagues who, for various reasons — geography, pregnancy, their own Covid-like symptoms — have not been able to provide frontline care despite their desire to help. Or the medical students itching to learn and contribute but who have been told to stay home.(119)*

The battlefield of the healthcare worker is a complexity that anyone who hasn't lived it cannot fathom:

The complex truths of their experiences — ones we might avoid considering and that the hero label lets us paint over — trail them home at the end of each shift like an unwelcome smell on their skin. If and when they are ready to tell their stories, the more space the hero label takes up, the harder it will be for them to authentically express themselves. It's as though we're saying, "Tell your story through the hero lens of our cultural imagination, or don't tell it at all.(119)

It's a lens that makes healthcare workers feel wrong for wanting more out of their professions.

It's a lens that makes healthcare workers feel wrong for wanting more out of life.

It's a lens that makes healthcare workers feel wrong for complaining about what has been construed as their duty.

It's a lens that makes healthcare workers feel wrong for wanting out. Yet, there is a growing schism between the direction that healthcare is moving and the capacity among healthcare workers to cope.

According to a 2020 survey:(120)

- 93% of health workers reported feelings of being stressed out and stretched thin
- 82% shared that they are exhausted
- 45% of nurses reported insufficient emotional support.

Other studies during the pandemic disclosed that:

- 22% of healthcare workers experienced moderate depression, anxiety, and post-traumatic stress disorder in a collective analysis of 65 studies(121)
- 69% of physicians experienced depression and 13% contemplated suicide.(122)

Frontline workers, including nurses, are more likely to experience and report severe psychological symptoms.(123) So are younger workers and those who identify as being female.(122, 123)

These challenges compound the growing shortage of available healthcare workers. One survey reported that nearly one in three nurses may leave their positions within a year.(124) Insufficient staffing, intensity of workload, and the emotional toll of their jobs have been cited as significant factors in job dissatisfaction.

The high expectations that healthcare workers place on themselves, combined with workplace expectations and family expectations, and perceived lack of social support at both work and at home have collectively created the perfect storm.

There is an ongoing crisis in healthcare, and it involves those we need to protect most of all: our workers.

11.5 Defining Burnout

Healthcare providers, including veterinarians, are burdened repetitively by a cycle of physical, mental, and emotional exhaustion. That cycle is often preceded by job dissatisfaction and paves the way for depersonalization and a sense of reduced personal accomplishment.

Those experiencing emotional exhaustion feel "used up" with nothing to offer.

Over time, this attitude breeds cynicism and diminished capacity to functionally perform. Collectively, these attributes are what we refer to as the syndrome, *burnout*.

According to Shanafelt:

Burnout happens when we are not able to recharge and recover between call nights or days in clinic; it is characterized by physical and emotional exhaustion, the development of a cynical and negative attitude toward patients, and a negative approach to work, which comes to feel meaningless. These feelings contrast with the positive approach to being a physician that characterized (and likely still does characterize) the early years of training in our profession, when we were enthusiastic, positive, fulfilled, and satisfied. We felt that our work truly made a difference and that our career, although busy and often stressful, was meaningful.(125)

The prevalence of burnout is rising within healthcare professions. Shanafelt discloses that:

A national study in 2011 found that at least 45% of a pool of 7288 physicians had symptoms of burnout, with many believing this percentage could easily exceed 50% if redone today. This increase in burnout stems from system, institutional, and individual recent trends in health care, including physician shortages and technology integration into hospitals (via electronic health records, patient portals, electronic prescriptions). Originally intended to help physicians with their day-to-day responsibilities, technology has inadvertently created an extra level of scrutiny, giving hospital leaders more metrics to critique medical professionals through patient satisfaction scores and closely monitored cost records. Physicians overall feel they have less control over medical decisions and are increasingly unhappy overall working in their professions.(125)

11.6 The Multifaceted Impact of Burnout

Burnout is significant because it adversely impacts physician health.(126) Physicians who experience burnout are more likely to experience:(126–137)

- depression
- motor vehicle accidents
- alcohol dependence/abuse
- suicidal ideation
- suicide attempts
- suicide completion
- decreased productivity
- job dissatisfaction
- intent to step down from their current position
- intent to resign from one's current place of employment
- intent to retire from practicing medicine.

Burnout also adversely impacts patient care.(126) Doctors who experience burnout are more likely to commit medical errors and/or experience an increased rate of near miss events.(126, 138–141) Patients of physicians who experience burnout report less satisfaction with care and perceive their care to be of lesser quality.(126, 142–149)

Those who are most prone to burnout were described by psychologist Harold Freudenberger, in 1974, as being the ones who:

Work in free clinics, therapeutic communities, hot lines, crisis intervention centers, women's clinics, gay centers, runaway houses, are people who are seeking to respond to the recognized needs of people. We would rather put up than shut up. And what we put up is our talents, our skills, we put in long hours with a bare minimum of financial compensation.(4)

Freudenberger explains that:

It is precisely because we are dedicated that we walk into a burn-out trap. We work too much, too long and too intensely. We feel a pressure from within to work and help and we feel a pressure from the outside to give. When the staff member then feels an additional pressure from the administrator to give even more, he is under a three-pronged attack.(4)

Healthcare workers are often told that they can avoid burnout by setting boundaries. Yet, it is not that simple. After all, healthcare is not just a "job" like any other. Healthcare workers are trained to prioritize others before themselves. They are trained to believe in duty and honor. They are trained to believe that this calling defines them.

This training initially strengthens their reserve. However, over time, such reserve is not sustainable. The system has been designed to exploit those who care most.(4) At the end of the day, healthcare workers sacrifice themselves, their health and well-being, and their relationships in the name of "work."(4) They may turn the other cheek when they experience dysfunction within their teams and when they encounter toxic learning environments because they elevate patient care above their own needs, even when in the process of doing so they suffer.(4)

11.7 Burnout Versus Compassion Fatigue

Burnout is increasingly prevalent among healthcare workers and is a function of work-related occupational stress. Stress may be associated with:

- job duties
- co-workers/colleagues
- supervisors/employers/practice managers/hospital directors
- poor work culture/toxic work environment.

Burnout takes time to develop. It is not associated with a single incident, but rather, multiple incidents sandwiched together over time in such a way that they wear someone down. It becomes "too much," "too often," and one begins to feel that it will never end.

There is a persistent feeling that the status quo is not amenable to change, and the instances of occupational stress will continue to bombard, and build, until nothing at all retains meaning. There is a gradual accrual of incidents that pave the way for apathy. At a certain point, nothing matters because it seems meaningless.

Those who are experiencing burnout tend to exhibit the following signs:

- fatigue
- anger
- frustration
- negativity
- cynicism
- social withdrawal.

Those who demonstrate the following tendencies are more apt to develop burnout:

- working extended hours
- inability to delegate
- declining breaks
- struggling to say no
- bottling up feelings
- demonstrating avoidance behaviors
- being a perfectionist
- taking work home
- allowing work to define them
- allowing work to spill over into home life
- prioritizing work over relationships
- allowing work to stamp out hobbies; there is no time to pursue anything outside of the office.

Initially, the employee may feel energized and a sense of added value. They are achieving the unachievable.

Over time, that achievement blurs into resentment and social withdrawal. There is a gradual consensus of "what's the point?" That attitude creeps into work like a stain and settles in for the long-haul.

It is hard to burn bright when one is effectively burnt out.

Burnout is not the only adverse mechanism to coping that healthcare workers may experience. Healthcare workers may also experience compassion fatigue.

Compassion fatigue has been defined as: "The emotional burden that health care providers may experience as a result of overexposure to traumatic events that patients are experiencing."(150)

Compassion fatigue is, in essence, the body's preoccupation with taking on the emotional stress that others are experiencing. Others' trauma in a sense becomes our own. Now we are traumatized by secondary exposure. For this reason, compassion fatigue was historically referred to as "secondary victimization."(151)

Signs of compassion fatigue may overlap with those of burnout. Those experiencing compassion fatigue may also become socially withdrawn. However, sadness and grief tend to predominate over anger and frustration. Rather than being overwhelmed by negativity and cynicism, those with compassion fatigue often express that they have a reduced capacity to feel, if they even feel at all.

Many with compassion fatigue become numb towards others, including patients and families. They often detach from those around them and may even go out of their way to avoid others. This includes those they love. Therefore, relationships outside of the office often suffer from decreased intimacy that stems from diminished connections between themselves and others.

Somatic symptoms are common with compassion fatigue. Physical signs include headaches, overwhelming fatigue, and frequent illness. Affected individuals may also exhibit changes in behavior, including, but not limited to:

- sleep disturbances
- appetite fluctuations
- fluctuations in weight
- increased irritability
- startling easily/hypervigilance.

It may be difficult for those with compassion fatigue to focus. They may arrive to work late or call out of work at the last minute. When they are on-site, they often lack concentration. Part of this may be owing to recurrent or unwanted thoughts. Their minds wander. This becomes a vicious cycle. Their lack of concentration, combined with their lack of attention to detail, produces poorer quality work. Because they remain unmotivated to change, their patterns of forgetfulness and inattention persist.

It may feel that they are digging themselves into a progressively deeper hole, one that lacks purpose and meaning. They may feel powerless, anxious, helpless, or distressed.

Alternatively, they may feel nothing at all.

11.8 Veterinary Well-being

Veterinarians and the healthcare teams within which they operate are not immune to compassion fatigue. If anything, they may be at greater risk because of continual exposure to traumatic events that they witness through the eyes of their patients.(151)

The Merck Animal Health Veterinary Wellbeing Study emerged on account of growing concerns about veterinarians with respect to published research about job dissatisfaction, work-related stress, psychological distress, burnout, compassion fatigue, and suicide.(152–154)

To assess the prevalence of mental health concerns and self-reported well-being among veterinarians, author John O. Volk and his research team reached out to a random sample of 20,000 veterinarians practicing within the United States to measure the prevalence of serious mental distress and determine the level of well-being within the profession. Almost 3,600 veterinarians responded to the survey invitation, with a net of 3,540 usable survey responses, representing a response rate of 17.7%.

According to Volk et al:

When respondents were presented with a list of 11 issues and asked to indicate how important each one was to the veterinary profession, the issues that were most frequently considered critically important were high student debt levels (67% indicated the issue was critically important), stress levels of veterinarians (53%), and suicide rate among veterinarians (52%).(152)

Volk et al disclosed that:

Two-thirds of respondents, including 79% of associate veterinarians in practice, reported experiencing feelings of depression, compassion fatigue or burnout, or anxiety or panic attacks within the past year. Overall, 5.3% of veterinarians experienced serious psychological distress within the past 30 days, which was similar to the percentage reported for the general population (4.7%), but significantly lower than the percentage for veterinarians reported by Nett et al (9.3%). Serious psychological distress occurred more frequently in younger (< 45 years of age) veterinarians and less frequently in older veterinarians. Only half of those with serious psychological distress indicated that they were receiving treatment.(152)

Veterinarians were more likely to experience serious psychological distress if they:(152)

- worked extended hours
- performed relief work
- were in debt from student loans.

With respect to availability and accessibility to mental health resources, Volk reported that: "Employee assistance programs (EAP) under which employees could receive treatment for mental illness were rare. Only 14% of respondents with serious psychological distress said their employer had an EAP."(152)

Outside of EAP, many veterinary organizations offer resources that are web-based for veterinarians who may be experiencing psychological distress. However, according to Volk et al.:

Of those respondents with serious psychological distress, only 16% had accessed any of those resources (10% of all respondents had accessed those resources).

The resources most frequently accessed were those of the AVMA (64%), followed by resources from the Veterinary Information Network (31%), state veterinary medical associations (29%), DVM360 (28%), the American Animal Hospital Association (13%), and other organizations (16%). Of those resources listed in the questionnaire, the [Veterinary Information Network, VIN] resources received the highest ratings, with 52% of users rating them as very or extremely useful.(152)

Accessibility with respect to mental health resources continues to be questionable. Volk et al. disclosed that:

One impediment to receiving treatment was that some respondents who needed treatment did not have confidence that they could find it. Only 46% of those with serious psychological distress agreed with the statement that 'mental health treatment is accessible' ... There was hesitancy seeking treatment because of concerns about being stigmatized. Sixty percent of those with serious psychological distress disagreed with the statement that 'people are caring towards those with mental illness' ... Veterinarians with serious psychological distress were much less likely to participate in the types of healthy activities mental health professionals typically recommend to prevent or mitigate psychological distress, compared with those without distress.(152)

With respect to suicidal ideation, Volk et al. reported that:

Overall, 25% of respondents had thought about suicide at some time in their lives, but only 1.6% of respondents reported having ever attempted suicide. That was similar to the percentage of veterinarians attempting suicide reported by Nett et al (1.4%), but substantially lower than the percentage reported for the general population (5.1%).(152)

11.9 Considering the Future of Veterinary Medicine Through an Alternate Lens

In 2017, Guest Editors Susan M. Rhind and Andrew Grant penned an editorial in the *Journal of Veterinary Medical Education* (*JVME*), titled: "From Studying the Rain to Studying the Umbrella: Mental Health and Well-Being of Veterinary Medical Students and Graduates." They express concern that the mental health and well-being of the veterinary profession is at stake. They suggest that:

Veterinary medical educators are positioned at the heart of this problem, taking students into intensive programs and sending them out as graduates into a profession featured regularly in the literature as having a problem with mental health and well-being and, at the extreme, with higher rates of suicidal ideation than other professions.(155)

Rhind and Grant acknowledge that significant strides have been made with respect to the following.(155–161)

- Identifying sources of stress and anxiety among veterinary students.
- Raising awareness about mental health among faculty and student bodies.
- Reducing the stigma associated with mental health.
- Uniting students, administrators, veterinarians, industry partners, social workers, and counselors to engage in constructive, collaborative dialogue about mental health and wellness issues.
- Identifying barriers to student access to mental health resources.
- Establishing support structures for students who experience mental health concerns.

However, Rhind and Grant suggest that we, as a profession, transition from a focus on "reporting the problem and reducing the stressors (the rain)" and instead focus on "how we can build resilience and nurture well-being (the umbrella)."(155) Their logic is that if we can design improved umbrellas, then we can better help students to protect themselves from the rain.

Those whom the profession tends to attract are often high-achievers who are performance driven perfectionists.(155) This ambition is a significant driving force that propels students to pursue long-held ambitions; however, ambition may come at a cost. It may predispose to anxiety and depression when goals are not reached and/or when the pursuer perceives that their expectations of self fell short.(155)

We may be able to better "care for our carers"(151) if we concentrate on those factors that are linked to healthcare professionals' ability to "bounce back."(162)

11.10 Building Resilience

The degree to which someone is able to effectively "bounce back" from stressors, including defeat and failure, is said to be that individual's resilience.(162) According to McArthur:(162) "Resilience is a dynamic and multifaceted process in which individuals draw on personal and contextual resources, and use specific strategies to navigate challenges and to work toward adaptive outcomes."

When we say that resilience is dynamic, what we mean is that it changes over time.(162) In that sense, it is temporal.(162) One who is resilient experiences that "bounce back" in stages that take time for the individual to navigate and ultimately process.(162)

Resilience is not all-or-none, nor is it "one size fits all."(162)

Resilience is not something one is either born with or without.(162)

Resilience can be acquired and learned.(162) Moreover, resilience can be cultivated, meaning that it can develop and strengthen over time. (162) Experience teaches one how to "bounce back" every time one has a setback.

It is not necessarily that the setbacks become easier to bear with time; it is that the learner begins to recognize that there is a way through what once might have felt like a dead end.

Some obstacles are harder than others to navigate, and each person's approach is unique. What for some might be an easy hill to climb might be Mount Everest to others. In this respect, resilience is contextual: some situations inspire more resilience from some than others. We cannot expect that everyone's path will be the same.

We also need to recognize that in those moments of hardship, it is not that others lack resilience. They may simply benefit from additional tools in that moment to see how to relate to and ultimately overcome the barrier.

As educators, we must commit ourselves to providing those tools and moreover, create a safe, supportive space that increases accessibility to a spectrum of learners who may have different needs in different instances.

As educators, we are used to cross-comparisons between students on the basis of assignments, projects, or exam scores.

When we evaluate resilience, we need to toss cross-comparisons to the side and draw upon our skills of unconditional positive regard (Refer to Section 10.6). In this way, we accept students as they are, and we meet them where they are at.

We can enhance resilience in our students by training mindfulness and self-compassion.(162) Both have their origins in Buddhist philosophy. (162, 163)

McArthur defines mindfulness as a "conscious and passive, real-time awareness and non-judgmental acceptance of an experience, including all its emotional, cognitive, and sensory components."(162) Mindfulness trains us to focus on the present, tuning into and accepting one's feelings, thoughts, and bodily sensations.

By focusing on the here and the now, we train ourselves to tune out distractions. What is going on around us becomes less essential than what is going on inside of us. Mindfulness is a way of moving our body from reaction to response. We dial back our inherent tendency to be overly reactive to the outside world, and we instead tune into our internal state of being. When we learn how to engage ourselves fully in the present, we can reduce tension and anxiety within ourselves. We also reduce our risk of developing depression and burnout.(162)

Self-compassion is an extension of unconditional positive regard, directed inwards.(162) Neff explains that: "Compassion can be extended towards the self when suffering occurs through no fault of one's own – when the external circumstances of life are simply hard to bear."(164)

Neff adds that: "Self-compassion is equally relevant … when suffering stems from our own mistakes, failures, or personal inadequacies."(164)

For self-compassion to be effective, we must make a conscious decision to choose self-kindness over self-judgment.(164) Just as we might accept a client's flaws when they present their pet to us, we attempt to accept the same of ourselves.(164) We accept that we are flawed. We accept that we are inadequate. We embrace ourselves when we need comfort, and we change the tone of language from harsh and critical to soft and compassionate.(164)

When we are kind to ourselves – when we change the language with which we speak of ourselves – we reframe our understanding of self-identity. We become more accepting of ourselves in a way that mirrors our acceptance of others.

We influence our own self-growth in a way that builds self-esteem and self-worth.(164) We also reduce anxiety and cortisol levels, depression, and heartrate variability.(162, 165–168)

Resilience does not appear overnight. It is a journey that we choose to take, step by step, day by day. Resilience does not mean that life is easy or that we are not presented with challenges. What it means is that we acknowledge and affirm those obstacles in our way and we commit to rising above as best we can. That doesn't mean we don't stumble. That doesn't mean we never fall.

We must normalize that falling isn't the problem.

We need to train ourselves, as much as we need to train our students, that life isn't about never failing.

It's about learning to live through failure and how to get back up.

As I once learned from my dance instructor, the one and only Lowell Fox: *"Today's failures are the brick and mortar of tomorrow's successes; they are the foundation of dreams that never would have come to fruition if they hadn't at first given us a fight."*

References

1. Ogunbanjo GA, van Bogaert KD. The Hippocratic oath: revisited. S Afr Fam Pract. 2009;51(1):30–1. https://doi.org/10.1080/20786204.2009.10873802.

2. Veterinarian's oath. American Veterinary Medical Association. Available from: https://www.avma.org/resources-tools/avma-policies/veterinarians-oath.

3. Cornett BS. A principal calling: professionalism and health care services. J Commun Disord. 2006;39(4):301–9. https://doi.org/10.1016/j.jcomdis.2006.02.005, PMID 16569412.

4. Stewart MT, Serwint JR. Burning without burning out: a call to protect the calling of medicine. Curr Probl Pediatr Adolesc Health Care. 2019;49(11):1–5. https://doi.org/10.1016/j.cppeds.2019.100655.

5. Cox CL. "Healthcare heroes": problems with media focus on heroism from healthcare workers during the COVID-19 pandemic. J Med Ethics. 2020;46(8):510–3. https://doi.org/10.1136/medethics-2020-106398, PMID 32546658.

6. Malm H, May T, Francis LP, Omer SB, Salmon DA, Hood R. Ethics, pandemics, and the duty to treat. Am J Bioeth. 2008;8(8):4–19. https://doi.org/10.1080/15265160802317974, PMID 18802849.

7. Clegg A. Occupational stress in nursing: a review of the literature. J Nurs Manag. 2001;9(2):101–6. https://doi.org/10.1046/j.1365-2834.2001.00216.x, PMID 11879452.

8. Sullivan P. Sullivan P. Stress and burnout in psychiatric nursing. Nurs Stand. 1993;8(2):36–9. https://doi.org/10.7748/ns.8.2.36.s46, PMID 8217684.

9. Munro L, Rodwell J, Harding L. Assessing occupational stress in psychiatric nurses using the full job strain model: the value of social support to nurses. Int J Nurs Stud. 1998;35(6):339–45. https://doi.org/10.1016/s0020-7489(98)00049-2, PMID 9871824.

10. Dolan SL, Van Ameringen MR, Corbin S, Arsenault A. Lack of professional latitude and role problems as correlates of propensity to quit amongst nursing staff. J Adv Nurs. 1992;17(12):1455–9. https://doi.org/10.1111/j.1365-2648.1992.tb02817.x, PMID 1474244.

11. Gou L, Ma S, Wang G, Wen X, Zhang Y. Relationship between workplace ostracism and turnover intention among nurses: the sequential mediating effects of emotional labor and nurse-patient relationship. Psychol Health Med. 2022;27(7):1596–601. https://doi.org/10.1080/13548506.2021.1905859, PMID 33784891.

12. Kim YT, Kim O, Cha C, Pang Y, Sung C. Nurse turnover: a longitudinal survival analysis of the Korea Nurses' Health Study. J Adv Nurs. 2021;77(10):4089–103. https://doi.org/10.1111/jan.14919, PMID 34118173.

13. Lavoie-Tremblay M, Gélinas C, Aubé T, Tchouaket E, Tremblay D, Gagnon MP, et al. Influence of caring for COVID-19 patients on nurse's turnover, work satisfaction and quality of care. J Nurs Manag. 2022;30(1):33–43. https://doi.org/10.1111/jonm.13462, PMID 34448520.

14. Li CC, Yamamoto-Mitani N. Ward-level nurse turnover and related workplace factors in long-term care hospitals: a cross-sectional survey. J Nurs Manag. 2021;29(6):1587–95. https://doi.org/10.1111/jonm.13293, PMID 33638892.

15. Suliman M, Aljezawi M, Almansi S, Musa A, Alazam M, Ta'an WF. Identifying the nurse characteristics that affect anticipated turnover. Nurs Manag (Harrow). 2020. https://doi.org/10.7748/nm.2020.e1956, PMID 33300318.

16. Warden DH, Hughes RG, Probst JC, Warden DN, Adams SA. Current turnover intention among nurse managers, directors, and executives. Nurs Outlook. 2021;69(5):875–85. https://doi.org/10.1016/j.outlook.2021.04.006, PMID 34148657.

17. Yun MR, Yu B. Strategies for reducing hospital nurse turnover in South Korea: nurses' perceptions and suggestions. J Nurs Manag. 2021;29(5):1256–62. https://doi.org/10.1111/jonm.13264, PMID 33486834.

18. Forde-Johnston C, Stoermer F. Giving nurses a voice through "listening to staff" conversations to inform nurse retention and reduce turnover. Br J Nurs. 2022;31(12): 632–8. https://doi.org/10.12968/bjon.2022.31.12.632, PMID 35736855.

19. Hughes A, Keys Y, Peck J, Garcia T. Reducing nurse practitioner turnover in home based primary care: a department of Veterans Affairs Quality Improvement Project. Home Healthc Now. 2021;39(6):327–35. https://doi.org/10.1097/NHH.0000000000001014, PMID 34738968.

20. Leontiou I, Papastavrou E, Middleton N, Merkouris A. Empowerment and turnover of nurse managers before and after a major health care reform in Cyprus: a cross sectional study. J Nurs Manag. 2022;30(5):1196–205. https://doi.org/10.1111/jonm.13606, PMID 35343017.

21. Muir KJ, Wanchek TN, Lobo JM, Keim-Malpass J. Evaluating the costs of nurse burnout-attributed turnover: a Markov modeling approach. J Patient Saf. 2022;18(4):351–7. https://doi.org/10.1097/PTS.0000000000000920, PMID 35617593.

22. Rutledge DN, Douville S, Winokur EJ. Chronic fatigue predicts hospital nurse turnover intentions. J Nurs Adm. 2022;52(4):241–7. https://doi.org/10.1097/NNA.0000000000001139, PMID 35348490.

23. Sawada S, Takemura Y, Isobe T, Koyanagi H, Kida R. Perceived impact of nurse turnover on the organization: a Delphi study on managers of nursing. J Nurs Manag. 2022;30(7):3168–77. https://doi.org/10.1111/jonm.13738, PMID 35815682.

24. Shapiro D, Duquette CE, Zangerle C, Pearl A, Campbell T. The seniority swoop: young nurse burnout, violence, and turnover intention in an 11-hospital sample. Nurs Admin Q. 2022;46(1):60–71. https://doi.org/10.1097/NAQ.0000000000000502, PMID 34860802.

25. Stemmer R, Bassi E, Ezra S, Harvey C, Jojo N, Meyer G, et al. A systematic review: unfinished nursing care and the impact on the nurse outcomes of job satisfaction, burnout, intention-to-leave and turnover. J Adv Nurs. 2022;78(8):2290–303. https://doi.org/10.1111/jan.15286, PMID 35533090.

26. Adriaenssens J, De Gucht V, Maes S. Causes and consequences of occupational stress in emergency nurses, a longitudinal study. J Nurs Manag. 2015;23(3):346–58. https://doi.org/10.1111/jonm.12138, PMID 24330154.

27. Araújo AF, Bampi LNDS, Cabral CCO, Queiroz RS, Calasans LHB, Vaz TS. Occupational stress of nurses from the mobile emergency care service. Rev Bras Enferm. 2020;73;Suppl 1:e20180898. https://doi.org/10.1590/0034-7167-2018-0898, PMID 32490952.

28. Basu S, Harris A, Mason S, Norman J. A longitudinal assessment of occupational stress in emergency department nursing staff. J Nurs Manag. 2020;28(1):167–74. https://doi.org/10.1111/jonm.12910, PMID 31756010.

29. Basu S, Yap C, Mason S. Examining the sources of occupational stress in an emergency department. Occup Med (Lond). 2016;66(9):737–42. https://doi.org/10.1093/occmed/kqw155, PMID 27852879.

30. Bauer H, Herbig B. Occupational stress in helicopter emergency service pilots from 4 European countries. Air Med J. 2019;38(2):82–94. https://doi.org/10.1016/j.amj.2018.11.011, PMID 30898289.

31. Carmassi C, Dell'Oste V, Bertelloni CA, Pedrinelli V, Barberi FM, Malacarne P, et al. Gender and occupational role differences in work-related post-traumatic stress symptoms, burnout and global functioning in emergency healthcare workers. Intensive Crit Care Nurs. 2022;69:103154. https://doi.org/10.1016/j.iccn.2021.103154, PMID 34895972.

32. de Wijn AN, Fokkema M, van der Doef MP. The prevalence of stress-related outcomes and occupational well-being among emergency nurses in the Netherlands and the role of job factors: a regression tree analysis. J Nurs Manag. 2022;30(1):187–97. https://doi.org/10.1111/jonm.13457, PMID 34448288.

33. Gholamzadeh S, Sharif F, Rad FD. Sources of occupational stress and coping strategies among nurses who work in admission and emergency departments of hospitals related to Shiraz University of Medical Sciences. Iran J Nurs Midwif Res. 2011;16(1):41–6. PMID 22039378.

34. Ilczak T, Rak M, Sumera K, Christiansen CR, Navarro-Illana E, Alanen P, et al. Differences in perceived occupational stress by demographic characteristics, of European emergency medical services personnel during the COVID-19 virus pandemic-an international study. Healthcare (Basel). 2021;9(11):1–10. https://doi.org/10.3390/healthcare9111582, PMID 34828627.

35. Lu DM, Sun N, Hong S, Fan YY, Kong FY, Li QJ. Occupational stress and coping strategies among emergency department nurses of China. Arch Psychiatr Nurs. 2015;29(4):208–12. https://doi.org/10.1016/j.apnu.2014.11.006, PMID 26165974.

36. Rajabi F, Jahangiri M, Molaeifar H, Honarbakhsh M, Farhadi P. Occupational stress among nurses and pre-hospital emergency staff: application of fuzzy analytic hierarchy process (FAHP) method. Excli J. 2018;17:808–24. https://doi.org/10.17179/excli2018-1505, PMID 30233280.

37. Santana RDS, Fontes FLL, Morais MJA, Costa GDS, da Silva RK, de Araujo CS, et al. Occupational stress among emergency and urgent care nurses at a public hospital in Teresina, Piaui, Brazil. Rev Bras Med Trab. 2019;17(1):76–82.

38. Wu H, Sun W, Wang L. Factors associated with occupational stress among Chinese female emergency nurses. Emerg Med J. 2012;29(7):554–8. https://doi.org/10.1136/emj.2010.094391, PMID 21680572.

39. Xu HG, Kynoch K, Tuckett A, Eley R, Newcombe P. Effectiveness of interventions to reduce occupational stress among emergency department staff: a systematic review protocol. JBI Database System Rev Implement Rep Rev implement rep. 2019;17(4):513–9. https://doi.org/10.11124/JBISRIR-2017-003955, PMID 30973525.

40. Yuwanich N, Sandmark H, Akhavan S. Emergency department nurses' experiences of occupational stress: A qualitative study from a public hospital in Bangkok, Thailand. Work. 2015;53(4):885–97. https://doi.org/10.3233/WOR-152181, PMID 26519019.

41. Abdulghani HM, Al-Harbi MM, Irshad M. Stress and its association with working efficiency of junior doctors during three postgraduate residency training programs. Neuropsychiatr Dis Treat. 2015;11:3023–9. https://doi.org/10.2147/NDT.S92408, PMID 26677329.

42. Aggarwal S, Kusano AS, Carter JN, Gable L, Thomas CR, Jr., Chang DT. Stress and burnout among residency program directors in United States radiation

oncology programs. Int J Radiat Oncol Biol Phys. 2015;93(4):746–53. https://doi. org/10.1016/j.ijrobp.2015.08.019, PMID 26530741.

43. Chesak SS, Morin KH, Cutshall S, Carlson M, Joswiak ME, Ridgeway JL, et al. Stress management and resiliency training in a nurse residency program: findings from participant focus groups. J Nurs Prof Dev. 2019;35(6):337–43. https://doi. org/10.1097/NND.0000000000000589, PMID 31651555.

44. Gülenç B, Yalçin S, Sürücü S, Mahiroğullari M, Erdil M, Bülbül M. Orthopedics and traumatology residency – working conditions, training, and psychological stress. Acta Chir Orthop Traumatol Cech. 2019;86(4):281–5. PMID 31524590.

45. Ha GQ, Go JT, Murayama KM, Steinemann S. Identifying sources of stress across years of general surgery residency. Hawaii J Health Soc Welf. 2020;79(3):75–81. PMID 32190839.

46. Lapointe R, Bhesania S, Tanner T, Peruri A, Mehta P. An innovative approach to improve communication and reduce physician stress and burnout in a university affiliated residency program. J Med Syst. 2018;42(7):117. https://doi.org/10.1007/s10916-018-0956-z, PMID 29808384.

47. McManus B, Galbraith JW, Heaton K, Mrug S, Ponce BA, Porterfield JR, Jr., et al. Sleep and stress before and after duty across residency years under 2017 ACGME hours. Am J Surg. 2020;220(1):83–9. https://doi.org/10.1016/j.amj-surg.2019.10.049, PMID 31757438.

48. Raimo J, LaVine S, Spielmann K, Akerman M, Friedman KA, Katona K, et al. The correlation of stress in residency with future stress and burnout: a 10-year prospective cohort study. J Grad Med Educ. 2018;10(5):524–31. https://doi.org/10.4300/JGME-D-18-00273.1, PMID 30386477.

49. Riall TS. Evaluating the feasibility of stress-resilience training in surgical residency: a step toward improving surgeon well-being. JAMA Surg. 2018;153(10):e182735. https://doi.org/10.1001/jamasurg.2018.2735, PMID 30167640.

50. Scudder DR, Sherry AD, Jarrett RT, Fernando S, Kuhn AW, Fleming AE. Fundamental curriculum change with 1-year pre-clerkship phase and effect on stress associated with residency specialty selection. Med Sci Educ. 2019;29(4): 1033–42. https://doi.org/10.1007/s40670-019-00800-7, PMID 34457581.

51. Sum MY, Chew QH, Sim K. Perceptions of the learning environment on the relationship between stress and burnout for residents in an ACGME-I accredited national psychiatry residency program. J Grad Med Educ. 2019;11(4);Suppl:85–90. https://doi.org/10.4300/JGME-D-18-00795, PMID 31428263.

52. Ahmed F, Baruch J, Armstrong P. Examining the constructs of burnout, compassion fatigue, secondary traumatic stress in physicians using factor analyses. Front Public Health. 2022;10:893165. https://doi.org/10.3389/fpubh.2022.893165, PMID 35602123.

53. Bock C, Zimmermann T, Kahl KG. The impact of post-traumatic stress on the mental state of university hospital physicians – a cross sectional study. BMC Psychiatry. 2022;22(1):1–9. https://doi.org/10.1186/s12888-022-03719-3, PMID 35114970.

54. Bulca Acar A, Nur Eke R, Özen M. An assessment of anxiety about the viral epidemic and work-related stress in family physicians in turkey: how does COVID-19 vaccination period affect anxiety and stress? Psychiatr Danub. 2022;34(1):139–47. https://doi.org/10.24869/psyd.2022.139, PMID 35467631.

55. Chang J, Ray JM, Joseph D, Evans LV, Joseph M. Burnout and post-traumatic stress disorder symptoms among emergency medicine resident physicians during

the COVID-19 pandemic. West J Emerg Med. 2022;23(2):251–7. https://doi.org/10.5811/westjem.2021.11.53186, PMID 35302461.

56. Groombridge CJ, Maini A, Ayton D, Soh SE, Walsham N, Kim Y, et al. Emergency physicians' experience of stress during resuscitation and strategies for mitigating the effects of stress on performance. Emerg Med J. 2022;39(11):839–46. https://doi.org/10.1136/emermed-2021-211280, PMID 34907004.

57. Jiang N, Zhang H, Tan Z, Gong Y, Tian M, Wu Y, et al. The relationship between occupational stress and turnover intention among emergency physicians: a mediation analysis. Front Public Health. 2022;10:901251. https://doi.org/10.3389/fpubh.2022.901251, PMID 35784222.

58. Nazik H, Çerçer Z, Özdemir F, Nazik E, Aygün E. Determination of attitude and stress levels of midwives, nurses and physicians working in obstetrics and gynecology clinics regarding COVID-19 pandemic. Psychiatr Danub. 2021;33;Suppl 13: 379–86. PMID 35150512.

59. Shikino K, Kuriyama A, Sadohara M, Matsuo T, Nagasaki K, Nishimura Y, et al. Work-related stress and coping methods of internists and primary care physicians during the COVID-19 pandemic in Japan: a mixed-method study. J Gen Fam Med. 2022;23(5):327–35. https://doi.org/10.1002/jgf2.560, PMID 35942469.

60. Urnberg H, Gluschkoff K, Saukkonen P, Elovainio M, Vänskä J, Heponiemi T. The association between stress attributed to information systems and the experience of workplace aggression: a cross-sectional survey study among Finnish physicians. BMC Health Serv Res. 2022;22(1): 1–10. https://doi.org/10.1186/s12913-022-08116-w, PMID 35641931.

61. Stress and burnout in the profession, part 3: veterinarians find peace after war against stress and burnout. J Am Vet Med Assoc. 1991;198(6):941–2. PMID 2032917.

62. Managing stress and avoiding burnout. A self-care primer for overly compassionate and overworked veterinarians. J Am Vet Med Assoc. 2004;225(4):492–3. PMID 15344350.

63. Harling M, Strehmel P, Schablon A, Nienhaus A. Psychosocial stress, demoralization and the consumption of tobacco, alcohol and medical drugs by veterinarians. J Occup Med Toxicol. 2009;4: 1–11. https://doi.org/10.1186/1745-6673-4-4, PMID 19243579.

64. Hatch PH, Winefield HR, Christie BA, Lievaart JJ. Workplace stress, mental health, and burnout of veterinarians in Australia. Aust Vet J. 2011;89(11):460–8. https://doi.org/10.1111/j.1751-0813.2011.00833.x, PMID 22008127.

65. Kahler SC. Moral stress the top trigger in veterinarians' compassion fatigue: veterinary social worker suggests redefining veterinarians' ethical responsibility. J Am Vet Med Assoc. 2015;246(1):16–8. PMID 25654818.

66. Kim RW, Patterson G, Nahar VK, Sharma M. Toward an evidence-based approach to stress management for veterinarians and veterinary students. J Am Vet Med Assoc. 2017;251(9):1002–4. https://doi.org/10.2460/javma.251.9.1002, PMID 29035658.

67. Ouedraogo FB, Lefebvre SL, Hansen CR, Brorsen BW. Compassion satisfaction, burnout, and secondary traumatic stress among full-time veterinarians in the United States (2016–2018). J Am Vet Med Assoc. 2021;258(11):1259–70. https://doi.org/10.2460/javma.258.11.1259, PMID 33978434.

68. Pohl R, Botscharow J, Böckelmann I, Thielmann B. Stress and strain among veterinarians: a scoping review. Ir Vet J. 2022;75(1):1–24. https://doi.org/10.1186/s13620-022-00220-x, PMID 35729648.

69. Smith DR, Leggat PA, Speare R, Townley-Jones M. Examining the dimensions and correlates of workplace stress among Australian veterinarians. J Occup Med Toxicol. 2009;4: 1–8. https://doi.org/10.1186/1745-6673-4-32, PMID 19995450.

70. Whiting TL, Marion CR. Perpetration-induced traumatic stress - A risk for veterinarians involved in the destruction of healthy animals. Can Vet J. 2011;52(7):794–6. PMID 22210948.

71. Whitnall VM, Simmonds JG. Occupational stress and coping strategies in experienced Australian veterinarians. Vet Rec. 2021;189(2):e202. https://doi.org/10.1002/vetr.202, PMID 33645680.

72. Nienhaus A, Skudlik C, Seidler A. Work-related accidents and occupational diseases in veterinarians and their staff. Int Arch Occup Environ Health. 2005;78(3):230–8. https://doi.org/10.1007/s00420-004-0583-5, PMID 15776262.

73. Gabel CL, Gerberich SG. Risk factors for injury among veterinarians. Epidemiology. 2002;13(1):80–6. https://doi.org/10.1097/00001648-200201000-00013, PMID 11805590.

74. Lucas M, Day L, Shirangi A, Fritschi L. Significant injuries in Australian veterinarians and use of safety precautions. Occup Med (Lond). 2009;59(5):327–33. https://doi.org/10.1093/occmed/kqp070, PMID 19468101.

75. Moses L, Malowney MJ, Wesley Boyd J. Ethical conflict and moral distress in veterinary practice: a survey of North American veterinarians. J Vet Intern Med. 2018;32(6):2115–22. https://doi.org/10.1111/jvim.15315, PMID 30320478.

76. Jameton A. What moral distress in nursing history could suggest about the future of health care. AMA J Ethics. 2017;19(6):617–28. https://doi.org/10.1001/journalofethics.2017.19.6.mhst1-1706, PMID 28644792.

77. Thomas TA, McCullough LB. A philosophical taxonomy of ethically significant moral distress. J Med Philos. 2015;40(1):102–20. https://doi.org/10.1093/jmp/jhu048, PMID 25503608.

78. Campbell SM, Ulrich CM, Grady C. A broader understanding of moral distress. Am J Bioeth. 2016;16(12):2–9. https://doi.org/10.1080/15265161.2016.1239782, PMID 27901442.

79. Burgart AM, Kruse KE. Moral distress in clinical ethics: expanding the concept. Am J Bioeth. 2016;16(12):1. https://doi.org/10.1080/15265161.2016.1253963, PMID 27901425.

80. Griffin BJ, Purcell N, Burkman K, Litz BT, Bryan CJ, Schmitz M, et al. Moral injury: an integrative review. J Trauma Stress. 2019;32(3):350–62. https://doi.org/10.1002/jts.22362, PMID 30688367.

81. Ducharlet K, Trivedi M, Gelfand SL, Liew H, McMahon LP, Ashuntantang G, et al. Moral distress and moral injury in nephrology during the COVID-19 pandemic. Semin Nephrol. 2021;41(3):253–61. https://doi.org/10.1016/j.semnephrol.2021.05.006, PMID 34330365.

82. Farrell CM, Hayward BJ. Ethical dilemmas, moral distress, and the risk of moral injury: experiences of residents and fellows during the COVID-19 pandemic in the United States. Acad Med. 2022;97(3S):S55–60. https://doi.org/10.1097/ACM.0000000000004536, PMID 34817403.

83. Hines SE, Chin KH, Glick DR, Wickwire EM. Trends in moral injury, distress, and resilience factors among healthcare workers at the beginning of the COVID-19 pandemic. Int J Environ Res Public Health. 2021;18(2):1–11. https://doi.org/10.3390/ijerph18020488, PMID 33435300.

84. Hines SE, Chin KH, Levine AR, Wickwire EM. Initiation of a survey of healthcare worker distress and moral injury at the onset of the COVID-19 surge. Am J Ind Med. 2020;63(9):830–3. https://doi.org/10.1002/ajim.23157, PMID 32677108.

85. Kellish A, Gotthold S, Tiziani M, Higgins P, Fleming D, Kellish A. Moral injury signified by levels of moral distress and burnout in health science clinical educators. J Allied Health. 2021;50(3):190–7. PMID 34495029.

86. Mackel CE, Alterman RL, Buss MK, Reynolds RM, Fox WC, Spiotta AM, et al. Moral distress and moral injury among attending neurosurgeons: a national survey. Neurosurgery. 2022;91(1):59–65. https://doi.org/10.1227/neu.000000000 0001921, PMID 35319531.

87. McAninch A. Moral distress, moral injury, and moral luck. Am J Bioeth. 2016;16(12): 29–31. https://doi.org/10.1080/15265161.2016.1239790, PMID 27901423.

88. Nichter M. From idioms of distress, concern, and care to moral distress leading to moral injury in the time of Covid. Transcult Psychiatry. 2022;59(4):551–67. https:// doi.org/10.1177/13634615221115540, PMID 35938212.

89. Papazoglou K, Chopko B. The role of moral suffering (moral distress and moral injury) in police compassion fatigue and PTSD: an unexplored topic. Front Psychol. 2017;8: 1–5. https://doi.org/10.3389/fpsyg.2017.01999, PMID 29187830.

90. Rashid S, Reeder C, Sahu S, Rashid S. Psychological distress and moral injury to oncologists and their patients during COVID-19 pandemic. Curr Psychol. 2022;41(11):8175–80. https://doi.org/10.1007/s12144-021-02128-1, PMID 343 41650.

91. Riedel PL, Kreh A, Kulcar V, Lieber A, Juen B. A scoping review of moral stressors, moral distress and moral injury in healthcare workers during COVID-19. Int J Environ Res Public Health. 2022;19(3):1–20. https://doi.org/10.3390/ ijerph19031666, PMID 35162689.

92. Ritchie EC. Reframing clinician distress: moral injury not burnout. Fed Pract. 2019;36(11):506–7. PMID 31892772.

93. Stanojević S, Čartolovni A. Moral distress and moral injury and their interplay as a challenge for leadership and management: the case of Croatia. J Nurs Manag. 2022;30(7):2335–45. https://doi.org/10.1111/jonm.13835, PMID 36194206.

94. Testoni I, Brondolo E, Ronconi L, Petrini F, Navalesi P, Antonellini M, et al. Burnout following moral injury and dehumanization: a study of distress among Italian medical staff during the first COVID-19 pandemic period. Psychol Trauma. 2022. https://doi.org/10.1037/tra0001346, PMID 35925698.

95. Xue Y, Lopes J, Ritchie K, D'Alessandro AM, Banfield L, McCabe RE, et al. Potential circumstances associated with moral injury and moral distress in healthcare workers and public safety personnel across the globe during COVID-19: a scoping review. Front Psychiatry. 2022;13:863232. https://doi.org/10.3389/fpsyt.2022.863232, PMID 35770054.

96. Moral distress and moral injury: recognising and tackling it for U.K. doctors. London: British Medical Association; 2021.

97. Kogan LR, Rishniw M, Hellyer PW, Schoenfeld-Tacher RM. Veterinarians' experiences with near misses and adverse events. J Am Vet Med Assoc. 2018;252(5): 586–95. https://doi.org/10.2460/javma.252.5.586, PMID 29461160.

98. Epp T, Waldner C. Occupational health hazards in veterinary medicine: physical, psychological, and chemical hazards. Can Vet J. 2012;53(2):151–7. PMID 22851776.

99. Rathwell-Deault D, Godard B, Frank D, Doizé B. Expected consequences of convenience euthanasia perceived by veterinarians in Quebec. Can Vet J. 2017;58(7):723–8. PMID 28698691.

100. Antelyes J. Convenience euthanasia revisited. J Am Vet Med Assoc. 1988;193(8):906–8. PMID 3192470.

101. Mitchell ME. A perspective on convenience euthanasia. Can Vet J. 1992;33(4):218. PMID 17423976.

102. Moats R. "Convenience" euthanasia – a comment. Can Vet J. 2012;53(11):1145. PMID 23633706.

103. Robertson S. "Convenience" euthanasia – a comment. Can Vet J. 2012;53(11):1145. PMID 23633707.

104. Rollin BE. An ethicist's commentary on characterizing of convenience euthanasia in ethical terms. Can Vet J. 2006;47(8):741–742. PMID 16933551.

105. Boller M, Nemanic TS, Anthonisz JD, Awad M, Selinger J, Boller EM, et al. The effect of pet insurance on presurgical euthanasia of dogs with gastric dilatation-volvulus: a novel approach to quantifying economic euthanasia in veterinary emergency medicine. Front Vet Sci. 2020;7:590615. https://doi.org/10.3389/fvets.2020.590615, PMID 33364255.

106. Weng HY, Hart LA. Impact of the economic recession on companion animal relinquishment, adoption, and euthanasia: a Chicago animal shelter's experience. J Appl Anim Welf Sci. 2012;15(1):80–90. https://doi.org/10.1080/10888705.2012.624908, PMID 22233217.

107. Salman MD, New JG, Jr., Scarlett JM, Kass PH, Ruch-Gallie R, Hetts S. Human and animal factors related to relinquishment of dogs and cats in 12 selected animal shelters in the United States. J Appl Anim Welf Sci. 1998;1(3):207–26. https://doi.org/10.1207/s15327604jaws0103_2, PMID 16363966.

108. Eagan BH, Gordon E, Protopopova A. Reasons for guardian-relinquishment of dogs to shelters: animal and regional predictors in British Columbia, Canada. Front Vet Sci. 2022;9:857634. https://doi.org/10.3389/fvets.2022.857634, PMID 35498734.

109. Scarlett JM, Salman MD, New JG, Jr., Kass PH. Reasons for relinquishment of companion animals in U.S. animal shelters: selected health and personal issues. J Appl Anim Welf Sci. 1999;2(1):41–57. https://doi.org/10.1207/s15327604jaws0201_4, PMID 16363961.

110. Englar RE. Using a standardized client encounter in the veterinary curriculum to practice veterinarian-employer discussions about animal cruelty reporting. J Vet Med Educ. 2018;45(4):464–79. https://doi.org/10.3138/jvme.0117-001r1, PMID 30285597.

111. Ascione F. Examining children's exposure to violence in the context of animal abuse. Brighton: Sussex Academic Press; 2009.

112. Flynn C. Acknowledging the 'zoological connection': a sociological analysis of animal cruelty. Spartanburg: University of South Carolina; 2001.

113. Paul ES. Empathy with animals and with humans: are they linked? Anthrozoos. 2000;13(4):194–202. https://doi.org/10.2752/089279300786999699.

114. Ascione FR. Enhancing children's attitudes about the humane treatment of animals – generalization to human-directed empathy. Anthrozoos. 1992;5(3):176–91. https://doi.org/10.2752/089279392787011421.

115. Ascione F. The abuse of animals and human interpersonal violence: making the connection. In: Ascione F, editor. Child abuse, domestic violence and animal abuse:

linking the circles of compassion for prevention and intervention. West Lafayette, IN: Purdue University Press; 1999. p. 50–61.

116. Arluke A, Luke C. Physical cruelty toward animals in Massachusetts 1975–1990. Soc Anim. 1997;5(3):195–204.

117. Pellegren J. The reality of owner-requested or convenience euthanasia: DVM360; 2016. Available from: https://www.dvm360.com/view/the-reality-of-owner-reque sted-or-convenience-euthanasia.

118. Taking action against clinician burnout: a systems approach to professional well-being. Washington, DC: National Academies Press; 2019.

119. Lewis M, Willette ZM, Park B. Calling health care workers "heroes" harms all of us; 2020. Stat [internet]. Available from: https://www.statnews.com/2020/05/21/ calling-health-care-workers-heroes-harms-all-of-us/.

120. The mental health of healthcare workers in COVID-19. Mental Health America; 2022. Available from: https://mhanational.org/mental-health-health care-workers-covid-19.

121. Li Y, Scherer N, Felix L, Kuper H. Prevalence of depression, anxiety and post-traumatic stress disorder in health care workers during the COVID-19 pandemic: a systematic review and meta-analysis. PLOS ONE. 2021;16(3):e0246454. https:// doi.org/10.1371/journal.pone.0246454, PMID 33690641.

122. Physician burnout & moral injury: the hidden health care crisis: National Institute for Health Care Management; 2021. Available from: https://nihcm.org/publications/ physician-burnout-suicide-the-hidden-health-care-crisis.

123. Vizheh M, Qorbani M, Arzaghi SM, Muhidin S, Javanmard Z, Esmaeili M. The mental health of healthcare workers in the COVID-19 pandemic: a systematic review. J Diabetes Metab Disord. 2020;19(2):1967–78. https://doi.org/10.1007/ s40200-020-00643-9, PMID 33134211.

124. Berlin G, Lapointe M, Murphy M. Surveyed nurses consider leaving direct patient care at elevated rates. McKinsey & Company; 2022. Available from: https:// www.mckinsey.com/industries/healthcare-systems-and-services/our-insights/ surveyed-nurses-consider-leaving-direct-patient-care-at-elevated-rates.

125. Shanafelt TD, Dyrbye LN, West CP. Addressing physician burnout: the way forward. JAMA. 2017;317(9):901–2. https://doi.org/10.1001/jama.2017.0076, PMID 28196201.

126. West CP, Dyrbye LN, Shanafelt TD. Physician burnout: contributors, consequences and solutions. J Intern Med. 2018;283(6):516–29. https://doi.org/10.1111/ joim.12752, PMID 29505159.

127. West CP, Tan AD, Shanafelt TD. Association of resident fatigue and distress with occupational blood and body fluid exposures and motor vehicle incidents. Mayo Clin Proc. 2012;87(12):1138–44. https://doi.org/10.1016/j.mayocp.2012.07.021, PMID 23218084.

128. Bianchi R, Schonfeld IS, Laurent E. Burnout-depression overlap: a review. Clin Psychol Rev. 2015;36:28–41. https://doi.org/10.1016/j.cpr.2015.01.004, PMID 25638755.

129. Shanafelt TD, Sloan JA, Habermann TM. The well-being of physicians. Am J Med. 2003;114(6):513–9. https://doi.org/10.1016/s0002-9343(03)00117-7, PMID 12727590.

130. Asai M, Morita T, Akechi T, Sugawara Y, Fujimori M, Akizuki N, et al. Burnout and psychiatric morbidity among physicians engaged in end-of-life care for cancer patients: a cross-sectional nationwide survey in Japan. Psychooncol. 2007;16(5): 421–8. https://doi.org/10.1002/pon.1066, PMID 16929464.

131. Brown SD, Goske MJ, Johnson CM. Beyond substance abuse: stress, burnout, and depression as causes of physician impairment and disruptive behavior. J Am Coll Radiol. 2009;6(7):479–85. https://doi.org/10.1016/j.jacr.2008.11.029, PMID 19560063.

132. Dewa CS, Loong D, Bonato S, Thanh NX, Jacobs P. How does burnout affect physician productivity? A systematic literature review. BMC Health Serv Res. 2014;14: 1–10. https://doi.org/10.1186/1472-6963-14-325, PMID 25066375.

133. Balch CM, Shanafelt TD, Sloan J, Satele DV, Kuerer HM. Burnout and career satisfaction among surgical oncologists compared with other surgical specialties. Ann Surg Oncol. 2011;18(1):16–25. https://doi.org/10.1245/s10434-010-1369-5, PMID 20953718.

134. Dyrbye LN, Varkey P, Boone SL, Satele DV, Sloan JA, Shanafelt TD. Physician satisfaction and burnout at different career stages. Mayo Clin Proc. 2013;88(12): 1358–67. https://doi.org/10.1016/j.mayocp.2013.07.016, PMID 24290109.

135. Garcia LC, Shanafelt TD, West CP, Sinsky CA, Trockel MT, Nedelec L, et al. Burnout, depression, career satisfaction, and work-life integration by physician race/ethnicity. JAMA Netw Open. 2020;3(8):e2012762. https://doi.org/10.1001/jamanetworkopen.2020.12762, PMID 32766802.

136. Kuerer HM, Eberlein TJ, Pollock RE, Huschka M, Baile WF, Morrow M, et al. Career satisfaction, practice patterns and burnout among surgical oncologists: report on the quality of life of members of the Society of Surgical Oncology. Ann Surg Oncol. 2007;14(11):3043–53. https://doi.org/10.1245/s10434-007-9579-1, PMID 17828575.

137. Miyasaki JM, Rheaume C, Gulya L, Ellenstein A, Schwarz HB, Vidic TR, et al. Qualitative study of burnout, career satisfaction, and well-being among US neurologists in 2016. Neurology. 2017;89(16):1730–8. https://doi.org/10.1212/WNL.0000000000004526, PMID 28931640.

138. Shanafelt TD, Balch CM, Bechamps G, Russell T, Dyrbye L, Satele D, et al. Burnout and medical errors among American surgeons. Ann Surg. 2010;251(6):995–1000. https://doi.org/10.1097/SLA.0b013e3181bfdab3, PMID 19934755.

139. Tawfik DS, Profit J, Morgenthaler TI, Satele DV, Sinsky CA, Dyrbye LN, et al. Physician burnout, well-being, and work unit safety grades in relationship to reported medical errors. Mayo Clin Proc. 2018;93(11):1571–80. https://doi.org/10.1016/j.mayocp.2018.05.014, PMID 30001832.

140. Trockel MT, Menon NK, Rowe SG, Stewart MT, Smith R, Lu M, et al. Assessment of physician sleep and wellness, burnout, and clinically significant medical errors. JAMA Netw Open. 2020;3(12):e2028111. https://doi.org/10.1001/jamanetworkopen.2020.28111, PMID 33284339.

141. West CP, Tan AD, Habermann TM, Sloan JA, Shanafelt TD. Association of resident fatigue and distress with perceived medical errors. JAMA. 2009;302(12): 1294–300. https://doi.org/10.1001/jama.2009.1389, PMID 19773564.

142. Halbesleben JR, Rathert C. Linking physician burnout and patient outcomes: exploring the dyadic relationship between physicians and patients. Health Care Manag Rev. 2008;33(1):29–39. https://doi.org/10.1097/01.HMR.0000304493.87898.72, PMID 18091442.

143. Sharma A, Sharp DM, Walker LG, Monson JR. Stress and burnout in colorectal and vascular surgical consultants working in the UK National Health Service. Psychooncol. 2008;17(6):570–6. https://doi.org/10.1002/pon.1269, PMID 17935146.

144. Shanafelt TD, Balch CM, Bechamps GJ, Russell T, Dyrbye L, Satele D, et al. Burnout and career satisfaction among American surgeons. Ann Surg. 2009;250(3):463–71. https://doi.org/10.1097/SLA.0b013e3181ac4dfd, PMID 19730177.

145. Siu C, Yuen SK, Cheung A. Burnout among public doctors in Hong Kong: cross-sectional survey. Hong Kong Med J. 2012;18(3):186–92. PMID 2266 5681.

146. Shanafelt TD, West CP, Sloan JA, Novotny PJ, Poland GA, Menaker R, et al. Career fit and burnout among academic faculty. Arch Intern Med. 2009;169(10):990–5. https://doi.org/10.1001/archinternmed.2009.70, PMID 19468093.

147. Haas JS, Cleary PD, Puopolo AL, Burstin HR, Cook EF, Brennan TA. Differences in the professional satisfaction of general internists in academically affiliated practices in the greater-Boston area. Ambulatory medicine quality improvement project investigators. J Gen Intern Med. 1998;13(2):127–30. https://doi.org/10.1046/j.1525-1497.1998.00030.x, PMID 9502374.

148. Haas JS, Cook EF, Puopolo AL, Burstin HR, Cleary PD, Brennan TA. Is the professional satisfaction of general internists associated with patient satisfaction? J Gen Intern Med. 2000;15(2):122–8. https://doi.org/10.1046/j.1525-1497.2000.02219.x, PMID 10672116.

149. DiMatteo MR, Sherbourne CD, Hays RD, Ordway L, Kravitz RL, McGlynn EA, et al. Physicians' characteristics influence patients' adherence to medical treatment: results from the Medical Outcomes Study. Health Psychol. 1993;12(2):93–102. https://doi.org/10.1037/0278-6133.12.2.93, PMID 8500445.

150. Schwam K. The phenomenon of compassion fatigue in perioperative nursing. AORN J. 1998;68(4):642–5, 7–8. https://doi.org/10.1016/s0001-2092(06)62569-6, PMID 9795719.

151. Huggard PK, Huggard EJ. When the caring gets tough: compassion fatigue and veterinary care 2008.

152. Volk JO, Schimmack U, Strand EB, Lord LK, Siren CW. Executive summary of the Merck Animal Health Veterinary Wellbeing Study. J Am Vet Med Assoc. 2018;252(10):1231–8. https://doi.org/10.2460/javma.252.10.1231, PMID 29701527.

153. Volk JO, Schimmack U, Strand EB, Reinhard A, Vasconcelos J, Hahn J, et al. Executive summary of the Merck Animal Health Veterinarian wellbeing Study III and Veterinary Support Staff Study. J Am Vet Med Assoc. 2022;260(12):1547–53. https://doi.org/10.2460/javma.22.03.0134, PMID 35943942.

154. Volk JO, Schimmack U, Strand EB, Vasconcelos J, Siren CW. Executive summary of the Merck Animal Health Veterinarian Wellbeing Study II. J Am Vet Med Assoc. 2020;256(11):1237–44. https://doi.org/10.2460/javma.256.11.1237, PMID 32412878.

155. Rhind SM, Grant A. From studying the rain to studying the umbrella: mental health and well-being of veterinary medical students and graduates. J Vet Med Educ. 2017;44(1):1–2. https://doi.org/10.3138/jvme.1116-170, PMID 28206839.

156. Bartram DJ, Baldwin DS. Veterinary surgeons and suicide: a structured review of possible influences on increased risk. Vet Rec. 2010;166(13):388–97. https://doi.org/10.1136/vr.b4794, PMID 20348468.

157. Milner AJ, Niven H, Page K, LaMontagne AD. Suicide in veterinarians and veterinary nurses in Australia: 2001–2012. Aust Vet J. 2015;93(9):308–10. https://doi.org/10.1111/avj.12358, PMID 26313208.

158. Nett RJ, Witte TK, Holzbauer SM, Elchos BL, Campagnolo ER, Musgrave KJ, et al. Risk factors for suicide, attitudes toward mental illness, and practice-related stressors among US veterinarians. J Am Vet Med Assoc. 2015;247(8):945–55. https://doi.org/10.2460/javma.247.8.945, PMID 26421408.

159. Turnwald GH. Theme: stress in veterinary students. J Vet Med Educ. 2005;32(2):169.

160. Baker HJ. Our troubled colleagues. J Vet Med Educ. 2012;39(4):311. https://doi.org/10.3138/jvme.0812.078, PMID 23169009.

161. Chew-Graham CA, Rogers A, Yassin N. "I wouldn't want it on my CV or their records": medical students' experiences of help-seeking for mental health problems. Med Educ. 2003;37(10):873–80. https://doi.org/10.1046/j.1365-2923.2003.01627.x, PMID 12974841.

162. McArthur M, Mansfield C, Matthew S, Zaki S, Brand C, Andrews J, et al. Resilience in veterinary students and the predictive role of mindfulness and self-compassion. J Vet Med Educ. 2017;44(1):106–15. https://doi.org/10.3138/jvme.0116-027R1, PMID 28206835.

163. Williams JMG, Kabat-Zinn J. Mindfulness: diverseperspectives on its meaning, origins, and multiple applications at the intersection of science and dharma. Contemp Buddhism. 2011;12(1):1–18.

164. Neff KD. Self-compassion, self-esteem, and well-being. Soc Pers Psychol Compass. 2011;5(1):1–12. https://doi.org/10.1111/j.1751-9004.2010.00330.x.

165. Körner A, Coroiu A, Copeland L, Gomez-Garibello C, Albani C, Zenger M, et al. The role of self-compassion in buffering symptoms of depression in the general population. PLOS ONE. 2015;10(10):e0136598. https://doi.org/10.1371/journal.pone.0136598, PMID 26430893.

166. Wong CCY, Mak WWS. Differentiating the role of three self-compassion components in buffering cognitive-personality vulnerability to depression among Chinese in Hong Kong. J Couns Psychol. 2013;60(1):162–9. https://doi.org/10.1037/a0030451, PMID 23088681.

167. Rees CS, Breen LJ, Cusack L, Hegney D. Understanding individual resilience in the workplace: the international collaboration of workforce resilience model. Front Psychol. 2015;6:1–7. https://doi.org/10.3389/fpsyg.2015.00073, PMID 25698999.

168. Rockliff H, Gilbert P, McEwan K. A pilot exploration of heart rate variability and salivary cortisol responses to compassion-focused imagery. Clin Neuropsychiatry. 2008;5(3):132–9.

Part Four

Developing Reflective Practice

CHAPTER 12

End-of-Chapter Reflection Questions

Written in partnership with Teresa Graham Brett, JD

We have provided end-of-chapter reflection questions for your thoughtful review.

As you work through these questions individually, consider that your gut reactions, thoughts, perspectives, and responses are valid and unique. Your past and present experiences have shaped the lens through which you view yourself and surrounding communities, and your voice in turn influences both your future self and your future interactions with clients.

Some, if not all, of these reflection questions can be transitioned into small group discussions with facilitation to promote learning from those outside of ourselves with respect to how others experience the world around us.

Other people serve many roles in our communities. Some are our colleagues. Some are our clients. Some are both.

To be successful as a veterinarian, you must find ways to connect to other people. Most people who we encounter day-to-day as veterinarians are our clients. Clients will enter your consultation room with their own unique blends of past and present life experiences, gut reactions, thoughts, feelings, concerns, and perspectives.

In my textbook, *A Guide to Oral Communication in Veterinary Medicine,* I wrote that "in the poker game of veterinary practice, your clients hold the cards. They determine whether to play [their cards] (commit to care), hold (consider care), or fold them (decline care altogether)."(1)

How you interact with, connect to, and communicate with your clients determines the level of care that you and your team can provide. Quality of life and end-of-life consultations require significant investment from the veterinary team as you work with and prepare your clients for what is to come.

These reflection questions, paired with their respective chapters, are intended to stimulate critical thinking about your own personal and professional growth journey through end-of-life considerations within the practice of veterinary medicine as you prepare to support the bereaved.

Clients may or may not be prepared for poor patient health outcomes, diagnoses, or prognoses. Even those clients who are experiencing anticipatory grief as they navigate chronic and/or terminal disease processes in their pets benefit from additional support from the veterinary team. Anticipating death is often very different from bearing witness to it.

The primary goal in working through each question is to identify, acknowledge, and solidify your own understanding, thoughts, and perspectives about the human–animal bond, death and dying, anticipatory grief, bereavement, and memorialization.

We intentionally are choosing to ask about you, your memories, your present-day experiences, your emotional ties to past and present, and your hopes, dreams, and aspirations for the future.

Before you can provide relationship-centered care to others, you must first care for and understand yourself. Therefore, within this subsection of the text, you, the learner, are often primed to consider and reflect upon your own unique frame of reference. You will be tasked with considering the origin of your world-view and how or why it may have shifted over time.

By asking questions of yourself, you develop an understanding of your own assumptions, beliefs, values, and experiences. This enriches your understanding of self. Having this secure foundation allows you to then engage in perspective taking to acknowledge, understand, accept, and bridge differences. The practice of veterinary medicine will require you to stretch beyond your own sense of self to recognize that our clients also operate from within their own distinct worldviews. The only way to make sense of another's worldview is to solicit and take on another's perspective in a way that inspires dialogue and partnership.

Reflecting on this process trains you to identify challenges, discover new meanings, and apply lessons learned to future encounters with others.

Reflections on Chapter 1

Beyond Self: Animal–Animal Interactions, Human–Animal Interactions, and the Evolution of the Human–Animal Bond

1. Perspectives and worldviews continue to evolve every day as we journey through life.
   a) In broad terms, what is your understanding of the term, *worldview*?
   b) What factors help to shape a person's worldview?

    c) How would you define *your* worldview?

    d) When you reflect upon *your childhood*, what and who do you consider to be most influential in the development of your worldview?

    e) What and who do you consider to be most influential in the development of your worldview as it stands *in the present day*?

    f) When you encounter someone whose worldview is distinct from yours, how do you approach the situation? Do you acknowledge differences? Do you ask questions to clarify your understanding? Do you feel a need to compare their worldview to yours and/or explain any distinctions?

    g) How open are you to exploring another's worldview? Does your relationship with the other person influence your curiosity?

    h) How might your present-day life be different if you had been born into another home, culture, continent, or faith?

    i) How has global communication and accessibility to international travel increased your awareness of others' worldviews?

    j) What are barriers to exploring another's worldview?

2. Socialization plays a critical role in how we develop our values, beliefs, attitudes, and worldviews.

    a) How would you define socialization with respect to people (as opposed to the socialization of puppies or kittens)?

    b) In what ways is socialization similar across species?

    c) In what ways is socialization different across species?

    d) What are your earliest memories from childhood about your interactions with *other people*?

    e) What are your earliest memories from childhood about your interactions with *non-human animals*?

Consider broadening the scope of your memories by including the following details:

- where you were
- what you were experiencing externally and internally
- what you saw
- what you smelled
- what you touched
- what you heard
- what you felt in the moment
- what feelings remained with you after the experience.

3. What are your earliest memories about interactions that you witnessed between your caregivers, parents, immediate or extended family members, and non-human animals?

4. Based upon what you have shared with respect to these earliest memories, what messages did you learn or receive about how to interact with animals and from whom?

5. Based upon what you have shared with respect to these earliest memories, what messages did you learn or receive about how *not* to interact with animals and from whom?

6. Did the messaging that you received from others surrounding human–animal interactions align with or contradict what you considered to be the social norms of the times? In what ways?

7. Do you recall ever questioning the messaging that you received from others surrounding human-animal interactions? If so, in what ways?

8. As you reflect upon your earliest memories surrounding human–animal interactions, do you *now* question the messaging that you received from others? If so, in what ways?

9. Before this reflective exercise, had you ever been prompted to think about your earliest memories and experiences? The prompt may have come internally or from someone else.
    a) If yes, describe in what ways you have thought about these experiences before this?
    b) If not, has anything surprised you about what these prompts have helped you to recall?

10. How have your interactions with animals – or your perceptions of those interactions – changed since those earliest memories?

11. What discoveries have you made about yourself, others, your family, community or even society, because of this guided reflection exercise?

12. In your own words, how do you define the human–animal bond?

13. Consider your own bonds with animals from your past and present-day life. Do you believe these relationships are connected to a desire to bond with nature, as is suggested by the biophilia hypothesis? Why or why not? Please elaborate.

14. The American Veterinary Medical Association's definition of the human–animal bond states that the relationship must be mutually beneficial.
    a) Broadly speaking, how do animals benefit *people?*
    b) Broadly speaking, how do people benefit animals?
    c) Considering companion animals specifically, how do pets benefit people?
    d) How do people benefit companion animals?

e) Are relationships between humans and companion animals always reciprocal?

f) In a mutually beneficial relationship, can one member benefit more? If so, in what ways?

> As we consider our past experiences with animals, we are also tasked with considering the value of those same experiences: what did we learn from those experiences and from whom? If we truly believe that we are learning from our interactions with animals, then we must also consider the value that they bring to the interactions that we collectively share.

15. What is value? How do you define it?

16. In broad terms, how do we decide what (and who) is of value to us? What makes the determination in our minds that something is inherently valuable?

> How we measure the value of animals depends upon the lenses through which we are looking. We each have our own unique perspectives to bring to the table.
>
> For instance, if we explore animal value from the lens of a biologist, we might consider that an animal's life has value to its own species, value to other species (for instance, as a food source or based upon other ecological contributions) and value to future generations through genetic fitness and reproductive success.
>
> As humans, we develop our own value systems. Through these systems, which are influenced by past experiences and perspectives as well as those around us, we confer values onto animals.

17. Do you value all species equally? Are there some species that you value more or less? Why or why not? Please expand upon your answer.

18. Has the value that you have assigned to a particular species changed over time? If so, which species and in which ways?

19. How has your present-day assigned value of animals been influenced by your socialization as a child? What, if any, correlation is there between your early socialization and what animals you value most now?

20. Based upon your own perceptions, which species are currently most valued by society?

21. Are the species you perceive to be most valued by society the same species that you value most?

a) Please expand upon any differences that you perceive.

b) What is the impact of those differences *on you as a person and in your life?*

c) What is the impact of those differences on what you perceive to be *your role as a veterinarian?*

As veterinarians, we are part of a healthcare team.

That team includes, but is not limited to, our colleagues (other Doctors of Veterinary Medicine), veterinary technicians, veterinary assistants, client service representatives (CSR), kennel or barn workers, administrative assistants, office managers, hospital directors, employers, and clients.

Teams are unique blends of abilities that work together to ensure the delivery of high-quality veterinary care for animals.

Collaboration is not without conflict.

There may be disparate views among team members, and tension, disagreements, and conflicts can and will arise.

Two potential areas of conflict are our perceptions surrounding the human–animal bond and/or what we consider to be appropriate case management.

We do not always agree with or clients; they do not always agree with us.

22. When you discover that your own worldview does not align with a client's, what tools might you use to learn more about your client, their perspective, and the role(s) that animals play in their lives?

23. When you discover that you disagree with decisions or actions that a client is taking based upon their worldview, what is your gut reaction?

24. How might you transition from gut reaction to response so that you are able to provide care that is *responsive to the realities for your clients and their animal(s)?*

25. When there is disagreement between you and your client, the disagreement may be rooted in differences in worldview or differences in levels of understanding of the medical aspects of a case. How might you discern which type of disagreement you are experiencing? Why is it important to consider this distinction? How does becoming aware of this information move stalled client interactions forward?

In our explorations of the relationships between humans and animals, we have touched upon the idea that how we perceive, describe, and think about human–animal relationships is a social construct. Different societies and cultures (both historically and in the present day) have built different conceptions of their relationships with animals. This building or construction of human–animal–environment relationships is connected to how groups, cultures and societies see, interact, define, value, and live out those relationships, which are passed down from generation to generation.

As part of this reflective work, we have been explicit in the process of exploring our own identities, perspectives, values, and socialization with the goal of bringing to conscious awareness the processes that have shaped who we are in the world and how we interact with others. Others includes other people and groups, the environment, and non-human animals.

Let's transition now to explore how our perceptions and definitions of intelligence impact our thoughts and ideas about the reasons that we may deeply connect to animals and how those connections shape our personal and professional lives.

Reflection Questions:

26. What are some of the differences between asking "How smart is this animal or species?" and "How is this animal or species smart?"

27. How do you define intelligence?

28. Does your perception of which species are intelligent influence your level of attraction to them and/or the degree to which you ascribe value to them?

29. In this chapter, we shared that companion animals are now considered to be members of the family by 85%–99% of pet owners.(2–7)

    a) How do these statistics resonate with you? Are pets truly family?

    b) What about companion animals might make your clients view them as family members? Is it their intelligence? Is it something else? Does it vary depending upon the animal and/or the owner?

    c) Do you currently own pets, or have you owned pets in the past? If so, do you consider your current pets (or did you consider your past pets) to be members of the family? Why or why not? If so, in what ways?

30. Some clients consider pets to be their children.

    a) What are your thoughts about this analogy? Are pets "fur kids"? Can childless people be "pet parents"? What about those with human kids?

    b) How might pet ownership be akin to having a child?

    c) In what ways might pet ownership be different than having a child?

    d) Should pets have the same rights as children? Why or why not?

31. In this chapter, we shared that 40% of pet owners within the U.S. felt that their pet was a better listener than their partner.(8)

    a) How does this statement resonate with you? Do you agree or disagree?

    b) What do you think that people who affirm this statement mean? What is it that they are looking for that they are not receiving from their partner?

    c) In what ways might a pet "hear" us more than our partner does?

As we alluded to in this chapter, the human–animal bond is not exclusive to companion animals. The human–animal bond also extends to non-companion animals. This broadening of the species to which we can be bonded has significant implications for animal welfare. The Veterinary Oath that is pledged at time of graduation assigns veterinarians the responsibility of making animal welfare assessments to determine if animal needs are being met. Interactions and bonds with animals in and of themselves do not guarantee the absence of welfare issues.(6) It is essential that we recognize when reciprocity does not exist and that we partner with our clients to address shortcomings with respect to relationship-centered care.

32. In broad terms, how would you define a *positive* human–animal relationship?

33. Does your definition of what constitutes a positive human–animal relationship change depending upon the species of animal? Why or why not? Please expand upon your answer.

34. Now let's specifically turn our attention to production animals. How would you describe the *relationships* between Animal Care Managers and the animals that are under their care?

35. What *benefits* do *production animals* bring to their relationship with Animal Care Managers?

36. What *benefits* do *Animal Care Managers* bring to their relationships with the animals that are under their care?

37. What kinds of *behaviors and/or actions* do you think Animal Care Managers might display toward the animal(s) they are responsible for that demonstrate *positive* human animal relationships?

38. Why might the relationship between Animal Care Managers and the animals that they are responsible for become *negative?* In other words, what factors might lead to a *breakdown* in that relationship?

39. What kinds of *behaviors and/or actions* do you think Animal Care Managers might display toward the animal(s) they are responsible for that demonstrate *negative* human animal relationships?

40. As we consider the potential for negative human–animal relationships, let's take our thoughts a step further. What do you think the impact of a *negative* human-animal relationship would be on each of the species below? In other words, what physiological and behavioral sequelae you might see in each of the following species?
    a) Poultry
    b) Swine
    c) Ruminants (dairy)
    d) Ruminants (beef)

 e) Farmed fur animals
 f) Farmed fish

In their 2010 article in the *Journal of Dairy Science*, Kielland et al. write that:(9)

Farm animal welfare is dependent on human care. Farmers decide on both the choice in housing systems and how the system is managed. Inadequately designed and badly maintained facilities can cause skin lesions and reduced welfare. Previous research suggests a direct relationship between farmers' attitudes and behavior(10, 11) and between farmers' behavior and their management decisions.(12) Their behavior affects dairy cattle management and the consequences of management decisions can be measured by defined variables related to production and health. Higher milk yield was reported in farms with positive indicators of human–animal interaction(11, 13, 14) Hanna et al (2009) reported that empathy was positively correlated with milk yield and that negative beliefs had a negative correlation with milk yield, and assessed negative beliefs using the response of farmers to statements such as "cows respond better to shouting than to a gentle voice."(15)

41. Based upon your past and present experiences, current perspective, and worldview, what are the most important factors that contribute to positive attitudes and empathy among farmers, ranchers, producers, and other Animal Care Managers?
42. Do you believe it is possible for an individual to shift their attitudes and increase empathy for animals under their care? Please elaborate.
43. What might contribute toward a *positive* shift in the direction of greater empathy among individuals who take care of animals?

Empathy has also been studied with respect to veterinary medical education because it:

… plays an important role in veterinarians' relationships with their patients, clients, and colleagues. Because it relates to greater clinical competence and facilitates the acquisition of information for diagnosing, prescribing therapies, and identifying and treating animal pain, empathy is an essential competence to be strengthened during professional training.(16)

Despite the documented need for empathy in clinical practice, empathy among human medical and veterinary medical students has been shown to decline after the first year of healthcare training programs.(17–19) Veterinary students in their final year of study also, on average, perceive animals to be less sentient than entry-level students.(20)

44. What might account for the reported decline in empathy among healthcare students as they progress through their respective training programs?
45. In your own experience, have you seen a decline in empathy in yourself or in your peers? If so, in what ways? Please elaborate.
46. Could this decline in empathy be protective? If so, to whom?
47. Could this decline in empathy be an indicator of compassion fatigue and/or burnout? If so, in what ways?
48. How might this decline in empathy impact the delivery of healthcare, veterinary–client–patient relationships (VCPRs), and patient outcomes?

In their 2021 publication, *Love, Fear, and the Human-Animal Bond: On Adversity and Multispecies Relationships*, Jennifer W. Applebaum, Evan L. MacLean, and Shelby E. McDonald write that:

> In contemporary society, love comes in many forms, including attachment bonds between people and their pets. Evidence of our close bonds and kinship with other species manifests in many ways. Particularly notable in the United States is the prevalence of cohabitation with pets and growing recognition of the modern, multispecies household ...(21)
>
> Love and strong social bonds are known buffers in the experience of adversity. However, the literature to date has failed to adequately consider how love that is characterized by the bond between a human and non-human animal (i.e., pet) impacts the lived experience of adversity. There is some evidence that strong bonds with pets may buffer stress and promote resilience in adverse social contexts. However, strong bonds with pets can also complicate adverse situations, and create barriers to meeting the social, emotional, and basic needs of both the individual and their pet.(21)

The authors define adversity as those: "life experiences (hardships, challenges, misfortunes) that have the potential to influence human development in a way that disrupts typical development, compromises an individual's adjustment, and/or has the potential to lead to undesirable outcomes."(21)

---

49. How do you define *adversity*? Is your definition similar or different from the authors and in what ways? Is there a portion of the authors' definition that you would like to adapt as your own? Is there a portion of the authors' definition that you feel could benefit from expansion with one or more of the concepts from yours?
50. How might the human–animal bond *overcome* adversity? Please include specific examples.

51. How might the human–animal bond *contribute to* adverse situations and create barriers for pet owners?
52. In those cases where the human–animal bond contributes to adversity, what are the roles and responsibilities of the veterinary team in helping the client to overcome barriers?
53. When cost of care is the primary barrier, what is the impact on the *patient* and the patient's outcome?
54. When cost of care is the primary barrier, what is the impact on the *client?*
55. When cost of care is the primary barrier, what is the impact on the *veterinary team?*
56. In what ways might financial constraints contribute to compassion fatigue and/or burnout within the veterinary field?
57. What solutions, if any, are there to reducing the impact of financial constraints on the veterinary team?
58. Some people believe that if you cannot afford to care for an animal, then you should not own one. How does this statement resonate with you? Is it accurate? Is it inaccurate? Are there some situations in which this is truer than others?
59. Is animal ownership a right or a privilege?

Reflections on Chapter 2

The Circle of Life and Loss: An Introduction to Grief and Grieving

> Understanding our own worldview is the first step to understanding others' worldviews. We must explore our own worldview first to increase our self-awareness, to understand where we are starting from in relationship to others. Exploring your own thoughts, beliefs, and values regarding grief and grieving, death and dying, and euthanasia will prepare you for cross-cultural explorations of this content with your colleagues.

1. Death is an inevitable part of life. Broadly speaking, do we talk about death in our society? If yes, in what ways?
2. Are there certain aspects of death that society does not typically discuss? Why do you think these subjects are "off-limits"?
3. Does your family talk openly about death? If yes, in what ways?
4. What are your family's customs or rituals surrounding death and dying?
5. How did you come to learn about your family's customs or rituals surrounding death and dying?

6. Do your family's customs or rituals surrounding death and dying resonate with you?

7. As you have grown older, do you find yourself leaning on your family's customs or rituals surrounding death and dying or do you find yourself creating your own? Please expand upon your answer.

8. Have you encountered any customs or rituals surrounding death and dying *outside of your family circle* that resonate with you? If so, what is it about these customs or rituals that resonate with you? How do they make you feel and why?

9. Some people's first awareness of and/or experience with death stems from television (news), movies, cartoons, music, and other elements of popular culture. How is death represented in these forums?

10. Consider an example of a *movie* that you have seen in which one of the main character dies.
    a) Identify the movie and the character.
    b) Discuss how death and dying is portrayed in the film.
    c) Is this portrayal of death useful, helpful, misleading, or unclear?
    d) Does this portrayal of death reflect your own thoughts, beliefs, views, perspectives, or values? Please expand upon your answer.

11. Consider an example of a *book* that you have read in which one of the main character dies.
    a) Identify the book and the character.
    b) Discuss how death and dying is portrayed in the text.
    c) Is this portrayal of death useful, helpful, misleading or unclear?
    d) Does this portrayal of death reflect your own thoughts, beliefs, views, perspectives, or values? Please expand upon your answer.

12. Does the media portray a diverse portrait of how society deals with death and dying? Why or why not? Please expand upon your answer.

13. Now that you have had an opportunity to consider your family's perspective – as well as the media's perspective – on death and dying, grief and grieving, what are your own core beliefs, views, perceptions, and perspectives about these topics?

14. What is your comfort level discussing death (broadly) with *colleagues*? Please expand upon your answer.

15. What is your comfort level discussing death (of patients) with *clients*? Please expand upon your answer.

16. In Chapter 2, we broach the subject of societal expectations about what it means to live and die well.
    a) Based upon your own thoughts, beliefs, and values surrounding death, dying, euthanasia, and grief, what are your expectations about what it means to *live* well?
    b) Based upon your own thoughts, beliefs, and values surrounding death, dying, euthanasia, and grief, what are your expectations about what it means to *die* well?
    c) Do you feel that your expectations align with how you were raised? Please expand upon your answer.
    d) Do you feel that your expectations match what you perceive to be societal expectations of you?
17. How would you define *good death*?
18. Is your definition of "good death" the same when you consider "good death" in people versus "good death" in animals? Why or why not?
19. Why might "good death" not be achievable to all patients? In other words, what are the barriers to "good death" in *people*?
20. What are the barriers to "good death" in *animals*?
21. Are the barriers to "good death" the same in animals as they are in people? Why or why not?
22. How might the concept of "good death" disregard diversity?
23. What can healthcare professionals do to acknowledge, comprehend, and honor diversity through death and dying, grief and grieving?
24. How would you define grief?
25. Make a list of living beings, events, places, etc. – anything you can think of that someone might grieve. Remember that the word grief can be used about any topic or situation. So, be open to many different ideas about what someone might grieve, even if it is something that is outside your own experience or context.
26. Is there a timeline for grief? In other words, how long does grief take? What factors influence the duration of grief?
27. Is there a *right* way to grieve? Please explain your answer.
28. What (and who) influences how we grieve? Please explain your answer.
29. Do clients grieve the same way when every animal that they own dies? Why or why not?
30. Do clinicians grieve the loss of their patients? If yes, do clinicians grieve the same way when every patient dies?
31. In Chapter 2, we presented several models of grief, beginning with the 5 Stages of Grief, as was first articulated by Kübler-Ross. In what ways might it be helpful to think of grieving as a staged

process? In other words, how might it be helpful to conceptualize grief as a series of stages?

32. In what ways might the stages of grief be an artificial construct? In other words, how might thinking of grief as a series of stages limit your scope of understanding?

33. In addition to Kübler-Ross' 5 Stages of Grief, we shared several other models of grief. Which model (including the one by Kübler-Ross) resonates most with you and why?

34. Do you prefer to think of grief in stages, phases, or tasks? Please expand upon your answer.

35. What have you found challenging about the stages, phases, and tasks regarding grief and grieving?

36. What, if anything, is missing in the models of grief and grieving that we have presented thus far? Is there any concept that you feel should be included in the grief stages, phases, or tasks that has not yet been discussed?

37. How might any of the stages, phases, and tasks regarding grief be helpful to you as a veterinarian? In other words, how might you draw upon them to aid you or your team in practicing veterinary medicine?

38. Why might the *veterinary team* be reluctant to ask about the client's beliefs and values concerning death and dying and/or euthanasia?

39. What specifically is important to know concerning the client's beliefs and values about death and dying and/or euthanasia?

40. Why it is important that the veterinary team understand the client's beliefs and values about death and dying and/or euthanasia? In other words, how does knowing the client's beliefs and values about death and dying and/or euthanasia facilitate case management?

41. How might you ask a client about their beliefs and values surrounding death and dying and/or euthanasia? What words specifically will you use?

42. What if your client's views surrounding death and dying are different from your own? How will you flex? In other words, how will you support your client in their grief journey if their views are different from your own?

43. Why might *the client* be reluctant to share their beliefs and values concerning death and dying and/or euthanasia?

44. What does the client need from you and the veterinary team to feel secure in sharing their beliefs and values about death and dying and/or euthanasia?

45. Can you think of a time when the client's beliefs and values about death and dying and/or euthanasia may complicate or otherwise

impede case management? In such a situation, how does one move forward? How does one find common ground?

Reflections on Chapter 3

The Multifaceted Impact of Grief: Normal Reactions and Responses Among the Bereaved

1. You might consider that the way we each grieve is like a fingerprint. No two people are alike in terms of needs, wants, and expectations.

    Describe broadly how *people* experience grief in the following ways:
    a) physically
    b) mentally
    c) socially
    d) emotionally
    e) spiritually.
    As you answer this question, expand your answer to include any and all types of grief – not solely that which is related to death of a loved one.
2. Tell us about a time in your life when you experienced grief of any sort.

    Include the following details as you share your experience with us:
    a) Was your grief expected or unexpected?
    b) Of the five areas that grief is impactful (physical, cognitive, social, emotional, and spiritual), what was its primary impact on you? Why do you suspect this to be so?
    c) Did your grief impact anyone else that you know, including friends and family? If so, what was the primary impact of grief on them?
3. With respect to the time that you shared in the preceding question, what has your experience with grief taught you about your wants and expectations when it comes to your own grief journey? Did you have access to what and who you needed for support?
4. Reflecting back upon that time of grief that you shared in Question #2, are there any aspects of your grief journey that you would have changed, knowing what you know now?
5. Think of a time when someone supported you in your grief. What, if any, words or statements, quotes or sayings helped you to navigate your grief?
6. Now think of a time when someone was *not* helpful in supporting you in your grief.

a) What did they say or do that did not resonate with you? In which aspects were they not supportive?
b) What was their intent in saying or doing what they did?
c) Describe the impact of their words or actions on you and your grief journey.
d) What would have been more helpful for you to hear in that moment?

7. In Question #1, you were asked to consider how people experience grief.
a) Choose a non-human animal.
b) Consider how the non-human animal that you have selected experiences grief.
c) Do non-human animals grieve the same way that humans do? Why or why not?
d) Do all five of the ways in which grief is impactful (e.g., physical, cognitive, social, emotional, and spiritual) apply to animals? Why or why not? Do some apply more than others? Please expand upon your answer.

8. We have now considered the impact of grief on the individual who is actively grieving. Let's now shift our focus to consider those who companion the bereaved through their respective grief journeys. What is the impact of manifestations of grief on those who companion us through grief?

9. Are you always aware of the impact that grief has on you? Why or why not?

10. How do you acknowledge and recognize grief in yourself?

11. How do you acknowledge and recognize grief in others?

12. Why might some people choose to hide grief?

13. Why might some non-human animals choose to hide grief?

14. Can we understand another's grief without having experienced their loss?

15. Can we understand another's grief without being them?

16. Do we need to understand another's grief in order to show support in the form of empathy or unconditional positive regard?

17. Is there a "right" way to grieve?

18. How do you acknowledge and affirm someone whose manner of grieving is the opposite of how you experience grief?

19. When you and someone else are both grieving the same loss, how do you support each another without losing the ability to experience your own unique grief journey?

20. When you and someone else are both grieving different losses, is it helpful to compare losses? When might it be appropriate? When

might it not be appropriate? What are the challenges that might be associated with such comparisons?

Reflections on Chapter 4

Children, Adolescence, and Grief

1. In what ways does childhood bereavement mirror the grief journey that adults navigate?
2. In what ways does childhood bereavement stand apart from the grief journey that adults navigate? In other words, in what ways is the grief that is experienced in childhood unique?
3. Childhood bereavement has can be subdivided into descriptive ranges that attempt to capture key developmental distinctions between age groups:
   - Stage 1: Children ages three to five
   - Stage 2: Children ages five through nine
   - Stage 3: Children ages ten and up.
   a) Describe children's conceptualization of death at each stage. Compare and contrast between the stages.
   b) Provide examples of ways that you can support each stage of children in their respective grief journeys.
4. What do infants and toddlers understand about death?
5. How do infants and toddlers react to the death of a loved one? In other words, what are they reacting to?
6. How might you provide comfort to an infant or toddler whose family unit has experienced the death of a loved one?
7. How might you describe death to a child who is between the ages of 3–5 years old?
8. What about death do you think is most concerning to a child who is between the ages of 3–5 years old?
9. What questions might a 4-year-old have about death and dying?
10. How might you choose to answer the child in the preceding question (Question #9)?
11. How might you describe death to a child who is between the ages of 5–9 years old?
12. What about death do you think is most concerning to a child who is between the ages of 5–9 years old?
13. What questions might a 6-year-old have about death and dying?
14. How might you choose to answer the child in the preceding question (Question #13)?

15. How might you describe death to a pre-teen?
16. What about death do you think is most concerning to a pre-teen?
17. What questions might a 12-year-old have about death and dying?
18. How might you choose to answer the pre-teen in the preceding question (Question #17)?
19. How might you approach conversations about death with a teenager?
20. What about death do you think is most concerning to a teenager?
21. What questions might a 17-year-old have about death and dying?
22. How might you choose to answer the teenager in the preceding question (Question #21)?
23. A family unit may include children of several different age groups. How might you ensure that all age groups are supported in their own respective grief journeys?
24. What and/or who influences the ways in which children react to grief?

> We have not yet considered pet loss as a significant type of bereavement. However, the next set of reflective questions will encourage you to brainstorm about this topic as it is one of the first ways in which children experience grief and grieving, death and dying.

25. What comes to mind when you read or hear the phrase "pet loss?"
26. The preceding question asked you to consider the phrase "pet loss." Did you approach your answer to this question from the perspective of a client, a clinician, as both, or as neither? Please explain your answer.
27. Is pet loss the same as or different from loss of a human?
    a) In what ways might they be similar?
    b) In what ways might they be different?
    c) What is the impact of pet loss on veterinary *client(s)*?
    d) What is the impact of pet loss on the *veterinarian*?
    e) What is the impact of pet loss on *other members of the veterinary team*?
28. Imagine that one of your veterinary clients telephones you because their geriatric cat died in their sleep at home while the children were at school. They ask you how they should explain the death of the cat to the children when they arrive home from school. What questions might you have for the veterinary client?
29. The same client in the preceding question (Question #28) asks if you will explain the death of the cat to the children.
    a) What is your response to the client? Please explain your answer.

b) If you choose to explain the death of the cat to your client's children, should the visit be in-person or via telephone?

c) What might the advantages be to an in-person visit?

d) What might the disadvantages be to an in-person visit?

e) What might the advantages be to a telephone conversation?

f) What might the disadvantages be to a telephone conversation?

g) Might one age group of children response better to the in-person versus telephone conversation? What are your thoughts surrounding the means by which an age-appropriate conversation takes place?

h) In order for you to feel comfortable explaining the death of the cat to your client's children, what specifically do you need to know from the client?

i) Should you, the veterinarian, touch upon the concept of an afterlife? Why or why not? In what circumstances might it be appropriate? In what circumstances might it be inappropriate?

30. Now let's rethink the example from Question #28. Instead of the geriatric cat dying a natural death at home, let's assume that the client asked you to humanely euthanize the cat while the children were at school. The client was present for humane euthanasia and will be taking the cat's body home with them for burial. Prior to the client departing from the clinic, the client asks you what they should tell the children. What do you say?

a) Would you explain that the cat was euthanized? Why or why not? Might it depend upon the age group?

b) How might you explain euthanasia to a child? Be specific. What words might you say and to which age group?

c) What questions might a child ask you after hearing that their pet was euthanized?

d) What concerns might the concept of euthanasia raise for the child?

e) What euphemisms should you avoid when discussing euthanasia with children and why?

Reflections on Chapter 5

Complicated Grief

1. In your own words, how would you define *complicated grief*?

2. Complicated grief is sometimes referred to as "prolonged grief." What is the implication of the word, "prolonged"?

3. How long is "too long" when it comes to grief?
4. Who gets to decide the duration of grief?
5. Complicated grief used to be referred to as "traumatic grief." In what ways can complicated grief be traumatic and for whom?
6. How does complicated grief differ from *acute grief?* How are the two types of grief similar?
7. How does complicated grief differ from *depression?* How are the two clinical conditions alike?
8. What are risk factors for the development of complicated grief?
9. What is the impact of complicated grief on the bereaved? In other words, why might companions of the bereaved concern themselves that grief may be taking "too long?"
10. If experts say that grief has no timeline, then why is complicated grief defined by duration of bereavement?
11. What factors might complicate pet loss *for the adult veterinary client?*
12. What factors might complicate pet loss *for the child of a veterinary client?*
13. What factors might complicate pet loss *for the veterinarian?*
14. What factors might complicate pet loss *for the veterinary team?*

Reflections on Chapter 6

Disenfranchised Grief: The Invisible Wound

1. How would you describe social norms in your own culture, religion, and/or community with respect to bereavement?
2. How did you learn what those social norms were for your culture, religion, and/or community with respect to bereavement?
3. How did you learn what was not socially "acceptable" within your culture, religion, and/or community with respect to bereavement?
4. Is it possible to be a part of two or more cultures, religions, and/or communities that have conflicting norms with respect to bereavement?
5. How might you reconcile conflicting norms with respect to bereavement if you find yourself to be a part of more than one culture, religion, and/or community?
6. How might you demonstrate openness and receptivity to learning about another person's culture, religion, and/or community with respect to bereavement?
7. If you aren't aware of how another person grieves based upon their culture, religion, and/or community, is it appropriate to ask them to share? Why or why not?

8. What might make another person *more* likely to share their cultural and/or religious views on grieving with you?

9. What might make another person *less* likely to share their cultural and/or religious views on grieving with you?

10. Is it okay to disagree with someone's cultural and/or religious views on grieving? If so, in what ways? Is it appropriate to voice your disagreement? Why or why not?

11. Which people or groups of people have been historically marginalized when it comes to experiencing and expressing their grief?

12. What do we mean, broadly, by the word, *disenfranchised*?

13. Can you think of what it means to be disenfranchised in any context *other than* grieving?

14. How would you define disenfranchised grief?

15. What are *physical* manifestations of disenfranchised grief?

16. What are *cognitive* manifestations of disenfranchised grief?

17. What are *social* manifestations of disenfranchised grief?

18. Have you ever felt that something or someone you grieved was discounted?
    - If yes, please share what that experience was like for you. What or who were you grieving and what happened to make you feel that your grief was not acknowledged or affirmed?
    - If not, please consider how such an experience would impact you.

19. What are examples of things that people might *say* that discount someone else's grief?

20. What are examples of things that people might *do* that discount someone else's grief?

21. Do those who discount others' grief mean to? What is their intent?

22. Are there circumstances in which discounting someone else's grief is appropriate?

23. In what circumstances is it *inappropriate* to discount someone else's grief?

24. How might discounting someone else's grief complicate their grief journey?

25. How might discounting someone else's grief affect their ability to trust others?

26. From the perspective of someone who is companioning a loved one through grief, why might you be tempted to discount grief? In other words, what is it that you are trying to achieve for your loved one?

27. As a follow-up to the preceding question (Question #26), Is there an alternate approach that would achieve the same means without discounting their grief?

Reflections on Chapter 7

When the Loss of a Companion Animal Is not Recognized: Pet Loss as a Unique Form of Disenfranchised Grief

1. Do you currently own one or more pets?
   a) If so, tell us about them.
   b) If not, was there ever a time in your life when you owned one or more pets? Tell us about that time in your life.
2. In broad terms, what are the functions of a pet?
3. Does a pet need to have a purpose?
4. Can you still value someone else's attachment to a pet if you do not perceive that pet to have purpose?
5. Is it rational for people to ascribe human qualities to pets?
6. Why might people see pets as miniature people?
7. Is it rational for people to see themselves as "pet parents" or to see their pets as "fur children?"
8. Why might people look to their bond with pets as a means of fulfilling the parent–child relationship?
9. Can a pet function as a surrogate child?
10. How might you come to learn the extent to which a pet means to a particular person? What might you ask that person to find out?
11. Why is it critical for the veterinary team to recognize the strength of the bond between humans and their companion animals?
12. Is everyone's bond with their companion animal the same? In what ways might there be similarities? In what ways might there be differences?
13. Does everyone who resides under the same roof feel the same way about their companion animals?
14. Does everyone who resides under the same roof ascribe the same purpose to their companion animals?
15. Does everyone who resides under the same roof grieve the same way when their companion animal dies?
16. Have you ever grieved the loss of a companion animal? Please share your experiences with us.
17. If you answered "yes" to the preceding question (Question #16), did you feel supported in your grief and, if so, by whom?
18. In what ways might culture, society, and/or community discourage outward expressions of grief for a deceased animal?
19. What actions might be taken by others that intentionally or unintentionally discourage outward expressions of grief for a pet?

20. What phrases/statements might be said to the bereaved that intentionally or unintentionally discourage outward expressions of grief for a pet?
21. How might hearing these phrases/statements complicate an *adult* veterinary client's grief process?
22. How might hearing these phrases/statements complicate the grief process for the *child* of a veterinary client?
23. How might we as veterinarians acknowledge, normalize, and validate the impact of pet loss so that grief is not diminished or devalued by the veterinary team?
24. What role might we play as veterinarians in helping communities to acknowledge, normalize, and validate the impact of pet loss so that grief is not diminished or devalued by society at large?
25. What assumptions might the veterinary team make about our clients' grief or support needs?
26. Why might the veterinary team make these assumptions about our clients' grief or support needs? In other words, what is it that leads us to make these assumptions?
27. What is the impact of our assumption-making if our assumptions about our clients' needs, wants, and/or expectations are wrong?

Reflections on Chapter 8

Suffering, Quality of Life, Anticipatory Grief, and Pet Loss: Preparing for the Ultimate Goodbye

1. There is no universal definition for quality of life (QOL). How do you define QOL?
2. Does your current definition apply to all species equally? Or is your current definition specific to certain species? Please explain your answer.
3. Does the definition of QOL for a particular patient depend upon their purpose/function? In other words, does the same definition of QOL apply to a cow in production agriculture as to a show heifer?
4. Does the definition of QOL for a particular patient depend upon their age? In other words, does the same definition of QOL apply to a geriatric patient as to a juvenile?
5. Does the definition of QOL for a particular patient depend upon their sex or sexual status? In other words, does the same definition of QOL apply to a steer as to a bull?

6. Has your definition for QOL changed over your lifetime? If so, in what way? What was your prior understanding of QOL, as compared with your current definition? To what or to whom do you attribute any changes?

7. What *objective* measures might we take into consideration (as clinicians) when determining a patient's QOL?

8. What *subjective* measures might we take into consideration (as clinicians) when determining a patient's QOL?

9. As *clinicians*, do we or should we value objective measures of QOL or subjective measures of QOL more, or less?

10. What do our *clients* measure when they assess their animals' QOL? Are they looking at the same things that we are, or are they emphasizing different qualities when they consider a patient's QOL?

11. Do you think that our *clients'* value objective or subjective measures of QOL more? Please explain your answer.

12. How might *physical health* contribute to or detract from QOL in animals? Can you think of an example?

13. How might *psychological health* contribute to or detract from QOL in animals? Can you think of an example?

14. How might *social well-being* contribute to or detract from QOL in animals? Can you think of an example?

15. Of the three contributing factors that have been suggested here (physical health, psychological health, and social well-being), do you feel that all three are of equal value in considering QOL in *companion* animals? Why or why not? If each contributes unequally to QOL, which carries the most value, and why?

16. Of the three contributing factors that have been suggested here (physical health, psychological health, and social well-being), do you feel that all three are of equal value in considering QOL in *production* animals? Why or why not? If each contributes unequally to QOL, which carries the most value, and why?

17. How might behavioral observations provide additional insight as to a particular animal's QOL?

18. Who is the expert when it comes to recognizing and understanding what constitutes normal behavior for a particular patient? Is it the veterinarian? Is it the client? Is it both? Please explain your answer.

19. What can the *veterinarian* teach the *client* about assessing a particular patient for normal versus abnormal behavior?

20. What can the *client* teach the *veterinarian* about assessing a particular patient for normal versus abnormal behavior?

21. When we talk about QOL, we often ask our clients to consider "good days" versus "bad days." What does "more good days than

bad days" mean to you, with respect to *your* life? What constitutes a "good" day for you? What constitutes a "bad" day for you?

22. What does "more good days than bad days" mean to you, with respect to your *patient's* life?

23. How do we know what constitutes a "good" or "bad" day for a particular patient? Who do we need to ask and how might we phrase those questions?

24. Coming back to the HHHHHMM QOL scale as a whole, what are the advantages and disadvantages of a decision aid such as this one from the perspective of the *clinician?*

25. What are the advantages and disadvantages of a decision aid such as this one from the perspective of the *client?*

26. What, if anything, is the HHHHHMM QOL scale missing? What might you add to, subtract from, and/or revise about it?

27. Why is QOL important from *the clinician's perspective?*

28. Why is QOL important from *the client's perspective?*

29. Do veterinarians and clients always see eye to eye in terms of their perceptions of QOL when they evaluate a particular patient? Please explain your answer.

30. What influences the client's perception of their animal's QOL?

31. What influences your perception of a patient's QOL in your role as a clinician?

32. What might make a client perceive that their animal's QOL is *better* than you, the clinician, may perceive it to be?

33. What might make a client perceive that their animal's QOL is *worse* than you, the clinician, may perceive it to be?

34. Whose responsibility is it to acknowledge and/or address QOL in the consultation room?

35. Should clinicians initiate dialogue about QOL in the consultation room? If so, in what context? When and why?

36. Are there instances when clinicians should wait for clients to initiate dialogue about QOL in the consultation room? If so, when and why?

37. Now let's transition to consider Goals of Care (GOC) conversations. What, if any, risks are associated with members of the veterinary team engaging in GOC conversations?

38. What is the risk to the *patient* if veterinarians and clients do *not* engage in GOC conversations?

39. What is the risk to the *client* if veterinarians and clients do *not* engage in GOC conversations?

40. What is the risk to the *clinician* if veterinarians and clients do *not* engage in GOC conversations?

41. Why is it essential to assess a client's understanding of where their animal is with regards to their disease process?
42. Why is it essential to gain an understanding of how much information a client wants to receive?
43. What constitutes a "good" prognosis? What constitutes a "poor" prognosis? Are these defined the same by both clinician and client?
44. Is patient prognosis an objective or subjective measure? Explain your answer.
45. How does euthanasia as an endpoint impact prognosis?
46. How might the client's emotional status complicate GOC conversations?
47. How might disagreements within the family about patient care complicate GOC conversations?
48. How might a client's prior traumatic experience with human/ animal death/loss complicate GOC conversations?
49. How might our own emotions, as the clinician, complicate GOC conversations?
50. What strategies might we take to separate our emotions from the medical aspects of case management to assist clients with decision-making?
51. What comes to mind when you read or hear the phrase, "anticipatory grief?"
52. Is anticipatory grief always about death and dying? In other words, can you think of any examples in which someone experiences anticipatory grief that is unrelated to death and dying?
53. In which specific situations might a veterinary client experience anticipatory grief?
54. How does anticipatory grief differ from the grief that results from sudden, traumatic, or unexpected loss?
55. How might veterinary clients be *emotionally* impacted by anticipatory grief? That is, what emotions might they feel as they engage in end-of-life decision-making on behalf of their pet?
56. Can anticipatory grief have physical manifestations? In other words, how might veterinary clients be impacted *physically* by anticipatory grief?
57. How are veterinary clients impacted *cognitively* by anticipatory grief? In other words, what thought processes might be going through their minds as they question whether they are doing enough to help their pets, whether their pet is suffering, and when it will be time to say goodbye?
58. Does anticipatory grief strengthen or weaken the human–animal bond?

59. Might anticipatory grief cause a client to prolong an animal's life beyond the point at which it is not in the animal's best interest?

60. Alternatively, might the strain of anticipatory grief cause a client to decide to euthanize earlier than you may have expected?

61. Can veterinarians also experience anticipatory grief with regards to their patients? Why or why not? Please explain your answer.

62. Since anticipatory grief occurs before the actual loss of a loved one, what are veterinary clients who experience anticipatory grief actually grieving?

63. What can you say or do as a clinician to acknowledge, normalize, and/or validate what your client with anticipatory grief is experiencing?

64. Why is it vital for you, the clinician, to acknowledge, normalize, and/or validate what your client with anticipatory grief is experiencing?

65. It is often said in veterinary practice that "planning" is part of the process of experiencing anticipatory grief. What is it that veterinary clients who experience anticipatory grief are actually planning?

66. What is the role of the veterinarian in helping the client to plan?

67. Why is it important that you, the veterinarian, include *all* caregivers in conversations about end-of-life?

68. When there is the anticipation of death, veterinary clients may ruminate about whether they are making the right decisions for their pet. Clients may ask:
    - What if I wait too long to say goodbye?
    - What if I say goodbye too soon?

    How might you respond to each of these questions?

69. Clients may rehearse end-of-life as they process anticipatory grief. They may be waiting for the "perfect" moment. Part of that "perfect" moment may include seeking the "right" time to let their pet go.
    a) Is there a "right" time for euthanasia?
    b) What can you say to a client who asks you:
       - "How will I know when it is the right time to let him go?"
       - "What would you do if my pet were yours?"

70. What additional questions might veterinary clients who are experiencing anticipatory grief ask of you as their pet approaches end-of-life?

71. What can your client do to help themselves cope with anticipatory grief?

72. What can you, the veterinarian, do to help your client cope with anticipatory grief?

Reflections on Chapter 9

Shared Decision-Making Before, During, and After Euthanasia

1. Euthanasia is derived from the Greek terms *eu* meaning good and *thanatos* meaning death. What does *good death* mean to you?
2. What are the veterinarian's roles and responsibilities with regards to the *patient* when performing euthanasia?
3. What are the veterinarian's roles and responsibilities with regards to the *client* when performing euthanasia?
4. Who evaluates euthanasia methods to determine which techniques are considered humane?
5. What are commonly employed methods of humane euthanasia in companion animal (canine/feline) patients?
6. In your opinion, what is or should be the role of *sedatives and/or immobilizing agents* in the euthanasia process?
7. In your opinion, what is or should be the role of *analgesics* in the euthanasia process?
8. In your opinion, what is or should be the role of *anesthetic agents* in the euthanasia process?
9. What criteria should determine whether euthanasia techniques are considered humane?
10. If more than one method of humane euthanasia is listed in the AVMA Guidelines, how do you determine which is most appropriate?
11. Other than method of euthanasia, which additional factors should be taken into consideration?
12. Who is allowed to perform euthanasia of companion animal patients?
13. What concerns about euthanasia do you think that clients have, particularly those clients who may never have been through the process before?
14. How likely do you think clients are to share their concerns about euthanasia with the veterinary team?
15. What may make clients *more* likely to express their concerns about the euthanasia process in advance of the procedure?
16. What may make clients *less* likely to express their concerns about the euthanasia process in advance of the procedure?
17. Imagine yourself as an associate veterinarian in companion animal practice. How can the design of your practice facilitate end-of-life

care, specifically the euthanasia process? In other words, what do clients want/need at their pet's end-of-life and how can we build that into the design of the building?

18. How do interactions between veterinary team members and the *client* before, during, and after euthanasia impact the *client's* experience?

19. How do interactions between veterinary team members and the *patient* before, during, and after euthanasia impact the *client's* experience?

20. Provide examples of what you might say to your client to acknowledge their emotions during end-of-life care.

21. Provide examples of what you might say to normalize, validate, and/or empathize with your client during end-of-life care.

22. Why might it be helpful to ask for permission from your client before broaching sensitive subjects?

23. How might you ask your client for permission? Provide at least one example. Write down exactly what you might say.

24. How does preparing a client for what to expect facilitate a positive experience?

25. Can you overprepare a client for what to expect during the euthanasia process? In other words, is there such a thing as preparing a client too much?

26. Should owners be given the *option* to be present or not to be present during the euthanasia of their pet?

27. Why might an owner *choose* to be *present* to witness the euthanasia process? Consider the perceived benefits to both the client and patient.

28. Why might an owner elect *not* to be present? Consider the perceived disadvantages to both the client and patient.

29. What are body aftercare options following companion animal euthanasia?

30. How might a client choose to memorialize their pet and how can we, the veterinary team, support them through this process?

31. What are your roles and responsibilities to the client *after* euthanasia? In other words, how (if at all) does the patient's death change the VCPR?

32. Should you reach out to the client after euthanasia with a telephone call or bereavement card? Why or why not?

33. What else, if anything, might you do to support the client through the grieving process?

Reflections on Chapter 10

When Loss is Sudden, Traumatic, or Unanticipated

In their 2007 publication in Veterinary Clinics of North America, Dr. Shane W. Bateman writes that:(22)

> *"Time is limited in the emergency department. Effective communication, however, is not a function of time but rather one of skill". Perhaps the biggest barrier for emergency veterinary care teams to overcome is the commonly held belief that they simply do not have time to communicate more effectively—the perception that good communication somehow requires a lot of time. Rather, when viewed in a more comprehensive way, poor communication may actually result in investment of more time because of inappropriate diagnostic evaluations, interpersonal conflicts, repeat visits, and poor adherence.*

1. What do you think that the author means when he says that "*Effective communication is not a function of time but rather one of skill.*"?
2. Do you agree with the author's statement in the preceding question? Why or why not?
3. What do you need to do or say – in other words, what skills are essential – for communication to be effective in emergency situations and why? Please expand upon your answer.
4. What might you do or say that could adversely impact or otherwise complicate communication between you and *the client* during an emergency scenario?
5. What might you do or say that could adversely impact or otherwise complicate communication between you and *the rest of the veterinary team (e.g., colleagues, support staff)* during an emergency scenario?
6. When communication challenges arise, particularly during emergency situations, how do you and the rest of the veterinary team recover from it in order to continue to prioritize patient care?

In "Client Communication in an Emergency," *Small Animal Emergency and Critical Care for Veterinary Technicians*, Jim Clark writes that:(23)
  "Veterinary emergency clients have three key desires":

  1. to understand their pet's medical condition
  2. to feel in control
  3. to feel "felt"

7. How does the client's understanding of their pet's medical condition facilitate case management?

8. How might the client's misunderstanding of their pet's medical condition hinder case management?

9. How do you help the client to understand their pet's medical condition when time is of the essence, and you need to act quickly to stabilize the patient?
   a) What can you tell the client now?
   b) What can you postpone telling the client until later?
   c) How do you prioritize aspects of information-sharing?

10. In an emergency, so much is outside of the client's control (and yours, too). How does *the client* feeling out of control have the potential to derail the clinical consultation?

11. How does *your team* feeling out of control have the potential to derail the clinical consultation?

12. How might *the client* react to bad news we must share if they are feeling out of control during an emergency?

13. Based upon your answer to the preceding question, what emotions might the client's reaction stir up inside of us and why?

14. How do we transition from reaction to response in an urgent situation so that we maintain leadership over and prioritize case management without getting derailed by emotion?

15. What do you think Jim Clark means when he says that veterinary emergency clients need to feel "felt?"

Often emergency patients require emergency procedures. These procedures frequently require anesthesia. Answer the following questions with respect to your baseline understanding of anesthetic risk.

16. Is any anesthesia 100% safe? In other words, is anesthesia ever without risk?

17. What are examples of anesthetic risk? Consider a broad range of examples, everything from what might be considered very minor to what might be catastrophic.

18. Are there breed-specific risks?

19. Are there patient-specific risks?

20. How concerned are clients about anesthesia?

21. How do we know if clients are concerned about anesthesia?

22. How do we elicit clients' concerns about anesthesia?

23. How much is typically conveyed to clients about anesthesia and anesthetic risk and by whom?

24. Does how much we choose to share about anesthesia and anesthetic risk depend upon the patient's health status and whether the procedure is elective or performed on an emergency basis? Please expand upon your answer.
25. What do you think most clients want to know about anesthesia?
26. How might we discuss anesthetic risks before they happen? In other words, what should we tell clients about anesthetic risk prior to procedures that require the use of anesthesia?
27. How do we disclose anesthetic risks to clients without scaring them away from having the procedure performed?

Consider a fictitious clinical scenario in which Alemana, an apparently healthy 4-month-old spayed female Devon Rex kitten, is presented for elective ovariohysterectomy by client Jovi.

Alemana's procedure went well. There were no surgical complications. Following skin closure, you hand her care over to the recovery team in the treatment area so that you can continue on with other surgeries.

You are knee deep in a Great Dane ovariohysterectomy when you hear chaos break out in the treatment area just outside of the Operating Room.

Your lead veterinary technician rushes in to share that Alemana has gone into cardiopulmonary arrest (CPA).

You instruct the team to initiate cardiopulmonary resuscitation (CPR) and you scrub out of surgery while another technician monitors the anesthesia of your current surgical patient so that you can assist. It's all hands on deck as you struggle to resuscitate Alemana.

Alemana never recovers and you pronounce her dead at 2:08PM.

You search everywhere on the Hospital Admittance Form for Jovi's emergency contact information, but it appears that Jovi left that item blank.

There is no way for you to contact Jovi until they arrive to pick Alemana up from surgery.

The client service representative (CSR) alerts you that "Jovi is here." They have arrived for their previously scheduled post-op appointment to have the kitten discharged to their care.

The CSR places Jovi in a consultation room. Jovi has no idea what transpired or that Alemana is deceased.

Please answer the following questions to help you to formulate your approach to this challenging conversation.

---

28. Jovi is expecting you to walk through the door to the consultation room with a cat carrier that contains a live kitten. How will you break the news to Jovi that Alemana has died? Write out exactly what words you may say to share this unexpected news with the client.
29. Put yourself in the client's shoes.

    a) How would you react to this news? In your response, please name the emotions that you anticipate you would feel in that moment and how these emotions may contribute to your response.

    b) How does the way in which the clinician delivers the news influence your reaction?

    c) What might the clinician do or say that would intensify your reaction? In other words, what might the clinician do or say that would make your reaction worse?

    d) As the client, what might the clinician say or do in that moment that could potentially help to deescalate the situation?

30. Even though we can anticipate what our reaction to this situation would be, we are not the client. The client will experience this news in their own way.

    Six potential reactions have been listed below. For each potential reaction, brainstorm an appropriate response that you, the clinician, might say:

    a) SHOCK – [Silence] Jovi says absolutely nothing.

    b) DENIAL – "There must be some mistake. You must be talking about a different cat. Not *our* cat, Alemana."

    c) SADNESS – "She was our whole life."

    d) GUILT – "I should never have agreed to have her spayed. She was too young and too tiny."

    e) ANGER – "We trusted you and you killed our cat. You are not going to get away with this!"

    f) BLAME – "You must have done something wrong during the surgery."

31. Which of the anticipated client reactions in the preceding question would be easiest for you personally and professionally to navigate? Why?

32. Which of the anticipated client reactions in Question #30 would be the most challenging for you personally and professionally to navigate? Why?

33. What can you offer to do for the client at this rather difficult time to help them journey through grief?

34. What factors influence how this client might grieve?

35. How might this scenario play out if the kitten were not a Devon Rex and instead were a Domestic Shorthaired cat? Would the change in breed influence the client's reaction? Why or why not?

Reflections on Chapter 11

When Caring Hurts: Acknowledging Burnout, Addressing
Compassion Fatigue, and Building Resilience

1. In broad terms, how would you define wellness or well-being?
2. In broad terms, what are the various components that make-up wellness or well-being?
3. How does personal wellness or well-being differ from professional wellness or well-being, or are they one of the same? Please expand upon your answer.
4. What do you require *as a person* in order to not just survive, but thrive?
5. What do you require as a *veterinarian* in order to not just survive, but thrive?
6. What are physical, emotional, and psychological obstacles to thriving as both a person and veterinarian?
7. What support systems are in place for individuals and/or organizations that help someone overcome the obstacles that you named in the preceding question?
8. How might needing to "care" for others – the people on the other end of the leash or carrier – inspire us as veterinarians?
9. Is continual "care" for others without respite sustainable? Please expand upon your answer beyond just "yes" or "no."
   a) How might needing to "care" for others – the people on the other end of the leash or carrier – deplete us in our roles as veterinarians?
   b) Is it possible for veterinarians to care "too much?" Please expand upon your answer beyond just "yes" or "no."
   c) Are there times when you might need to "turn off" or "dial back" your capacity to care for others in your role as veterinarian? Please expand upon your answer.
   d) What are potential risks associated with not "turning off" or "dialing back" your capacity to care?
10. What mental health challenges concern you most as you prepare to enter or maintain your standing within the profession of veterinary medicine? How can *educators* help?
11. What mental health challenges concern you most as you prepare to enter or maintain your standing within the profession of veterinary medicine? How can *other veterinarians* help?

12. What mental health challenges concern you most as you prepare to enter or maintain your standing within the profession of veterinary medicine? How can *employers* help?

13. How do you think that more recent graduates differ from more established (seasoned) veterinarians in terms of their perceptions of well-being? In what ways might their perspectives align?

14. How might time spent on social media contribute to (help or hinder) our perceptions of well-being?

15. Not all veterinarians recommend that others follow in their footsteps and select the same career choices that they have.

   a) What do you think is their intent behind *not* recommending the profession? In other words, why do you think they are providing younger generations with this warning?

   b) Is this strategy supportive or helpful? In what ways yes? In what ways no? In other words, are they helping or hurting the next generation of veterinary leaders?

   c) What is the impact when DVMs make recommendations that others should *not* pursue this profession?

   d) Does their recommendation carry weight? In other words, how influential do you think these DVMs are when they make recommendations that others should *not* pursue this profession?

   e) Have you ever been told by anyone (the person doesn't have to be a DVM) not to join this profession? If so, how did you respond?

   f) What do you think it would take for these DVMs to change their minds and start recommending this profession again?

   g) How can you, as part of the next generation of veterinary leaders, re-inspire current professionals?

16. Is mental health treatment accessible where you live? Is mental health treatment accessible in your country of residence?

17. Why might mental health treatment be inaccessible?

18. How might we make mental health treatment more accessible?

19. Do you feel that people are free to discuss mental health as openly as they discuss physical health? Why or why not?

20. Is there a stigma associated with mental health?

   a) How would you define *stigma* broadly?

   b) What types of stigma surround mental illness?

   c) Where does stigma around mental illness come from? In other words, why does stigma exist? What emotions may perpetuate stigma?

   d) What is the impact of stigma around mental illness on those who are affected by mental health challenges?

    e) What is the impact of stigma around mental illness on loved ones of those who are affected by mental health challenges?

    f) How might stigma around mental illness become a major barrier to people accessing mental health services?

21. What do we as veterinarians need to understand about colleagues who may be facing mental health challenges?

22. Many hypotheses have been proposed as to why veterinarians are at increased risk of contemplating, planning, or attempting suicide. Why do you think the risk is greater for us than the general population?

23. The stigma associated with suicide has been a barrier to discussing the issue. How do we – as teachers and learners – acknowledge a topic that historically was not addressed or even acknowledged?

24. What are the risk factors for suicide?

25. What are myths about suicide?

26. How can we – as teachers and learners – support each other through this challenging topic?

> Let's shift our focus now to consider *burnout*.

27. Prior to reading this chapter, had you ever before heard the term, "burnout?" If so, in what context?

28. Without consulting any resources, how would you define *burnout*?

29. What factors in general might contribute to burnout in *any* profession?

30. What factors might contribute to burnout in *healthcare* broadly?

31. What factors (in addition to those you identified in the preceding question) might contribute to burnout specifically within the *veterinary* profession?

32. How do you think that the COVID-19 pandemic has contributed to burnout among veterinarians?

33. What obstacles stand in the way of overcoming burnout?

34. How can we as a profession overcome the obstacles that you named in the preceding question?

35. How might *veterinary college* precipitate and/or hasten burnout among new graduates?

36. How might *veterinary college* guard against and/or protect new graduates from burnout?

37. What are the consequences of burnout with respect to patient care?

38. What is the impact of burnout on healthcare costs?

39. What are the consequences of burnout with respect to physician wellness?

40. What *work-specific* factors might contribute to burnout?

41. Which *personal* characteristics might contribute to burnout?
42. Which *organizational factors* might contribute to burnout?
43. What *strategies* might we employ to mitigate some of these contributing factors?
44. What do pet owners expect of us? Are pet owners' expectations of us realistic? Why or why not?
45. What are your own expectations for yourself about how much to care and whether that degree of caring is "enough?"
46. Are there times/circumstances or patients/clients that you may care more about than others? Please expand upon your answer.
47. Is it okay to emotionally invest in your cases? When, how, and why? Please expand upon your answer.
48. When might caring be "too much" for us? In other words, what internal and/or external factors might fatigue us and our ability to care?
49. What "critical incidents" do you anticipate will be the most challenging for you to navigate as a veterinarian?
50. When caring is "too much," how do we proceed with case management?

> Let's revisit our consideration of quality of life (QOL). As a profession, we are used to discussing QOL in the context of our patient. Yet how often do we consider our own QOL?

51. What does QOL mean to you, for you? In other words, what do you consider to be quality living when it comes to living your own life?
52. What *internal* influences impact your own personal QOL?
53. What *external* influences impact your own personal QOL?
54. What do you think is meant by the term, *professional QOL?*
55. Does your *personal* QOL differ from your *professional* QOL?
56. How might your perception of professional QOL differ from a colleague's perception? Please provide examples and/or expand upon your answer.

> Now let's transition to consider *compassion fatigue.*

57. How do you define *compassion fatigue?*
58. Based upon the definition that you provided, how is compassion fatigue similar to burnout?
59. Based upon the definition that you provided, how is compassion fatigue distinct from burnout?

60. How are the signs and symptoms of compassion fatigue *related to or consistent with* the signs and symptoms of grief?
61. How are the signs and symptoms of compassion fatigue *distinct from* the signs and symptoms of grief?
62. Overcoming compassion fatigue requires coping skills.
    a) How would you describe your coping style? In other words, what coping skills do you default to during times of stress?
    b) On a scale of 1–10, 1 being *least* effective and 10 being *most* effective, how would you rate the efficacy (effectiveness) of your current coping strategies?
    c) What works well (WWW) about your current coping strategies?
    d) What are opportunity areas for growth (OAG) with respect to your current coping strategies?
63. What can *employers* do to assist you with navigating critical incidents and traumatic stressors to mitigate the risk of developing compassion fatigue?
64. What can *employers* do to help you build compassion *satisfaction*?

Now let's consider *resilience*.

65. How do you define *individual resilience*?
66. How do you define team *resilience*?
67. How important is the role of *leadership* in cultivating *individual* resilience? In other words, what kind of impact does leadership have on individual team members developing resilience? Please elaborate. If you have examples from your own experiences, please share those.
68. How important is the role of *leadership* in cultivating *team* resilience? In other words, what kind of impact does leadership have on team resilience? Please elaborate. If you have examples from your own experiences, please share those.

In Chapter 11, we included the following excerpt from the 2017 editorial in *Journal of Veterinary Medical Education* by Guest Editors Susan M. Rhind and Andrew Grant:(24)

Several of the articles in this issue [of the Journal of Veterinary Medical Education*] are moving from the focus on identification of the problem and the associated factors to the positive psychology approach, which seeks to "focus on adaptation and thriving, rather than disorder and deficit." It is this approach that explains the title of our editorial: "From Studying the Rain to Studying the Umbrella." While* for obvious reasons much of the published research in the area of mental health and well-being focuses on reporting the problem and reducing stressors (the rain), an alternative approach is to focus on how we can build resilience and nurture well-being (the umbrella)—that is, how can we develop better umbrellas and help students protect themselves from the rain?

69. How does the analogy that the authors used to identify stressors (rain) and resilience/well-being (umbrella) resonate with you?
70. When working towards problem-solving to navigate mental health challenges, what are the benefits of focusing on the stressors (the rain)?
71. When working towards problem-solving to navigate mental health challenges, what are the benefits of shifting focus onto building resilience and well-being (the umbrella)?
72. Is it ever truly possible to protect you (as students and colleagues) from the rain?
73. Should we (as veterinary medical educators) protect you (as students and colleagues) from the rain?
74. How do we balance acknowledging the harsher realities of veterinary medicine (compassion fatigue) against the sunnier realities of veterinary practice (compassion satisfaction)?
75. How can we better prepare you for experiencing both?
76. How does one bounce back from adversity in their *personal* life?
77. How does one bounce back from adversity in their *professional* life?
78. Is the ability to bounce back innate? In other words, is resilience something we either just naturally have or not?
79. Is the ability to bounce back teachable? In other words, can we teach resilience? Please expand upon your answer.
80. How would you define *mindfulness*?
81. How would you define *self-compassion*?
82. How might either mindfulness or self-compassion influence, inspire, or enhance resilience?

References

1. Englar RE. Preface. In: Englar RE, editor. A guide to oral communication in veterinary medicine. Great Easton: 5m Books; 2020. p. xvii–xx.
2. Brown JP, Silverman JD. The current and future market for veterinarians and veterinary medical services in the United States. J Am Vet Med Assoc. 1999;215(2):161–83. PMID 10416465.

3. Martin F, Ruby KL, Deking TM, Taunton AE. Factors associated with client, staff, and student satisfaction regarding small animal euthanasia procedures at a veterinary teaching hospital. J Am Vet Med Assoc. 2004;224(11):1774–9. https://doi.org/10.2460/javma.2004.224.1774, PMID 15198261.

4. Bustad LK, Hines LM, Leathers CW. The human-companion animal bond and the veterinarian. Vet Clin North Am Small Anim Pract. 1981;11(4):787–810. https://doi.org/10.1016/s0195-5616(81)50086-6, PMID 6977933.

5. Voith VL. Attachment of people to companion animals. Vet Clin North Am Small Anim Pract. 1985;15(2):289–95. https://doi.org/10.1016/s0195-5616(85)50301-0, PMID 3872510.

6. Wensley SP. Animal welfare and the human-animal bond: considerations for veterinary faculty, students, and practitioners. J Vet Med Educ. 2008;35(4):532–9. https://doi.org/10.3138/jvme.35.4.532, PMID 19228905.

7. Lagoni L, Hetts S, Butler C. The human-animal bond. In: Lagoni L, Hetts S, Butler C, editors. The human-animal bond and grief. Philadelphia: Saunders; 1994. p. 3–28.

8. Silcox D, Castillo YA, Reed BJ. The human animal bond: applications for rehabilitation professionals. J Appl Rehabil Couns. 2014;45(3):27–37. https://doi.org/10.1891/0047-2220.45.3.27.

9. Kielland C, Skjerve E, Osterås O, Zanella AJ. Dairy farmer attitudes and empathy toward animals are associated with animal welfare indicators. J Dairy Sci. 2010;93(7):2998-3006. https://doi.org/10.3168/jds.2009-2899, PMID 20630216.

10. Coleman GJ, Hemsworth PH, Hay M. Predicting stockperson behaviour towards pigs from attitudinal and job-related variables and empathy. Appl Anim Behav Sci. 1998;58(1–2):63–75. https://doi.org/10.1016/S0168-1591(96)01168-9.

11. Breuer K, Hemsworth PH, Barnett JL, Matthews LR, Coleman GJ. Behavioural response to humans and the productivity of commercial dairy cows. Appl Anim Behav Sci. 2000;66(4):273–88. https://doi.org/10.1016/s0168-1591(99)00097-0, PMID 10700627.

12. Hemsworth PH. Human-animal interactions in livestock production. Appl Anim Behav Sci. 2003;81(3):185–98. https://doi.org/10.1016/S0168-1591(02)00280-0.

13. Hemsworth PH, Coleman GJ, Barnett JL, Borg S. Relationships between human-animal interactions and productivity of commercial dairy cows. J Anim Sci. 2000;78(11):2821–31. https://doi.org/10.2527/2000.78112821x, PMID 110 63304.

14. Waiblinger S, Menke C, Coleman G. The relationship between attitudes, personal characteristics and behaviour of stockpeople and subsequent behaviour and production of dairy cows. Appl Anim Behav Sci. 2002;79(3):195–219. https://doi.org/10.1016/S0168-1591(02)00155-7.

15. Hanna D, Sneddon IA, Beattie VE. The relationship between the stockperson's personality and attitudes and the productivity of dairy cows. Animal. 2009;3(5):737–43. https://doi.org/10.1017/S1751731109003991, PMID 22444453.

16. Romero MH, Escobar L, Alberto Sánchez JA. Empathy levels among veterinary medicine students in Colombia (South America). J Vet Med Educ. 2022;49(6):740–7. https://doi.org/10.3138/jvme-2021-0048, PMID 34499579.

17. Calderón-Amor J, Luna-Fernández D, Tadich T. Study of the levels of human-human and human-animal empathy in veterinary medical students from Chile. J Vet Med Educ. 2017;44(1):179-86. https://doi.org/10.3138/jvme.0216-038R, PMID 28206834.

18. Nunes P, Williams S, Sa B, Stevenson K. A study of empathy decline in students from five health disciplines during their first year of training. Int J Medical Education;2:12–7. https://doi.org/10.5116/ijme.4d47.ddb0.

19. Colombo ES, Pelosi A, Prato-Previde E. Empathy towards animals and belief in animal-human-continuity in Italian veterinary students. Anim Welf. 2016;25(2):-275–86. https://doi.org/10.7120/09627286.25.2.275.

20. Paul ES, Podberscek AL. Veterinary education and students' attitudes towards animal welfare. Vet Rec. 2000;146(10):269–72. https://doi.org/10.1136/vr.146.10.269, PMID 10749039.

21. Applebaum JW, MacLean EL, McDonald SE. Love, fear, and the human-animal bond: on adversity and multispecies relationships. Compr Psychoneuroendocrinol. 2021(Aug):1–12. https://doi.org/10.1016/j.cpnec.2021.100071, PMID 34485952. Erratum in: Compr Psychoneuroendocrinol. 2022(Jan 20);9:100112. PMCID: PMC8415490.

22. Bateman SW. Communication in the veterinary emergency setting. The veterinary clinics of North America. Small animal practice. 2007;37(1):109–21. https://doi.org/10.1016/j.cvsm.2006.09.005.

23. Clark, J. Client communication in an emergency. In: Battaglia A, Steele AM, editors. Small animal emergency and critical care for veterinary technicians. St Louis, MO: Elsevier, Inc; 2022. p. 385–390.

24. Rhind SM, Grant A. From studying the rain to studying the umbrella: mental health and well-being of veterinary medical students and graduates. Journal of veterinary medical education. 2017;44(1):1–2.

Part Five

Using the Literary Arts to Explore Grief: *Poems and Stories of Bereavement*

CHAPTER 13

Poems

Please be Gentle: An After Loss Creed

Please be gentle with me for I am grieving.
The sea I swim in is a lonely one
and the shore seems miles away.
Waves of despair numb my soul
as I struggle through each day.

My heart is heavy with sorrow.
I want to shout and scream
and repeatedly ask 'Why?'
At times, my grief overwhelms me
and I weep bitterly,
so great is my loss.

Please don't turn away
Or tell me to move on with my life.
I must embrace my pain
before I can begin to heal.

Companion me through the tears
And sit with me in loving silence.
Honor where I am in the journey,
Not where you think I should be.

Listen patiently to my story.
I may need to tell it over and over again.
It's how I begin to grasp the enormity of my loss.

Nurture me through the weeks and months ahead.
Forgive me when I seem distant and inconsolable.
A small flame still burns within my heart,
And shared memories may trigger
both laughter and tears.

I need your support and understanding.
There is no right or wrong way to grieve.
I must find my own path.
Please, will you walk beside me?

© Jill Englar, 1999

Please Be Patient

Please be patient, as I am still grieving.
The sea I swim in remains turbulent
And unexpected grief riptides
Pull me further from shore.

The numbing fog which enveloped me has lifted
And I am faced with the cold,
Stark reality of my loss.
Adrift in the deep end of the ocean,
I founder in unfamiliar waters – lost in uncharted territory.

I cry for help in a world that
Has already moved on.
"Stop wallowing," they say, "Buck up –
It has already been three months."
To me, three months seems like yesterday,
When the world I knew ended
And I was left drowning in my despair.
I cannot recall the funeral –
Only a blur of faces and the endless condolences.

"Be brave – make her proud."
"Be grateful for the time you had – she lived a long life."
"Call me if there is anything I can do."

I am calling now,
Seeking a lifeline, a listening ear.
A hug. A cup of tea.
Someone to hear my story,
And help me make sense of this tragedy.

© Jill Englar, 2009

A Time to Mourn

I am lost in grief, numb with shock,
Filled with disbelief and at times, rage –
Besieged by an army of rebellious emotions,
My instinct is to retreat.

I want to hide under a blanket and sleep,
Awakening only to your smiling face.
But the nightmare is real –
And you are not coming back.

I am a worry to my family
And a stranger to our friends,
Adrift in a sea of despair
And marooned in an unwelcome reality.

Please don't rush my grief
Or tell me to move on with my life.
I need time.
My loss must be processed, my pain must be healed.

Please be gentle and kind.
Offer a hot meal – not advice!
Share a cup of tea.
Understand my silence may be from fatigue and emptiness within.
Please don't shy away when I vent anger and frustration.
I may even seem bitter and envious of those around me.

Have patience as I reminisce and gaze fondly at old photographs.
Speak my beloved's name and smile as we reflect shared memories.
I am not afraid of tears –
Only the loneliness each day brings.

Grieving takes time. Grieving requires support.
Embrace me with love. Companion me with hope.
My faith gets me out of bed –
Your support keeps me going.

Thank you for being my friend.

© Jill Englar, 2002

Graveside

Alone
and feeling abandoned
at your graveside I weep.

Tears of despair and anguish
make me tremble
and my knees buckle
into newly turned earth.

I kneel, consumed with grief.
I want to shout and wail in sorrow.
Yet no sound escapes my lips
beyond the whisper of your name.

So profound is my yearning –
I dream of your return
or a sign you haven't really left me,
without hope, without your love
or comforting presence.

For a moment I am quiet.
I hush my tears
and strain to hear your voice
or any sign that would make
this tragedy bearable.

The sun shines warmly on my back
and slowly I stop trembling.
I notice the nearby hillside and lone tree.

The sky is vibrant blue and the
white clouds billow above me.

The smell of honeysuckle drifts by
and raspberries ripen in the distance.
Wildflower petals dance in the breeze
and a woodthrush begins his evening song.

A gentle calm fills the air
and my soul is momentarily at peace.

The Day You Died

The day you died, something inside of me died, too.
With no inner flame to light the way,
I am greeted by an endless night,
dampened in your absence,
and darkened by the lack of light.

The day you died, I lost a part of me forever.
I wander aimlessly with no direction.
I am a broken compass, all alone
on a journey without end,
on a path that leads me far from home.

The day you died, I lost a listener and a friend.
I search for understanding and warmth,
but my cries are hushed by distanced stares,
An empty room, an empty silence,
An overwhelming lack of care.

The day you died, I lost my zest for life.
I am passionless, hopeless, listless.
I trudge through days, weeks, years,
Frozen solid, dazed, in constant fog
Living, breathing, fighting tears.

The day you died, I lost a world I thought I knew.
I drown myself in the question, "Why?"

I know that you are gone forever,
But still I expect you to return to me,
To restore the bond that death did sever.

The day you died, I lost my voice.
I want to scream and shout
And explain the emptiness I feel inside.
But I am silenced by my disbelief,
And have been since the day you died.

© Ryane E. Englar, 2010

CHAPTER 14

Stories

Harvey: A Story of Disenfranchised Grief

Jill B. Englar

Some pet deaths haunt you throughout your entire life. Looking back, Harvey's sudden death was unexpected and never "validated." The word "disenfranchised" hadn't been coined yet and as a ten-year-old girl, I wanted someone – anyone – to say that they were sorry. That didn't happen in the late 1950s. Pets were pets.

Harvey came into my life the summer I turned ten because my Sunday school teacher's son had won him in the end-of-year class raffle. Harvey was a young male, all white rabbit with beautiful pink eyes. We did not initially build a hutch for him as he was content to stay around our house in the country with our two cats and dog Dusty.

As fall approached, my father built a hutch as he was concerned about possible predators, and Harvey's life changed. He lost his freedom, but looked forward to me feeding him and taking him out after school. He enjoyed having his ears scratched. He enjoyed eating clover. My father had built a large hutch with a shingled roof and a sizable log that Harvey could hide behind, with lots of straw to burrow under on cold winter's nights. The hutch backed up against our house, next to the fireplace where it was warm and dry. His comfort and safety were important to me, and I find myself needing to tell my story that I tried my best.

One Friday night in December, relatives visited, and my father wanted to show off Harvey. I protested as it was night and I was afraid my father might not lock the cage securely. It was secured by a soft metal strip, which he promised to replace the next day with a padlock. I agreed reluctantly, and my father put Harvey back, but somehow failed to lock the cage.

The next morning as I was getting his pellets and carrots ready to feed him, my brother called that Harvey was lying on the snowy ground with our dog Dusty nuzzling him. I screamed because Harvey was dead, and the soft lock was nowhere in sight. Harvey must have seen Dusty outside and pushed against the cage. He had fallen to the ground. He broke his neck. I sobbed and cried, but my mother said, "It was no one's fault—accidents happen." I blamed Dad. Mom called my father at his office. He said he had forgotten to re-lock the cage and assumed Harvey would be fine. He said I had spoiled Harvey, and this was the reason he pushed the door open. My father said he would buy me a new rabbit. I cried. I did not want another rabbit. Harvey could not be replaced. My parents said I was being "over-dramatic." No one said, "You must be so sad, and we are very sorry."

A week later I was walking up Lathe Lane after seeing my friend, and my Sunday school teacher drove by. She said she was surprised that I had not come to Sunday school, and I told her that Harvey died. She said, "Well, you can always get another rabbit." I said, "But not Harvey" and she said that I needed to "grow up and understand that all things die." I said that his cage was not locked. She said not to be unkind and to accept that mistakes were made. I remember clearly saying that no one even said they were sorry or that it had been a sad accident. She said again that I was being selfish and was acting childish. I said, "But I am a child," And so she shook her head and drove off, and the next Sunday school lesson was about forgiveness. I remember saying, "But doesn't there need to be an 'I'm sorry' first?" I never received an answer.

Today, hopefully pet loss is validated and acknowledged. I am 70 and still remember Harvey so clearly in my heart and mind. Children were forgotten mourners back then, and sometimes still are today.

Max

Jill B. Englar

Max came to us as a three-month-old scrappy barn cat. A short-haired gray, he had the most beautiful long fur tail that fanned out as he ran down the lawn. Raised in a barn for three months, he allowed us to "rescue" him by providing food and a warm house to sleep in when the weather turned cold.

Max always made us laugh. He loved to hide behind our sofa; when strangers entered, he would race out and nip them on the leg and run proudly away. No one was fond of his antics except us. We laughed at his ability to outrun a mockingbird swooping down to peck him on the head. If a dog entered our yard, Max leaped upon his back and rode him until he scurried off our property. Then Max would jump off and proudly saunter home.

Max never missed dinner. One Thursday night, four years after he first "adopted" us, he failed to come home. Our property bordered a field and farm, and I walked up, thinking he had wandered off. Despite repeated calls, he did not answer or return home. On Friday, Mom sent me, protesting, off to school, and when I came home I raced up the field and called and called – no answer. I came home in tears. It was fall and people were hunting. Mom promised to look with me on Saturday, so bright and early we scoured the fields. I walked a half mile and heard a faint cry in response to my calls. As I ran calling, I found Max lying in the field, with his left leg shattered. Someone had shot him and left him to die. I took off my jacket, and Mom helped me put him in it so we could carry him home. He cried and snarled at the pain of being lifted, but allowed us to walk the half mile home. Mom called the local veterinarian, who told her to bring Max in.

I knew my widowed mother did not have the money to pay for Max's surgery. I told her I would pay, since I had saved $300 from house-cleaning jobs for college. Mom said to stay home and start dinner, and although I protested, she took Max by herself. I told him I would see him soon. Mom came home an hour later; Max had been euthanized and I was in shock. The vet said amputation wasn't the answer – a cat couldn't walk on three legs. I could only think that Max had waited for us to find him, and that we killed him. He trusted us, and in my adolescent mind we had let him down.

I called the vet, but Max had already been euthanized. I said I could have paid, and he told me cats couldn't live on three legs – especially outdoor cats. I cried that I didn't get to say goodbye and wasn't with him when he died. We did not get to bring him home to be buried. I wrote an article in the local paper about the person who shot him and left him to die.

I have never forgotten Max and how I felt we had failed him. Today as an adult, I know I finally found him and ended his pain, but that is little consolation.

Boo

Jill B. Englar

It has been six years since Boo's death and yet I still mist up at the traumatic experience I felt when he was being euthanized. But I need to back up 17 years, when Boo first appeared on our porch one snowy, cold night, afraid, feral, and starving.

I heard what sounded like a cat outside, and when I opened our door, I saw huddled up in the corner of our porch a bedraggled young cat with frightened, wary eyes. I said, "Wait, and I will get you something to eat." Luckily, we had eaten roast chicken and rice for dinner, and had leftovers. I cut some up in a bowl and put the meal outside.

He watched me and jumped down as I pushed the dish further from the door. Calling to my husband, I closed the door and we watched him from a window as he devoured the food.

Shelter? He wouldn't come near us, so we quickly fashioned my plastic laundry basket with foam duct-taped on the outside and piles of old rugs on top. Inside, we put more rugs and covered the top so there was only a small entrance. I put more food in his bowl all the while, telling him the shelter was for him.

We closed the door slowly and he approached the dish with caution, ate again, and crawled into the makeshift shelter.

The next morning, we fed him warmed chicken and rice and knew he was here to stay.

He refused to come inside the house and jumped off the porch each time the door was opened and the offer was made. So, my husband bought cat food and I bought a small cat igloo for the sheltered corner of our porch and a bale of straw to keep him warm inside.

He survived the winter on our porch but would never approach us.

By early summer, he allowed us to sit next to him on the porch and I was able to place drops on his neck to kill the fleas. We had hoped to bring him inside, but he was so afraid.

When mid-July came, my husband was home for the summer as a high school teacher. We agreed he needed to work on getting Boo to come in. We chose the name Boo, because he was so afraid and over the 11 years we had Boo, no one ever saw him except for our daughter who happened to be a veterinarian.

It took weeks of Richard laying on his stomach every day with our front door open trying to coax Boo to come in.

Finally, Boo came just inside the door to eat, but refused to allow the door to close.

By September, I said, "Boo, you need to come inside so I can close this door." I showed him the litter box near the door much to my chagrin, and Boo slept inside at night but insisted on going out in the daytime.

Everything was his way – maybe because my mother had died in a motor vehicle accident the summer before Boo found us. I was grieving and understood his pain of abandonment.

By late fall, he was trusting enough to be taken to the vets for neutering and shots. We had come to an understanding. He was a part of our family if he chose to be.

Two incidents are recalled with humor now. I looked out our back porch two summers later and saw Boo sleeping in the sun under our bird feeder. Ready to call out to him to leave my birds alone, I saw a fox 9 feet away, ready to pounce on Boo as he slept. I opened the door and yelled, "Boo, Boo, a fox!" and I waved my arms like an insane woman as I ran down the stairs towards him. The fox gave up his meal of Boo and ran off. Boo looked up at me and closed his eyes again as if to say he thought I was nuts! He never saw the fox. I got him to come in by shaking his bag of treats.

The other incident was the following spring when Boo was under the feeder sleeping again and my husband said, "Look, a doe is in our yard stomping her front leg and hoof in Boo's direction."

Boo had looked up but didn't move. The doe approached slowly, but stopped repeatedly and stomped and stomped.

I went outside with his treats and he came running in – all we could think was that the doe saw Boo as a "fox" or predator to her newborn fawn.

Nothing ever pleased Boo.

No one believed we had a cat as no one ever saw him. We lived at the end of a lane.

Several years before Boo died, we moved to another house again with the woods all around us. We kept Boo inside for three days until his yowling to go out each day made us give in. We walked him around the property several times and he stayed close by and then took off into the wood.

Night came and no Boo. We stayed up all night walking around the yard with flashlights calling him. We kept our floodlights on all night and at 6A.M. in the morning, I heard him at the front porch.

He came in and ate and stayed inside while we trudged off to work.

Boo got sick about three years later and when our daughter came home for Christmas, she examined him and felt a palpable mass in his abdomen. We decided to euthanize him a week later as he was no longer the Boo we knew and loved. He was sick, incontinent, and crying for us to help him.

Our daughter went with us and perhaps our vet thought the sedative was enough or that Ryane would explain it.

But it wasn't enough and Boo became restless. He kept trying to look up at me in this daze.

The vet had left us alone for 10 minutes and Ryane went to get her to explain it wasn't enough. She said, "I guess he's a bigger guy than I thought."

I said, "I think I made a mistake. I can't do this."

Ryane talked me through my fears that Boo was not seeking help, but in a drugged hallucinatory state. He was not upset with me. He probably felt like he was coming out of anesthesia.

When he calmed down and was properly sedated, I still questioned what we were doing and if he was not ready to die.

He couldn't speak and trusted me to do the right thing.

Ryane was compassionate and took her time explaining everything.

I was able to cry and sob that this feral cat had lived life his way and we were there as his "keepers."

I loved Boo more than I could ever imagine and my initial guilt was acknowledged, respected, and made better by our daughter's open dialogue with me.

When our own vet said after his death, "Do you want to take him home with you?" I cried and said "yes."

She said he had a good life for a feral cat.

But he was much more to me than a "feral" cat.

He was a survivor and he had learned to love us in his own way.

Derrick

Jill B. Englar

Out of all the cats I have rescued in my lifetime, Derrick is the one that still brings tears to my eyes. Perhaps tears of sadness that it was too late to save him despite our family's attempts over a two-year period.

Derrick showed up in the city one day at our son's place of business. Hungry, dirty, and very leery of humans, yet desperate enough to cry out for food and perhaps help. He was emaciated – skin over bones – and seemed to be at least 14.

Our son started feeding Derrick and we had a cat outdoor igloo that he was allowed to put in a sheltered area with straw. Derrick survived the first winter but would never come close enough to be petted. Over time, Derrick trusted our son, Brent, and was in need of more than food and shelter. He wanted companionship.

As Brent's mom, I was willing to pick Derrick up in a cat carrier and wash him in our home. Tired and trusting, Derrick allowed it and changed from grey to snowy white as the years of dirt and grime washed away. Our son had taken him to a vet nearby the year before and had ruled out feline leukemia, but found a massive ear infection.

I treated the ear infection twice a day for three months and fed Derrick a high protein cat food. But he did not improve and when our daughter, a veterinarian, came home for Christmas from out-of-state, she determined that Derrick had cancer in the ear that was incurable. She sadly recommended euthanasia and explained that Derrick had been given good end-of-life care and the chance to be loved.

I made the appointment and was taken into an examination room. Through the closed door, I heard the tech tell the vet why I was there, only to have him complain loudly that he had missed his lunch and now had to work through his break.

As he opened the door and recognized me, I apologized for making him lose his lunch break. He apologized and we started over.

Derrick was gently euthanized and the vet was kind and compassionate as he listened to Derrick's life story. He said I did the best I could and gave Derrick the best three months of his life. He looked at his emaciated body and said Derrick had lived a hard life and had been rescued before he died on the street.

I never forgot the vet's kindness, and realized how brave Derrick had been. Alone, hungry, and lost for possibly his entire life. But he seemed to be happy to have been taken in and fed and loved. He never minded the ear drops. I never minded him flicking out the pieces of skin and debris.

I am sorry we found him too late.

I am sorry he was abandoned years ago. But I am at peace with how we took him in and in his dying, he taught me to be strong.

Bereavement Resources

Resources for Young Children

- *Always and Forever* by Alan Durant
- *A Terrible Thing Happens* by Margaret Holmes
- *Badger's Parting Gift* by Susan Varley
- *Bottled Sunshine* by Andrea Spalding & Ruth Ohi
- *Goodbye Mog* by Judith Kerr
- *Healing Your Grieving Heart for Kids* by Alan D. Wolfelt
- *I Miss You: A First Look at Death* by Pat Thomas
- *"I Wish I Could Hold Your Hand … ": A Child's Guide to Grief and Loss* by Pat Palmer
- *Lifetimes: The Beautiful Way to Explain Death to Children* by Bryan Mellonie & Robert Ingpen
- *Rudi's Pond* by Eve Bunting
- *Sad Isn't Bad: A Good-Grief Guidebook for Kids Dealing with Loss* by Michaelene Mundy
- *Saying Goodbye to Lulu* by Corinne Demas
- *The Bug Cemetery* by Frances Hill
- *The Fall of the Freddie Leaf: A Story of Life for All Ages* by Leo Buscaglia
- *The Giving Tree* by Shel Silversteen
- *The Tenth Good Thing About Barney* by Judith Viorst
- *Today I Feel Silly & Other Moods That Make My Day* by Jamie Lee Curtis
- *When A Pet Dies* by Fred Rogers
- *When Dinosaurs Die: A Guide to Understanding Death* by Laurie Krasny Brown & Marc Brown
- *When Someone Very Special Dies: Children Learn to Cope with Grief* by Marge Heegaard
- *Where Do Balloons Go? An Uplifting Mystery* by Jamie Lee Curtis

Resources for Middle School/Teens

- *All Rivers Flow to the Sea* by Allison McGhee
- *Healing Your Grieving Heart for Teens* by Alan D. Wolfelt
- *Helping Children Cope with Death* by The Dougy Center
- *Helping Teens Cope with Death* by The Dougy Center
- *How It Feels When a Parent Dies* by Jill Krementz
- *Mick Harte Was Here* by Barbara Park
- *Missing May* by Cynthia Rylant
- *Remembering Mrs. Rossi* by Amy Hest
- *Safe at Home* by Sharon Robinson
- *Sarah's Journey: One Child's Experience with the Death of Her Father* by Alan D. Wolfelt
- *Sun and Spoon* by Kevin Henkes
- *What Is Goodbye?* by Nikki Grimes
- *What on Earth Do You Do When Someone Dies* by Trevor Romain
- *You Are Not Alone: Teens Talk About Life After the Loss of a Parent* by Lynne Hughes

Workbooks

- *Fire In My Heart, Ice in My Veins: A Journal for Teenagers Experiencing a Loss* by Enid Samuel-Traisman
- *Good Grief Rituals: Tools for Healing* by Elaine Childs-Gowell
- *Communication Activities for Adults* by Jayne Commins
- *My Grieving Journey Book* by Shavatt
- *The Understanding Your Grief Journal: Exploring the Ten Essential Touchstones* by Alan Wolfelt
- *Waving Goodbye: An Activities Manual* by The Dougy Center
- *Someone I Love Has Died* – Coloring Book for Young Children
- *Why Did You Die?* by Erika Leewenburgh & Ellen Goldring
- *Get Rid of the Hurt* by Madeleine Brehm & Rachel Wenslaff
- *Why did you Die? Activities to Help Children Cope with Grief & Loss* by Erika Leeuwenburgh & Ellen Goldring

Resources for Adults

- *Living with Loss: Hope & Healing for the Body, Mind & Soul* – magazine: www.livingwithloss.com
- *A Broken Heart Still Beats* by Anne McCracken and Mary Sewel
- *A Decembered Grief: Living with Loss While Others are Celebrating* by Harold Ivan Smith
- *After the Death of a Child: Living with Loss Through the Years* by Ann Finkbeiner
- *A Grief Recovery Handbook: The Action Program for Moving Beyond Death, Divorce, and Other Losses* by John W. James & Russell Friedman
- *A Journey Through Grief: Gentle, Specific Help to Get You Through the Most Difficult Stages of Grieving* by Alla Bozarth
- *Answers to a Child's Question About Death* – pamphlet by Novak-Thurston
- *A Time to Grieve: Meditations for Healing After the Death of a Loved One* by Carol Staudacher
- *A Time to Mourn, a Time to Comfort: A Guide to Jewish Bereavement* by Dr. Ron Wolfson
- *Chicken Soup for the Grieving Soul* by Jack Canfield & Mark Hansen
- *Children Mourning, Mourning Children* by Kenneth Doka
- *Companion Through the Darkness: Inner Dialogues on Grief* by Stephanie Ericson
- *Final Gifts: Understanding the Special Awareness, Needs, and Communications of the Dying* by Maggie Callanan & Patricia Kelley
- *Grief, Dying, and Death: Clinical Interventions for Caregivers* by Therese Rando
- *Grieving Mindfully: A Compassionate and Spiritual Guide to Coping with Loss* by Sameet M. Kumar
- *Guidelines for Life Beyond Loss* – pamphlet by Brookline Home Care and Hospice
- *Handbook of Thanatology* by Association for Death Education and Counseling
- *Healing After Loss: Daily Meditations for Working Through Grief* by Martha Whitmore Hickman
- *Healing the Adult Child's Grieving Heart* by Alan D. Wolfelt
- *Help for the Hard Times: Getting Through Loss* by Earl Hipp
- *Helping the Grieving Student* by The Dougy Center
- *Helping Your Child Grieve* – pamphlet by the National Hospice Organization
- *How To Go On Living When Someone You Love Dies* by Therese Rando

- *I Wasn't Ready to Say Goodbye: Surviving, Coping & Healing After the Sudden Death of a Loved One* by Brook Noel & Pamela D. Blair
- *Letting Go: Morrie's Reflections on Living While Dying* by Morrie Schwartz
- *Life Lessons: Two Experts on Death and Dying Teach Us About the Mysteries of Life and Living* by Elizabeth Kubler-Ross and David Kessler
- *Live and Learn and Pass It On* by Jackson Brown
- *Living When a Loved One Has Died* by Earl A. Grollman
- *Living With Grief* by Hospice Foundation of America
- *Losing a Parent: Passage to a New Way of Living (A Guide to Facing Death and Dying)* by Alexandra Kennedy
- *Maze of Life: Discovering Your Path to Health, Happiness and Inner Peace* by Barry Bittman & Anthony DeFail
- *Motherless Daughters: The Legacy of Loss* by Hope Edelman
- *On Death and Dying: What the Dying Have to Teach Doctors Nurses, Clergy, and their Own Families* by Elizabeth Kubler-Ross
- *Parental Loss of a Child* by Therese Rando
- *Perfect Balance: Create Time and Space for all Parts of Your Life* by Paul Wilson
- *Remembering Well: Rituals for Celebrating Life and Mourning Death* by Sarah York
- *Swallowed by a Snake: The Gift of the Masculine Side of Healing* by Thomas R. Golden
- *Talking About Death: A Dialogue between Parent and Child* by Earl A. Grollman
- *Talking with Your Children About Death* – pamphlet by Fred Rogers
- *Tear Soup: A Recipe for Healing After Loss* by Pat Schwiebert & Chuck DeKlyen
- *The Courage to Grieve: Creative Living, Recovery, & Growth Through Grief* by Judy Tatelbaum
- *The Grieving Child: A Parent's Guide* by Helen Fitzgerald
- *The Loss that Is Forever: The Lifelong Impact of the Early Death of a Mother or Father* by Maxine Harris
- *The Mourning Handbook: A Complete Guide for the Bereaved* by Helen Fitzgerald
- *The Orphaned Adult: Understanding and Coping with Grief and Change After the Death of Our Parents* by Alexander Levy
- *The Understanding Your Grief Support Group Guide: Standing and Leading a Bereavement Support Group* by Alan Wolfelt
- *The Year of Magical Thinking* by Joan Didion
- *Treatment of Complicated Mourning* by Therese Rando
- *Triumph Over Grief* by Joyce Williams

- *Understanding Your Grief: Ten Essential Touchstones for Finding Hope and Healing Your Heart* by Alan Wolfelt
- *When Death Impacts Your School* by The Dougy Center
- *When Your Pet Dies* by Alan Wolfelt

Bereavement Cards

Written by a veterinarian for all members of the veterinary team, this unique line of cards recognizes that those who are grieving often must mask their grief. Being seen by others offers support as they navigate grief in a world that does not allow space for loss to be recognized and understood. Check out Dr. Englar's growing collection of empathy cards today at www.intheirpaws.com.

Index